Music Therapy with Autistic Children in Aotearoa, New Zealand

"For many music therapists in the global community, work with autistic children can often be at the very core of their practice. Rickson's passion for the work shows through in this book. Readers will be drawn close into the therapy experience through the rich exploration of ten case studies of music therapy with autistic children in Aotearoa, New Zealand. They will gain a real understanding of the importance of the work to the children, their families, and educational and healthcare professionals. The book provides compelling reading; it is well-crafted and elegantly written. It truly brings music therapy practice to life and will be a resource for music therapy students and practitioners to return to time and time again throughout their professional career."

—Dr. Liz Coombes, *Lecturer, University of South Wales*

"This is a fascinating book centred around ten individual music therapy case studies with autistic children. The children are seen by ten different New Zealand music therapists in a variety of settings. Each case tells an engaging and varied story primarily through the eyes of family members and multi-disciplinary professionals who have 'witnessed' the music therapy via video excerpts and detailed stories of the practice written by the child's music therapist. Rickson draws these wide-ranging perspectives together in an honest and skilful way, commenting on the different music therapy approaches and key areas of progress. In later chapters, she reflects on what she considers to be characteristic and essential in the work. This book is a 'must read' for music therapists working with autistic children not just in New Zealand but all over the world."

—Emeritus Professor Amelia Oldfield, *Anglia Ruskin University, Cambridge Institute for Music Therapy Research (CIMTR)*

"This very approachable book gives an overview of the role and effectiveness of music therapy with autistic children in New Zealand. Case studies with commentaries from family, friends, and commentators from other disciplines, medical and educational, give both life and insight into the work. Rickson's critique of each case, providing supportive commentary and alternative suggestions for the work, is particularly interesting. She is very open about her familial experience of autism and refers to the challenges of cultural differences found in the New Zealand population. This timely book will appeal not only to music therapists but also to other practitioners and, most importantly, to families with children on the autistic spectrum and to autistic people themselves."

—Auriel Warwick, *Co-author, Alvin & Warwick (1992) Music therapy for the autistic child, Oxford University Press, UK*

"This is a valuable and inclusive text from Daphne Rickson, a highly experienced music therapist, educator, researcher, and passionate advocate of music in schools for children and young people. By inviting a team of music therapists and people with a keen interest in the well-being of takiwātanga tamariki to be part of a research project, Rickson has been able to present the stories of ten autistic children and to critically review the practice of music therapy. This comprehensive text offers the reader valuable insight into the research origins, process, and findings of the study. The different contributions and perspectives from the various experts are effectively woven and integrated with the author's reflections, creating a fully collaborative and honest account. This book will be useful for all persons interested in music and the wellbeing of children with Autism. It offers a wealth of information on music and music therapy for children with Autism, with literature to turn to and pointers to research that has been undertaken around the world. This is an essential text for people interested in person-centred research. It outlines research methods and data presentation in depth and is bold and innovative in its pursuit of person-centred values and participant-led perspectives."

—Dr. Philippa Derrington, *Senior Lecturer and Programme Leader, Music Therapy, Queen Margaret University, Edinburgh*

Daphne Rickson

Music Therapy with Autistic Children in Aotearoa, New Zealand

Haumanu ā-Puoro mā ngā Tamariki Takiwātanga i Aotearoa

Foreword by Dr. Grace Thompson

palgrave macmillan

Daphne Rickson
New Zealand School of Music
Victoria University of Wellington
Wellington, New Zealand

ISBN 978-3-031-05232-3 ISBN 978-3-031-05233-0 (eBook)
https://doi.org/10.1007/978-3-031-05233-0

This Palgrave Macmillan imprint is published by the registered company Springer Nature Switzerland AG

The registered company address is: Gewerbestrasse 11, 6330 Cham, Switzerland

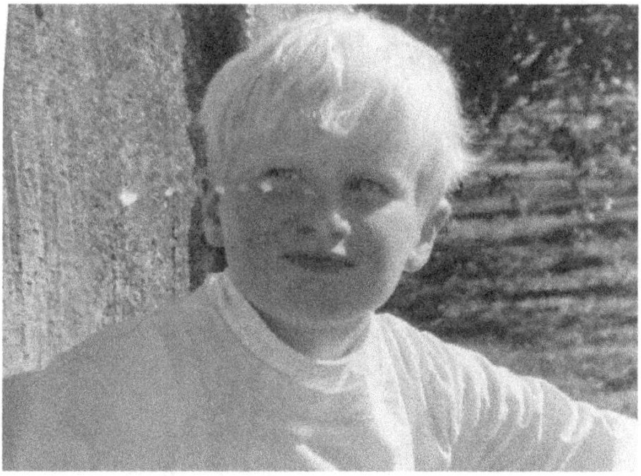

In Loving Memory of Tim McIlroy Humphrey

1 February 1984–3 July 2005

Takiwātanga—He lived in his own time and space

Foreword by Dr. Grace Thompson

A love for stories is a common connection point for people across generations and experiences. Stories of people's lives, whether they are based on everyday moments or grand adventures, provide a framework for us to resonate with others, be inspired, gain a new perspective, and so much more. Stories can fuel our understanding, our compassion, our knowledge, and our curiosity. Some extraordinary or exceptional stories have provided evidence that has challenged the status quo or revealed new possibilities for understanding. Stories are therefore often shared with the intention to actively engage and affect the reader.

From a research standpoint, case stories can challenge widely held beliefs, lead to new paths of inquiry, and convey a richness of complexity that was otherwise concealed. Researchers can thoughtfully structure case study designs in such a way that broader commentary and perspectives are actively sought. The case story can therefore expand to become a dynamic dialogue that might reveal deeper layers of insight and fuel reflection in subsequent readers.

In this book, Daphne Rickson skilfully narrates the story of a research project that is based on ten case studies with autistic children who engage in music therapy. The music therapists who facilitated the sessions prepared a Narrative Assessment of each child's therapy process in the way that felt most relevant and meaningful for their context. Each case story was then presented to commentators; some who knew the child well, and six who had a professional or personal understanding of autistic children. The commentators shared their subjective responses to the case through multiple qualitative descriptions and by rating their level of agreement with key statements devised by Rickson (see Chapter 4). The different data streams were subsequently woven together by Rickson and infused with her own critical reflections and lived experiences, along with perspectives from the music therapists. The research aim to "explain the complex process of music therapy, rather than 'prove' that it is effective" (see p. 65) is powerfully met by Rickson's innovative study design and wise insights. Chapters 17–24 methodically describe and discuss the various important learnings revealed through the synthesis of perspectives from these ten case studies, including the powerful affordances of working from a child-centred and strengths-based stance, and the therapists' respect for each child's unique musicality.

Music therapists have described their work with autistic children since the 1950s (Reschke-Hernandez, 2011) and have applied various research designs to evidence the outcomes, including case studies, qualitative enquiries, controlled studies, and meta-analyses (see Chapter 3). Over this time, researchers have documented numerous promising results, and yet building the evidence base for music therapy with autistic children seems to be an increasingly complex endeavour. As a music therapy researcher, I am frequently faced with multiple layers of complexity concerned with the ways we might understand the nature of music, the nature of autism, and the nature of therapy. The way researchers understand each of these complex phenomena will drive their research in profound ways. Perhaps I can best explain some of my own understandings by sharing my story of being a music therapist. Or at least, by telling a condensed version of that story.

My relationship with music began early on, as is the case for most people. I have fragmented memories of my mother singing an Italian play song to me, where the combination of melody and dipping movements would build my anticipation of being hugged or tickled. I remember laughing with my whole body, feeling close to my mother, and asking for multiple repetitions of this song, even perhaps when I was a little too big for my mother to manage the dipping movements. This was my first experience of musical forms of expression being embedded within relationship and culture. As a person with a physical disability who experienced numerous surgeries during childhood which involved lengthy hospital stays that separated me from my family, I also came to understand how music engagement could provide personal comfort and expression. Learning piano and singing provided a creative outlet, and I remember playing different versions of pieces to change the mood by altering the dynamics (volume), or tempo (speed), or register on the keyboard (pitch). I could become lost in my own musical world. As I grew in musical ability, I played the piano for a church music group and quickly learnt that I also needed to listen to the other musicians and singers and support the flow of the music. These intra- and interpersonal experiences with music were themes threaded throughout my childhood.

When I came to study music therapy, I felt the same strange paradox of being lost in the music making but needing to remain aware of the response of the person I was working with. I was trying to musically attune to the other person/people, and over time I developed a deeper understanding of the mutuality within this process. By that I mean, it was not only important to follow the person I was working with, but also to invite them to try something different, and be open to their forms of expression. I started to understand the notion of balance within a healthy relationship; that both leading and following are important, that misattunements might strengthen relationship, and that understanding is co-created. When the music therapy session was really flowing, I could "feel" the connection with the other person through a goosebump-like tingling or a wave of emotion and sensed that the other person also seemed to be immersed in the experience in their own way. When improvisations or play songs would come to an end, children might exclaim "that was fun!", others might laugh or smile, while others might have a moment of incredible calm and stillness.

Over time, there were two key concepts from the literature that guided my music therapy practice. Firstly, that through these musical interactions we are co-creating a history of meaning (Holck, 2004) and that within the process of intentionally attuning to a child the adult is enculturing that child into the social norms of their society (Stern, 1977, 1985, 2010). Secondly, this process is playful, and the act of playing invites play partners to surrender to a spontaneous, freely unfolding, and mutual experience (Kenny, 1989; Winnicott, 1971). Each play partner must be genuinely committed to the play and open to the influences of the other, i.e., there is no rigid script to follow. It is this "not knowing" exactly what might happen next that gives life to the interaction. I have therefore come to understand that therapy processes are about the "we," the space between people, that each person is interconnected, and therefore the experience is mutually dependent.

For me, the highlight of being a music therapist who works with autistic children and their families is sharing in moments when there is a "sparkle in the child's eye." This sparkle doesn't have to be literally in the child's eye though! It can be a facial expression, or a perfectly timed cymbal crash at the end of a phrase, or a giggle, or a vocal sound. It's something that tells me that the child is "in" the experience, or that they "get" the game, or they realise that they can influence others and/or the music through their response. These seemingly humble and small moments are what I understand to be the foundation of a therapeutic process.

Reading Rickson's descriptions of the ten music therapists in these case stories as being child-led and strengths-focused therefore resonated deeply with me. At the heart of these case stories is a deep respect for the children's ways of being in the world. Indeed, the research commentators variously noticed that the music therapists provided "safe spaces where [the] children feel comfortable to engage in play, try out new ideas, take leadership and express themselves, verbally, musically, and physically" (see Chapter 18, p. 234). I was impressed with the commentators' perceptiveness, and entirely agree that creating spaces where children can "be themselves" is essential for healthy personal and social development.

Within the autism literature, creating space for children to "be themselves" is not a common theme. Instead, there is often an emphasis on developing normative skills and changing the child's behaviours (Leza, 2020; Ne'eman, 2021; Pickard et al., 2020). I have often found myself reflecting on the distinction between "impairment" versus "difference," and even "treatment" versus "therapy". Rickson helpfully discusses the different approaches to defining autism, and how different models of disability inform a person's world view (see Chapter 2). For too long, autistic people have been told, either overtly or covertly, that their ways of being needed to change so that they can fit in with others, play with others, and communicate with others. Far from engaging in mutual understanding or embracing interconnectedness, the neurotypical majority has, under the belief of best intentions, sought to make autistic people appear, well, less autistic (Cage & Troxell-Whitman, 2019). Despite these sometimes-good intentions, autistic people report that they still experience discrimination and social isolation (Jones et al., 2018). Autistic scholar and researcher Damian Milton (2012) highlights a disturbingly obvious "double empathy problem" in society where autistic people are expected to understand and relate to non-autistic people, but non-autistic people do not seek to understand autistic forms of expression. I take these critiques seriously as a non-autistic therapist, educator, and researcher, and have committed to seek out autistic perspectives and collaborations within my work (Thompson et al., 2020).

Rickson's research findings are therefore radical in the most human and humbling way. The commentators noticed the music therapists' sincere efforts to engage with any form of expression that the children offered to them. As the music therapists got to know the children better, the children's interactions seemed to become more communicative and creative. Most surprising to me, the commentators highlighted that the music therapists seemed to genuinely like the children and wanted to build a relationship with them (see Chapter 19). My hopes for the autistic children I have worked with resonate with these humble human qualities; I hope that through our musical interactions the child feels valued and respected. From these relational foundations, I believe children flourish. They might feel brave enough to try new things, spirited enough to persist when things are difficult, and proud enough to show their strengths and interests. As Rickson's data suggests, children can then develop more resources to support their emotional, sensory, and cognitive regulation. They can manage their own comfort levels when they are with others who are attuned to them and supportive of their needs.

They can more clearly communicate when they can use their whole self to express, and others are curious enough to try to understand.

In my own research in this field, I have interviewed dozens of parents of young children on the autism spectrum and the qualitative findings complement those reported here by Rickson. Following music therapy, many parents experienced a deepening of their relationship with their child, more positive perceptions of their child's abilities, and a flow-on change in the way they responded to their child (Thompson & McFerran, 2015). When they looked back on their experiences in music therapy, some parents recognised that opportunities for mutual enjoyment with their child were rare and that musical play offered a distinct space for this to occur (Thompson, 2017). While understanding the perceptions of parents in my own research has been useful, and Rickson's innovative approach to case study design that includes the views of a panel of experts is undoubtedly valuable, perspectives of autistic children are yet to be included heartily in qualitative research. While in this text the children's experiences are ever present throughout the respectful discussion of the case stories, I still yearn to better understand their perspective of the musical play space and their relationship with the music therapist. Future perspectives from autistic children may help us to more deeply understand the potential ripple effects of sharing a mutually enjoyable musical play experience. Until then, Rickson's rich case study research can guide the reader through a reflective consideration of the nature of music therapy through engaging with stories that are at once both extraordinary and humbly human.

Grace Thompson
Associate Professor in
Music Therapy
The University of Melbourne
Melbourne, VIC, Australia

References

Cage, E., & Troxell-Whitman, Z. (2019). Understanding the reasons, contexts and costs of camouflaging for autistic adults. *Journal of Autism & Developmental Disorders, 49*(5), 1899–1911. https://doi.org/10.1007/s10803-018-03878-x

Holck, U. (2004). Interaction themes in music therapy: Definition and delimitation. *Nordic Journal of Music Therapy, 13*(1), 3–19.

Jones, S., Akram, M., Murphy, N., Myers, P., & Vickers, N. (2018). *Community attitudes & behaviours towards autism; and experiences of autistic people and their families: General awareness, knowledge and understanding of autism and social isolation.* AMAZE website http://www.onethingforautism.com.au/wp-content/uploads/2018/05/Autism-research-report-General-awareness-knowledge-and-understanding-of-autism-and-social-isolation-1.pdf

Kenny, C. B. (1989). *The field of play: A guide for the theory and practice of music therapy*. Ridgeview.

Leza, J. (2020). Neuroqueering music therapy: Observations on the current state of neurodiversity in music therapy practice. In D. Milton (Ed.), *The neurodiversity reader* (pp. 210–225). Pavilion.

Milton, D. E. (2012). On the ontological status of autism: The 'double empathy problem'. *Disability & Society, 27*(6), 883–887. https://doi.org/10.1080/09687599.2012.710008

Ne'eman, A. (2021). When disability is defined by behavior, outcome measures should not promote "passing". *AMA Journal of Ethics, 23*(7), 569–575. https://doi.org/10.1001/amajethics.2021.569

Pickard, B., Thompson, G., Metell, M., Roginsky, E., & Elefant, C. (2020). It's not what's done, but why it's done': Music therapists' understanding of normalisation, maximisation and the neurodiversity movement. *Voices: A World Forum for Music Therapy, 20*(3), 19.

Reschke-Hernandez, A. E. (2011). History of music therapy treatment interventions for children with autism. *Journal of Music Therapy, 48*(2), 169–207. https://doi.org/10.1093/jmt/48.2.169

Stern, D. N. (1977). *The first relationship: Infant and mother*. Billing & Sons Ltd.

Stern, D. N. (1985). *The interpersonal world of the infant*. Basic Books.

Stern, D. N. (2010). *Forms of vitality*. Oxford University Press.

Thompson, G. A. (2017). Families with preschool aged children with autism spectrum disorder. In S. L. Jacobsen & G. Thompson (Eds.), *Music therapy with families: Therapeutic approaches and theoretical perspectives* (pp. 92–115). Jessica Kingsley Publishers.

Thompson, G. A., & McFerran, K. S. (2015). Music therapy with young people who have profound intellectual and developmental disability: Four case studies exploring communication and engagement within musical interactions. *Journal of Intellectual & Developmental Disability, 40*(1), 1–11. https://doi.org/10.3109/13668250.2014.965668

Thompson, G., Raine, M., Hayward, S., & Kilpatrick, H. (2020). Gathering community perspectives to inform the design of autism-friendly music-making workshops for wellbeing. *International Journal of Wellbeing, 10*(5), 117–143. https://doi.org/10.5502/ijw.v10i5.1497

Winnicott, D. W. (1971). *Playing and reality*. Tavistock.

Acknowledgements

I offer my sincere thanks to the IHC Foundation and Victoria University of Wellington—Te Herenga Waka for their financial support, and to all music therapists, families, and other experts who have contributed to this research.

Thank you to music therapy colleagues and students, and other team members, in New Zealand and abroad, who have stimulated my professional growth in a variety of exciting ways.

My heartfelt gratitude goes to the many tamariki takiwātanga and whānau I have worked with, over the past three decades.

From all of you I have learnt.

> Ehara taku toa i te toa takitahi, engari he toa takitini
> Success is not the work of one, but the work of many

Acknowledgements

Contents

List of Figures

1

Introduction

The Nature of This Text

This book is grounded in my experiences practising as a New Zealand Registered Music Therapist (NZ RMTh) and my teaching and research in music therapy at the New Zealand School of Music—Te Kōkī, Victoria University of Wellington, New Zealand. Over my 30-year career I have been lucky enough to work with many autistic children (tamariki takiwātanga) and their families. My beautiful nephew Tim, who was takiwātanga and to whom this book is dedicated, gave me the initial confidence I needed, as a newly graduated music therapist, to develop what has become a lifelong passion for sharing music with tamariki takiwātanga. However, while I have drawn on all my experiences when writing the book, the content is based primarily on one research project investigating music therapy with autistic children in New Zealand as well as the exploratory project that preceded it. The purpose of both these exploratory and qualitative studies was to learn more about the processes involved in music therapy with tamariki takiwātanga, and how they might be understood by families and other stakeholders.

D. Rickson, *Music Therapy with Autistic Children in Aotearoa, New Zealand*, https://doi.org/10.1007/978-3-031-05233-0_1

This book is therefore not a manual. It does not tell readers "how to work" with tamariki takiwātanga and it does not try to prove that "music therapy works." What it does do, uniquely I believe, is to share the views of people who are *not* practising music therapists, who have carefully examined case studies and video extracts of music therapy processes, and who are, in essence, "looking in from the outside." In sharing their perceptions of what they have viewed, these thirty-two family members and other experts have not only provided rich descriptions of music therapy processes that I trust readers can relate to; but have also offered opinions that are at times powerfully consistent, and at times considerably diverse. As a reader of this book, you are therefore encouraged to engage with the commentators' views and to evaluate them in the context of other writing and, crucially, your own experiences of working or living with tamariki takiwātanga.

As a qualitative researcher, I have been committed to being "reflexive." In other words, as I was going through the research process, I continually wondered how my personal experiences were impacting on the research, and how the research may have been impacting on me. And when talking or writing about the research I have used many direct quotes from participants, to ensure their voices are brought to the fore. These processes increased the potential for me to represent the views of participants clearly, rather than generating the findings I wanted to see. I have explained more about this, the concept of reflexivity, on Sect. "Reflexivity."

Qualitative researchers often outline their position and assumptions before beginning the research to indicate their point of departure, sometimes with the idea of "bracketing" their experiences; putting behind them so they can engage with the work from a more objective position. However, the researcher can never be fully detached from the research. As we go through research processes, we are constantly influencing and being influenced by what we are hearing, seeing, and feeling (Berger, 2015; Probst, 2015; Walshaw, 2010). *Positioning ourselves socially* and emotionally in relation to participants is therefore an important aspect of the research process and writing about ourselves in a research project emphasises the negotiated nature of the work (Berger, 2015; Coffey, 2003; Walshaw, 2010).

Therefore, at the risk of "romanticising the self" (Walshaw, 2010), I have included the following paragraphs to help the reader to understand something of what I bring to this research and this text, what prompted my interest in the topic, my personal investment in the study, and to determine whether the findings presented in other chapters seem credible.

Author Context

A Musical Background

I was brought up in a home surrounded by informal music making. We had no "proper" musical instruments in our house when I was very young, but my mother playfully sang and danced with me and my three siblings, and another brother who was born when I was 12. We would listen to the radio and my mum would whistle and sing, and it seemed that music was always "just there." I was drawn to music at school, loved the regular classroom music sessions, and was keen to join the school choir when I was old enough to do so. When I was about eight years old, I moved to a classroom where there was a piano and where our teacher would accompany our classroom singing. I became enthralled with the piano and would try to play it at every opportunity.

I am extremely grateful to that classroom teacher, for valuing my "tinkling of the ivories" and for suggesting to my mother that it would be beneficial for us to have a piano at home. It took four years before mum had saved enough, and the piano arrived. I was in my element, taking formal lessons, playing duets with fellow students, working through Trinity College grade exams, and accompanying hymns for the school assembly. But what I loved most of all was playing popular songs "by ear," being able to play for family singalongs, and eventually joining duos and bands. The joy of music for me was in the sharing; being together in music.

An Introduction to Music Therapy

So, when my daughter was born profoundly deaf in 1984, one of my first instincts was to learn how to share music with her. Thankfully, we were privileged to have the opportunity to attend the preschool programme at van Asch Deaf Education Centre (VADEC) in Christchurch, New Zealand. Several autistic children also attended the centre because there were, and still are, no specialist facilities for this population in New Zealand, and it was assumed they would benefit from being in an environment where multiple modes of communication were being offered.

Staff members at VADEC were aware and appreciative of the therapeutic potential of music to support children with additional learning needs. Some had attended workshops with music therapy pioneers Paul Nordoff and Clive Robbins and were skilled at introducing music activities that would help the children to develop their listening, speech, and language. My experiences as a musician, mother of a deaf child, and aunt of tamariki takiwātanga, were highly valued and I was invited to facilitate music sessions, initially group sessions, for the preschoolers. My collaborations with staff were exciting and enlightening and led me to music therapy training at the earliest opportunity.

At the time it was not possible to study music therapy in New Zealand at a tertiary institution. However, the New Zealand Society of Music Therapy (now known as Music Therapy New Zealand) had developed an accreditation system, which involved modular learning. In addition to ongoing individualised supervised learning, students attended "live in" block courses facilitated by international experts including Clive and Carol Robbins. Clive and Carol's interest in working with autistic as well as Deaf children, led them to spend a generous amount of time with me at VADEC, and naturally I have been highly influenced by their approach to music therapy.

In 2002 I was invited to be a mentor for a Ministry of Education participatory action research team. This exciting initiative involved collaborations with educators who were working with tamariki takiwātanga in early childhood centres and schools and wanted to improve an aspect of their teaching practice. While this project did not focus on music therapy, I developed valuable research skills and insight into the lives of teachers, families, and learners who were striving to build inclusive school communities.

Over the years my clinical work expanded to include work with children who had a wide range of diagnoses at various special education facilities for children with intellectual disabilities, physical disabilities, and a residential school for adolescents with social and emotional difficulties. But my primary interest in working with tamariki takiwātanga remained, and I highly valued a contract, offered by a parent support group, to work with autistic children after school.

My Academic Career

I began my work in academia when the first New Zealand Master of Music Therapy programme began in 2004, initially at Massey University, but latterly at Victoria University of Wellington. My research has continued to focus on music therapy to support children who have learning support needs, including autistic children. My PhD study, completed in 2010, involved action research to support teams of educators in their use of music, including three teams who were working with autistic children. Following that, in 2015, I led a team of investigators exploring the practice of music therapy with autistic children in New Zealand (Rickson et al., 2015a, 2015b), in order to design a study that would be suitable for the New Zealand context (Rickson et al., 2016). Funding from the IHC Foundation and Victoria University of Wellington enabled this latter project to come into fruition in 2018. This book is therefore grounded in this practice and research knowledge as well as, importantly, my personal experiences of living and working with autistic children.

Am I Autistic Too?

Autism is known to be familial. That is, several members of one family might be autistic, or "on the spectrum." My nephew, Tim, required very substantial support to manage daily life whereas I and all other members of my family have not required any additional supports that might be related to autism. Yet when I look at myself closely, I recognise that I have differences that might not be considered "neurotypical" and, although these differences might not necessarily be visible to others, I have been comfortable for a long time with the idea that I might be on the spectrum too.

Many people who would meet the diagnostic criteria for autism spectrum disorder remain undiagnosed because their differences are less pronounced (Kim et al., 2011) or they have developed coping skills that mask their autism (Lai et al., 2011). As Bakan (2018) writes, "the question of just what the autism spectrum is - and by extension, who is 'on' it - is anything but self-evident" (p. 7). I like to imagine that this inclusive diagnosis describes the behaviours that all humans engage in, and that those who have the diagnosis could be described as having "well-developed" typical behaviours. For example, my "dedication to task," "excellent eye for detail," and "impeccable work ethic," serve me well; and for now, I feel no need to pursue a diagnostic label. Moreover, while I am comfortable being a person on the spectrum I am, like some of Bakan's collaborators, certainly not comfortable with claiming "I am autistic." Does it matter?

Autistic Identities and the "Problem" of Language and Labels

> When Bakan (2014) asked one of his musical collaborators "Are you an autistic kid or a kid with autism?", she replied "It doesn't matter. It's like asking a zebra, 'Are you black with white stripes or white with black stripes?'" (No page number)

On the other hand, many people do prefer to say they are "autistic" rather than a "person with autism" or "person on the spectrum" because they believe "autism" cannot be separated from their personhood. That is, they believe autism is fundamental to who they are. Importantly, they would argue that while autistic people function differently to "neurotypical" people, this does not necessarily mean they are "disordered." Neurodiversity and disability rights advocates argue that it is important for people to be able to make an informed choice regarding identity, prevention, and cure in relation to autism (Kapp et al., 2013). Autistic people can find themselves in difficult positions of needing to choose whether to seek support to adapt and appear like others, and/or use their energies towards the fight for acceptance. The diversity among autistic people, or people "on the spectrum," calls for acceptance of multiple agendas, and people need to be supported to make informed choices regarding what might work best for them, as well as for their wider communities. I will return to this topic in Chapter 2.

People who are not discriminated against based on their neurological differences arguably benefit from neurotypical privilege (Kapp, 2020). It is important for individuals to carefully consider their position in relation to autism culture, and as researchers to consider whether and at what points we might be positioned as "insiders" or "outsiders." Deaf, Autistic, Māori, and other identities invite others who are respectful and supportive of their cultures, into their communities. While I might not choose to claim autism as an identity marker, my personal and family experiences, music therapy practice with autistic children, and my research and teaching have, at various times, given me the privilege of being part of the autism community; and I have also had privileges which have enabled me to successfully navigate neurotypical landscapes.

Terminology and an Introduction to Tamariki Takiwātanga

I have long been a strong advocate for the use of strengths-based language which is mindful of the preferences of autistic individuals and communities. However, no singular term can meet the preferences of all people who have autistic traits. It is easy to respect individuals' choice regarding how they wish to be identified. We can refer to them as being Autistic, or having Autism, Autism Spectrum Disorder (ASD), Autism Spectrum Difference (ASD), or an Autism Spectrum Condition (ASC) for example, according to their personal wishes. It is much more difficult however, to decide how we might write about autistic people in a book. Further, as you read on, you will notice variations in language I have used as I refer to *other* people's writing, because I have used the words that they would use in their contexts.

In my recent writing and presentations, I have been constantly wavering between various terms which have been proposed by others, and which consider the meanings that labels impose, and the impact they can have on readers, listeners, and most of all the people we are referring to. The person-first language I used for a long time, such as a "child who has autism," seemed important because it took the focus from the condition and emphasised the value and worth of the individual. Recent research suggests that "person on the autism spectrum" is still a preferred term by many autism community members in Australia (Bury et al., 2020) and the UK (Kenny et al., 2016). In contrast, however, when an individual claims autism as part of their being, the "person-first" label can feel dismissive of their identity.

I have also recently been introduced to the te reo Māori word for autism—takiwātanga (Opai, 2020)—and I like it a lot. Takiwātanga is a derivation of the phrase "tōku/tōna anō takiwā"—"my/their own time and space," and it builds nicely on one of my favourite quotes from autistic author Donna Williams (2002) who explained: "Mind and consciousness are like a gradual sunrise that takes time to come up. […] Some of us stay longer (in the realm of sensing) than others" (p. 11). During the process of research and consultation with Māori to develop the term, Keri found that takiwātanga rarely, if ever, referred to themselves or others as "having" takiwātanga (i.e., a "condition" or "disorder" that led them to work in their own time and space). Rather, they claimed takiwātanga as part of their identity—they were takiwātanga. Those who live, work, and play respectfully with takiwātanga would typically be accepted members of the "takiwātanga community."

Kerri also noted the evolving nature of language and acknowledged that while the term takiwātanga is currently in use in Aotearoa and elsewhere, it is not yet well established locally or internationally. However, it works very well in music therapy contexts. The understanding that takiwātanga tend to have their own timing, spacing, pacing and life-rhythm (Opai, 2020), provides reinforcement for the practice of music therapy which focuses on "attunement." Music therapists using child-centred improvisational approaches connect with their participants by tuning in to the timing and rhythm of their musical and other communications. By attuning to children's emotional, physiological, creative, and playful qualities, they can "create a shared experience between the child and therapist that supports the child's regulation, continuity, organization, and vitality within the play" (Epstein et al., 2020, p. 81). The child feels understood, and reciprocal communication becomes possible (Stern, 1985).

The te reo Māori (Māori language) word for the practice of music therapy is "haumanu ā-puoro" (Opai, 2020). Hau means wind while manu is a bird—so therapy is understood as wind beneath the bird's wings that helps it to fly and prosper. So, kia ora (greetings), welcome to Haumanu ā-puoro mā ngā Tamariki Takiwātanga, music therapy with autistic children! I hope you enjoy this book and find it useful in supporting the well-being of tamariki takiwātanga.

Project Context

As noted earlier, the book draws heavily on rich findings from multiple case study research. The research aimed to uncover the perspectives of experts in the autism field; to find out whether they believe music therapy is beneficial for autistic children (tamariki takiwātanga) and if so, how, and why it might be helpful. The project began in response to a call for more evidence to underpin the potential employment of music therapists to work with takiwātanga in New Zealand. Specifically, the New Zealand Autism Guideline (Ministries of Health & Education, 2016) listed music therapy as an intervention option yet suggested evidence for its effectiveness was unclear.

Initial exploratory research indicated that rigorous but innovative designs would be needed to accommodate the diverse practices of music therapy with tamariki takiwātanga, while meeting the demands of evidence-based practice (Rickson et al., 2015a, 2015b). In 2015 there were approximately 60 Registered Music Therapists (NZ RMTh) in this country, and the 29 who participated in the exploratory research employed naturalistic, flexible, improvisational approaches when working with tamariki takiwātanga, which allows them to respond to the needs of their participants in the moment (Rickson et al., 2015a, 2015b). While numbers of NZ RMThs are gradually growing (85 at the time of writing), the small numbers of music therapists and heterogeneity of practice, which also reflects heterogeneity among tamariki takiwātanga, means the potential for large-scale positivist research was, and remains, limited.

It can be a difficult task for clinicians to convey whether, how, and why complex improvisational music therapy processes are beneficial for autistic children. Progress in music therapy can sometimes be slow and "intangible," and while anecdotal evidence abounds, acceptable "proof" such as that obtained from behavioural analyses do not necessarily capture the benefits of music therapy. On the other hand, music therapists are interested in knowing whether their participants and others close to them are satisfied with the music therapy process, whether it has some benefit in participants' lives, and whether institutions, agencies, and communities can also see those benefits (Aigen, 2015; Rickson et al., 2016). They are also aware that people who witness music therapy develop significant understanding and appreciation of the practice, and new perspectives of what children can achieve (Rickson et al., 2015a, 2015b; Rickson et al., 2016; Warwick, 2019). These premises underpinned the decision to invite teams of "commentators" to provide critical reflections on ten case studies of music therapy with tamariki takiwatanga. As Ansdell (2020) notes, while progress may be hard to measure the messy music therapy process is rich and colourful and yields plentiful data for analysis (Ansdell, 2020), and thus can lead to the production of an exciting text!

The main project began in 2018 when research funding enabled ten music therapists to work with individual children who had not experienced music therapy before, for up to a year. The music therapists, with informed consent, provided case reports of their work in Narrative Assessment form (Ministry of Education, 2009) for the commentators to critique. Narrative Assessments capture and document learning in authentic contexts, using text, video, photographs, and other media that can make the child's learning visible to interested parties. The diversity within the population of people diagnosed with ASD suggests it is important to understand children in context; to focus on the things that are meaningful to them and their families, and on the individual progress that they make rather than comparing them to their peers. The use of Narrative Assessment therefore felt highly appropriate because it is an ipsative approach, recommended by the Ministry of Education, and has similarities to the descriptive evaluation methods used by New Zealand music therapists (Rickson et al., 2016). The rich qualitative case reports with video examples would give observers good insight into what happens in music therapy and enable them, in turn, to convey their understanding of the music therapy processes in detail. Further information about the research design and Narrative Assessment is included in Chapter 4.

Music therapists often write of feeling constrained by research processes (Warwick, 2019). In contrast, this project enabled music therapists to engage in typical and naturalistic music therapy practice unhampered by research protocols. Only when the practice had ended, did they present case materials to be examined by the commentators. Then, two-four people who knew the child well, and six "other" autism experts who did not know the child, examined, and commented on the materials. Their rich descriptions of ten individual cases will give readers a view of the unique nature of each music therapy process, while findings from the cross-case analysis will communicate the ways in which commentators viewed music therapy more broadly.

Chapters 2–5 introduce the work. In Chapter 2, the concept of autism is discussed beginning with etiological and neurological perspectives through a medical lens. This is followed by a critique of the medical model and the introduction of the concept of neurodiversity, and cultural perspectives of autism particularly as they relate to Māori and Pacifika populations. Chapter 3 focuses on music therapy research and practice as it is represented in the international literature base. In Chapter 4 I return to my own project, to discuss the research design and processes in depth, and in Chapter 5 I draw on findings from the exploratory study (Rickson et al., 2015a, 2015b) to outline the way music therapy with tamariki takiwātanga is practiced in this country, and I explain how the case studies will be presented in subsequent chapters.

Chapters 6–15 contain ten case studies of music therapy with individual tamariki takiwātanga. In each of these chapters readers are given a brief introduction to a child and music therapist, and a summary of the music therapy intervention, followed by the main content—descriptions of each child's music therapy process from the observers' (commentators) perspectives. Subsequent Chapters 16–23 are grounded in themes from the cross-case analysis and include the commentators' overall perceptions of the ways in which music therapy helped the children, the resources that were utilized, goal setting and planning, child-centred processes, the individual nature of the sessions, and the evaluation and reporting procedures particularly as they related to Narrative Assessment. The final chapter examines the ways their observations align with good practice as outlined in the NZ Autism Spectrum Disorder Guideline (Ministries of Health & Education, 2016) and the Enabling Good Lives approach (Ministries of Health, Education, & Social Development, 2021).

References

Aigen, K. (2015). A critique of evidence-based practice in music therapy. *Music Therapy Perspectives, 33*(1), 12–24. https://doi.org/10.1093/mtp/miv013

Ansdell, G. (2020). *Shining some (gentle) light on ecological validity in music therapy research.* 2020 Online World Congress of Music Therapy, University of Pretoria.

Bakan, M. B. (2014). Ethnomusicological perspectives on autism, neurodiversity, and music therapy. In *Voices: A world forum for music therapy* (Vol. 14, No. 3). https://doi.org/10.15845/voices.v14i3.799

Bakan, M. B. (2018). *Speaking for ourselves.* Oxford University Press. https://doi.org/10.1093/oso/9780190855833.003.0005

Berger, R. (2015). Now I see it, now I don't: Researcher's position and reflexivity in qualitative research. *Qualitative Research, 15*(2), 219–234. https://doi.org/10.1177/1468794112468475

Bury, S. M., Jellett, R., Spoor, J. R., & Hedley, D. (2020). "It defines who I am" or "It's something I have": What language do [autistic] Australian adults [on the autism spectrum] prefer? *Journal of Autism and Developmental Disorders.* https://doi.org/10.1007/s10803-020-04425-3

Coffey, A. (2003). Ethnography and self: Reflections and representations. In T. May (Ed.), *Qualitative research in action* (pp. 313–331). Sage.

Epstein, S., Elefant, C., & Thompson, G. (2020). Music therapists' perceptions of the therapeutic potentials using music when working with verbal children on the autism spectrum: A qualitative analysis. *The Journal of Music Therapy, 57*(1), 66–90. https://doi.org/10.1093/jmt/thz017

Kapp, S. K. (2020). Introduction. In S. K. Kapp (Ed.), *Autistic community and the neurodiversity movement: Stories from the frontline* (pp. 1–19). Springer Singapore. https://doi.org/10.1007/978-981-13-8437-0_1

Kapp, S. K., Gillespie-Lynch, K., Sherman, L. E., & Hutman, T. (2013, January). Deficit, difference, or both? Autism and neurodiversity. *Developmental Psychology, 49*(1), 59–71. http://dx.doi.org/10.1037/a0028353

Kenny, L., Hattersley, C., Molins, B., Buckley, C., Povey, C., & Pellicano, E. (2016). Which terms should be used to describe autism? Perspectives from the UK autism community. *Autism: The International Journal of Research and Practice, 20*(4), 442–462. https://doi.org/10.1177/1362361315588200

Kim, Y. S., Leventhal, B. L., Koh, Y.-J., Fombonne, E., Laska, E., Lim, E.-C., Cheon, K.-A., Kim, S.-J., Kim, Y.-K., Lee, H., Song, D.-H., & Grinker, R. R. (2011, September 1). Prevalence of autism spectrum disorders in a total population sample. *American Journal of Psychiatry, 168*(9), 904–912. https://doi.org/10.1176/appi.ajp.2011.10101532

Lai, M.-C., Lombardo, M. V., Pasco, G., Ruigrok, A. N. V., Wheelwright, S. J., Sadek, S. A., Chakrabarti, B., & Baron-Cohen, S. (2011). A behavioral comparison of male and female adults with high functioning autism spectrum conditions. *PLoS ONE, 6*(6), e20835. https://doi.org/10.1371/journal.pone.0020835

Ministries of Health and Education. (2016). *New Zealand autism spectrum disorder guideline* (2nd ed.). Ministry of Health. https://www.health.govt.nz/publication/new-zealand-autism-spectrum-disorder-guideline

Ministries of Health, Education, & Social Development. (2021). *Enabling good lives.* Ministries of Health, Education, & Social Development. Retrieved November 10 from https://www.enablinggoodlives.co.nz/

Ministry of Education. (2009). *Narrative assessment: A guide for teachers.* Learning Media. http://www.throughdifferenteyes.org.nz/a_guide_for_teachers

Opai, K. (2020). *From autism to takiwātanga:* ASfAR 2020 Conference, Wellington, New Zealand.

Probst, B. (2015). The eye regards itself: Benefits and challenges of reflexivity in qualitative social work research. *Social Work Research, 39*(1), 37–48. https://doi.org/10.1093/swr/svu028

Rickson, D. J., Castelino, A., Molyneux, C., Ridley, H., & Upjohn-Beatson, E. (2016). What evidence? Designing a mixed methods study to investigate music therapy with children who have autism spectrum disorder (ASD), in New Zealand Contexts. *The Arts in Psychotherapy, 50*, 119–125. https://doi.org/10.1016/j.aip.2016.07.002

Rickson, D. J., Molyneux, C., Ridley, H., Castelino, A., & Upjohn-Beatson, E. (2015a). *Music therapy for children who have autism spectrum disorder ASD: Exploring the potential for research in New Zealand using a mixed methods design*. Victoria University of Wellington.

Rickson, D. J., Molyneux, C., Ridley, H., Castelino, A., & Upjohn Beatson, E. B. (2015b). Music therapy with people who have autism spectrum disorder—Current practice in New Zealand. *New Zealand Journal of Music Therapy, 13*, 8–32. https://www-proquest-com.helicon.vuw.ac.nz/docview/1897698669?accountid=14782

Stern, D. N. (1985). *The interpersonal world of the infant*. Basic Books Inc.

Walshaw, M. (2010, July 3–7). *The researcher's self in research: Confronting issues about knowing and understanding others*. Annual Meeting of the Mathematics Education Research Group of Australasia, Freemantle, WA.

Warwick, A. (2019). Prelude: The unanswered question. In H. Dunn, E. Coombes, E. Maclean, H. Mottram, & J. Nugent (Eds.), *Music therapy and autism across the lifespan: A spectrum of approaches* (pp. 15–34). Jessica Kingsley.

Williams, D. (2002). Foreword. In D. S. Berger (Ed.), *Music therapy, sensory integration and the autistic child* (pp. 11–12). Jessica Kingsley.

2

Autism—Takiwātanga

Autism Spectrum Disorder (ASD)

Autism Spectrum Disorder (ASD) is a broad medical term used to describe a range of developmental conditions that impact on the way people see, hear, and feel the world; and in turn on their ability to relate to and communicate with others. According to the Diagnostic and Statistical Manual of Mental Disorders (DSM-5) (American Psychiatric Association, 2013), people who have this diagnosis experience difficulties with social communication and interaction, and restricted interests and/or repetitive behaviours. Differences can be observed in early childhood.

Children who are diagnosed with ASD are presumed to require support (Level I), substantial support (Level 2), or very substantial support (Level 3). The number of people diagnosed with this condition is increasing rapidly, estimated to be one in 160 children worldwide (World Health Organisation, 2019). Boys are four times more likely to have a diagnosis (Alagoz et al., 2019). The New Zealand Health Survey (NZHS) (Ministry of Health, 2019) suggests that prevalence in children aged between 2 and 14 years in this country might be as high as

D. Rickson, *Music Therapy with Autistic Children in Aotearoa, New Zealand*, https://doi.org/10.1007/978-3-031-05233-0_2

1.6%, and a recent study (Bowden et al., 2020) reinforced these estimates. There is therefore a corresponding need for research that supports management and/or promotes understanding.

While autistic children (tamariki takiwātanga) are a heterogeneous group, there is a general agreement that important learning outcomes include the development of positive relationships, engagement in meaningful and valued activities, independence, and achieving personal fulfilment (Ministry of Education, 2009b). More specifically, a child might need support to initiate or respond to social communication; to share their interests; or to recognise, understand, or share emotions. They might not understand and/or use typical non-verbal communicative behaviours such as eye contact, facial expression, body language, or gestures; and they might have no or limited verbal communication. It can be difficult for some tamariki takiwātanga to engage in or share imaginative play. They might even appear disinterested in other children or adults and prefer solitary play.

Their solitary play might include intense engagement with favoured objects, and they might use these objects in unusual and repetitive ways. For example, rather than beating a cymbal they might become engrossed in spinning it, or they might put all the beaters in the music room in a line. They might also engage in repetitive movements such as flicking their hands, or rocking. These adaptive responses often increase when the children are anxious or stressed. Tamariki takiwātanga are often distressed when circumstances change, or during times of transition, perhaps because they don't understand the context of, or need for, the change. It is also common for them to have over, under, or unusual reactions to sensory input. They may become distressed when specific sounds are too loud and/or disturbing for them; or, in contrast, they might not respond overtly to sound at all and have the appearance of being deaf.

Many tamariki takiwātanga also have narrow interests and may become fixated on a topic. This can be restrictive because, as noted above, they may have difficulty sharing their interests with others and/or have difficulty attending to and learning about other subjects. On the other hand, their intense interest in a topic can be a resource to support their development in other areas. Some have significant cognitive strengths, including the ability to attend to and remember detail, and can have a strong drive to detect patterns (or "systemising") (Baron-Cohen, 2017) such as those that are inherent in music. They often have a special interest in music, and demonstrate superior skills particularly with pitch (Bergmann, 2016; Janzen & Thaut, 2018), timbre, melodic memory, the rules of Western musical harmony, and rhythm synchronisation (Janzen & Thaut, 2018). These musical responses will be discussed further on Sect. "ASD and the Potential of Music." In the introductory chapter, I touched on the idea that takiwātanga can be viewed through various, often contrasting lens. Using the terminology which seems appropriate to each viewpoint, the following paragraphs contrast "Autism Spectrum Disorder" (through a medical lens) with "Autism" or "Takiwātanga" (through a neurodiversity lens).

Autism Spectrum Disorder Through the Medical Lens

Autism spectrum disorders (ASDs) are known to have epigenetic, genetic, and environmental origins, yet the exact aetiology of ASDs still remains unknown (Alagoz et al., 2019; Ansel et al., 2017; Lang et al., 2016). Hundreds of diverse genes that are thought to predispose ASD have been identified (Ansel et al., 2017) and neuroimaging studies have identified cortical differences in people with ASD. For example, medical researchers have observed increased cortical thickness in children diagnosed with ASD from six years onwards, with differences diminishing during adulthood (Khundrakpam et al., 2017). Khundrakpamet and colleagues found that these cortical abnormalities were related to the severity of symptoms in social affect and communication domains. However, evidence of cortical abnormality is inconsistent, due to small sample sizes, differences in participant characteristics such as age, and the heterogeneity of ASD (Khundrakpam et al., 2017).

Drawing on data from social neuroscience, Trevarthen and Delafield-Butt (2013) locate the origin of autism spectrum disorders in early prenatal failure of development and systems that programme timing, serial coordination, and prospective control of movement, that in turn regulate affective evaluations of experiences. They argue that communication is enacted by transfer of dynamic forms of intention and feeling through movement. Mirror neurons activate when we are moving or watching the movements of others and support us to predict and imitate their actions. However, it has long been argued that children with ASD not only find it difficult to understand the actions of others but also lack "Theory of Mind"; the ability to understand the thoughts and feelings of others, and to recognise that not everyone shares our mental state. There are differences in brain activity (both in terms of location and connectivity) between neurotypical and autistic individuals, when they are asked to think about other people's mental state (Peterson, 2014).

Connectivity, specifically dysfunctional cerebro-cerebellar connectivity, might explain the large spectrum of symptoms that comprise ASD (Janzen & Thaut, 2018; Ronconi et al., 2016). Hypersensitivity to some sounds and loud noises for example, might not be associated with hypersensitivity of the auditory pathways but with differences in higher cortical processing systems (Bakan, 2018; Baron-Cohen, 2017; Funabiki et al., 2012; Janzen & Thaut, 2018). If children have higher levels of synaptic connectivity and responsiveness and are receiving stronger and potentially less predictable information than their neurotypical peers, they will expend considerable energy trying to attend to and process this information (Bakan, 2018; Stavropoulos & Carver, 2018). Their social development can be affected by the difficulty they have filtering out irrelevant information, attending to tasks, sharing attention, and engaging in reciprocal interaction with others.

Janzen and Thaut (2018) also argue that there is compelling research evidence indicating that motor and attention deficits are deeply implicated in the development of socio-communication skills. Structural imaging shows differences in the structure and function of the cerebellum which controls motor movement coordination, balance, equilibrium, and muscle tone. Children with ASD often display delay in motor development, and significant and pervasive motor impairments that are not associated with motor stereotypies, such as clumsy gait, poor balance and postural control, manual dexterity, and coordination (Janzen & Thaut, 2018). Unusual motor development is often evident as early as 6–9 months and, if persisting at two years of age, can be one of the best predictors of a later social communication difficulties and ASD diagnosis (Janzen & Thaut, 2018). Music-based developmental training for attention and motor control might therefore become critical in the treatment of autism due to the significant effect of auditory-motor entrainment on motor and attention functions and brain connectivity (Janzen & Thaut, 2018).

Observations that children with ASD lack motivation for social interaction and experience hyper- or hypo- sensitivity to sensory stimulation have also been linked to the reward system. The "Social Motivation Hypothesis" (Chevallier et al., 2012) is supported by studies which demonstrate differences in the development of the neural reward system in children with ASD compared to neurotypical children. It seems they might experience greater reward when anticipating their restricted interests and non-social stimuli, than when they are anticipating social information (Stavropoulos & Carver, 2018). Thus, it could be argued that social isolation, socio-emotional and cognitive delay, and language disorders in autistic children and adults could all be secondary consequences of poor sensorimotor control and affective regulation (Trevarthen & Delafield-Butt, 2013, p. 2). Atypical sensory experience is estimated to occur in as many as 90 per cent of autistic individuals (Robertson & Baron-Cohen, 2017) and is now included as a diagnostic feature of autism (American Psychiatric Association, 2013).

ASD and the Potential of Music

As noted earlier, children diagnosed with ASD often have musical strengths, including "absolute" or "perfect pitch" and enhanced melodic memory (Molnar-Szakacs & Heaton, 2012; Sharda et al., 2018; Stanutz et al., 2014); and have intact emotional responsiveness to music (Sharda et al., 2018). Researchers interested in a neurological approach to music therapy are concerned with the ways music can influence the brain, to support the development of speech, language, and movement.

To recap, the brains of autistic people are characterised by particularly high levels of synaptic connectivity and responsiveness in many areas, e.g., between auditory and visual regions, (Bakan, 2018; Bergmann,

2016; Sharda et al., 2018) and there is also evidence of under-connectivity in some areas, e.g., between auditory and motor regions (Sharda et al., 2018). Musical activities trigger a "widespread network of brain regions, in both cerebral hemispheres, and subcortically as well, including the brain stem, pons, and cerebellum" (Levitin, 2013, p. 20) which are involved in hearing, movement, emotion, pleasure, and memory (Sharda et al., 2018). Janzen and Thaut (2018) note that virtually all music-related tasks demand substantial cerebellum involvement, activating different cortical and subcortical regions in an organised and synchronised way. This suggests the therapeutic effects of music can be transferred to non-musical domains through structural and functional brain changes.

The elaborate, distributed, and reciprocal connectivity between the auditory and motor systems provides explanation for the success of auditory-motor entrainment approaches (Janzen & Thaut, 2018) and why music therapy can support social communication (Sharda et al., 2018) and speech and language development or rehabilitation (Lai et al., 2012; Sharda et al., 2015). For example, children diagnosed with ASD experience increased cortical activation when listening to songs, compared with speech (Lai et al., 2012; Yinger & Gooding, 2014), and active musical participation engages more areas of the brain than passive listening (Yinger & Gooding, 2014). "Music intervention alters functional brain activity in ASD leading to functional communication gains [...] (and) engaging in musical activities can directly influence auditory-motor connections in the brains of children diagnosed with ASD" (Sharda et al., 2018, pp. 8–9). Sharda et al.'s (2018) findings support the hypothesis that the bottom-up integration of sensorimotor brain networks leads to social functioning, rather than top-down music-based reward.

Rhythmic training is also considered to be effective in language rehabilitation (Janzen & Thaut, 2018) and speech production (Wan et al., 2011) because the rhythm of music provides a continuous time reference which primes the motor system into a state of readiness by providing anticipatory time cues that support movement anticipation and motor planning (Janzen & Thaut, 2018). The Neurologic Music Therapy technique, Developmental Speech and Language training through Music

(DSLM) uses a combination of music, speech, and movement (singing, chanting, playing musical instruments) (Thaut et al., 2014). Janzen and Thaut (2018) suggest evidence demonstrating the effects of auditory-motor entrainment on motor and attention functions and brain connectivity strongly points to music-based developmental training taking a critical role in supporting children diagnosed with ASD.

Some researchers have begun to suggest that music therapy may be able to improve brain function if it is specifically targeted to known impaired functions and tailored to the needs of individual children (Marquez-Garcia et al., 2021; Sharda et al., 2018). However, Bergman (2016) notes that neurological research has predominantly focused on the special abilities that people on the autism spectrum display, such as absolute pitch detection. They suggest emotionality, empathy, and affective regulation, and their relationships to music reception and active music playing, may be more relevant for music therapy practice.

Autism Spectrum Disorder: Disability or Neurodiversity?

Medicine has emphasised many deficits or abnormalities associated with the diagnosis of ASD and has, until recently at least, assumed that people who have the "disorder" would want to be different, to be other than as they are (Swain & French, 2000). The medical model, and medical approaches to music therapy such as those described above, therefore aim to ameliorate or cure the behaviours or traits that people with autistic conditions portray. Many people consider this to be a disempowering model because it suggests autistic people are reliant on experts to find answers to their "problems" rather than being able to find their own solutions. Over recent decades however, people have begun to develop self-advocacy; to challenge the ways societies understand and value human differences; and to agree that "disability" is the result of complex interactions between biological, psychological, cultural, and socio-political factors (Anastasiou & Kauffman, 2012).

This rejection of the medicalisation of difference has led to the emergence of various models of disability. Proponents of the "social model" for example argue that "disability" is the consequence of increased demands for productivity within uncaring and aggressive capitalistic societies (Anastasiou & Kauffman, 2012; Snyder & Mitchell, 2006). Political, social, and environmental norms result in misunderstandings and the mistreatment of individuals who are different and are said to *create* disability by preventing their participation and personal growth (Hemingway, 2008; Kapp, 2020). In the social model the focus turns from medical interventions and rehabilitation to valuing diversity and achieving social change to ensure every person has equal opportunities to participate fully in their communities.

Baron-Cohen (2017) argues that genetic, neural, behavioural, and cognitive evidence suggests that autistic people are different, and live with a disability, but not a disorder. Disorder is usually taken to require cure or treatment, whereas "disability requires societal support, acceptance of difference and diversity, and societal 'reasonable adjustment'" (p. 745). This acknowledgement of the interrelationship between bodily and social challenges led to the current predominant biopsychosocial model (World Health Organisation & World Bank, 2011). "Affirmative," "cultural," and "biopsychosocial" understandings of disability not only recognise biological difference but also celebrate it as important and natural human variation (Kapp et al., 2013). Natural human variation has been increasingly referred to as "neurodiversity" (Kapp, 2020; Kapp et al., 2013), and autistic people (takiwātanga) and others who function in a significantly different way to neurotypical people, as neurodivergent.

Acceptance of neurodiversity does not necessarily mean supporting the social model of disability and opposing the medical model. People who understand takiwātanga as neurodiversity are likely to observe and accept diagnostic criteria, and to conceptualise autism as biological, natural, and essentially innate (Kapp, 2020). However, they recognise that difference is not necessarily undesirable and reject the suggestion that takiwātanga is a disorder which can or should be cured. Instead, autistic forms of communication and self-expression are celebrated, and it is acknowledged that being takiwātanga can be valuable, exciting, and intrinsically satisfying (Campbell, 2008). The concept of neurodiversity therefore enables takiwātanga to develop a sense of pride in their minority group identity. As noted in the introduction of this book, many autistic people believe that "autism" is fundamental to their being, and they have no desire to be neurotypical (Jaarsma & Welin, 2012). They often understand and describe autism as an internal process, referring to thoughts, emotions, and sensations rather than external behaviours. This "inside-out view of autism" (Kapp, 2020) helps neurotypical people to understand that many of the atypical behaviours that takiwātanga engage in are adaptive responses to their environment.

When takiwātanga is explained as an identity marker, the importance of applying a framework that values the range of human differences and rights, including the rights to non-discrimination, inclusion, and autonomy, is highlighted (Kapp, 2020). The neurodiversity movement is therefore a social justice movement with takiwātanga fighting for improved attitudes and services, and to ensure that practices and research interests serve their needs, and the needs of parents (Kapp, 2020; Kapp et al., 2013). Neurotypical people are encouraged to learn from takiwātanga's experiences, draw on their "insider knowledge," and involve them in all issues that concern them (Bakan, 2018; Kapp, 2020). Acceptance of neurodiversity therefore involves neurotypical people being in autistic spaces and worlds, just as autistic people are invited into neurotypical spaces and worlds.

Neurodiversity and the Potential of Therapy

Importantly, neurodiversity and disability rights advocates are mostly accepting of informed choice regarding whether people choose to value their autistic identity or look towards prevention and cure (Kapp et al., 2013). Many proponents of neurodiversity acknowledge the value of appearing to be more neurotypical and may choose adaptation over the longer process of socio-political change (Kapp et al., 2013). For many too, having a medical diagnosis of Autism Spectrum Disorder is important because it is the only way they can obtain the services and support they need; rejection of the medical model could leave them with severe disadvantage. This is unfortunate. As Garcia (2020) argues, societies should "welcome neurodivergent people and give them the tools necessary to live a life of dignity [...] Instead of the world trying to make us be more 'neurotypical,' the world should celebrate our atypicality and accommodate accordingly" (p. 234).

Many of the therapeutic approaches used with takiwātanga may support them to develop behaviours and coping mechanisms that "mask" their autism. However, therapies that utilise Takiwātanga's strengths and interests, such as music, are important because the careful harnessing of "restricted" interests can foster social communication (Kapp et al., 2013; Savarese & Savarese, 2010). Kapp (2020) argues that more successful approaches involve educating others to respectfully understand takiwātanga's differences and to communicate on their terms rather than attempting to make them "less autistic." Therapeutic approaches that align with neurodiversity theories therefore typically focus on subjective well-being and adaptive functioning such as reliable (not necessarily verbal) forms of communication (Bakan, 2018); rather than normative performances such as the development of eye contact, reduction of repetitive movements, or speech (Kapp et al., 2013). Kapp's argument was reinforced in findings from a music therapy study (Low, 2021) in which autistic adults identified desired outcomes in the areas of anxiety reduction, self-advocacy, self-acceptance, self-expression, and musical skills. Positive interventions that accept, encourage, and support tamariki takiwātanga to communicate and be more flexible, are highly valued.

Takiwātanga: A Cultural Perspective

Like many ethnic minority groups, Māori and Pacific Island people are considered at risk of disadvantage across economic, health, and education domains (Bowden et al., 2020; Eggleston et al., 2019). While autistic people are found in all cultures and ethnicities and across socio-economic levels (American Psychiatric Association, 2013), various cultural understandings and practices, and access to resources, can have an influence on the prevalence, assessment, diagnosis, and understanding of takiwātanga.

For example, evidence suggests that rates of diagnosis of indigenous children are lower than in non-indigenous populations (Bailey & Arciuli, 2020; Bevan-Brown & Moldovanu, 2016; Bowden et al., 2020).

Systemic barriers can make healthcare systems inaccessible (Bowden et al., 2020) and minority groups experiencing socio-economic disadvantage might not seek diagnosis or support because of language, economic or geographic barriers; paucity of knowledge about autism; lack of diagnostic services; and/or because they perceive risks associated with increased marginalisation (Bailey & Arciuli, 2020; Bevan-Brown & Moldovanu, 2016; Bowden et al., 2020). On the other hand, there may be disinterest in diagnosis because "historical poverty, marginalisation, and racism have led some Indigenous communities to perceive disability as just one aspect of more general post-colonisation disadvantage" (Bailey & Arciuli, 2020, p. 1039).

However, a recent regional study in New Zealand (Drysdale & van der Meer, 2020) found the rate of takiwātanga diagnosis for Māori (23%) to be ***higher*** than the population rate (17.4%) in the city region in which their study was located. The authors suggested Māori may have good access to assessment in this location, because higher rates of identification can be anticipated in urban areas compared to rural areas (Antezana et al., 2017; Bowden et al., 2020).

> Geographic distance to healthcare providers, reduced ASD awareness, including within schools and healthcare providers, and potentially cultural characteristics such as lower levels of education and socioeconomic status, are all postulated to contribute to the diminished identification of ASD in rural areas. (Bowden Et Al., 2020, P. 2222)

A recent national study of parent satisfaction with the diagnostic process in New Zealand (Eggleston et al., 2019) included 516 parents/caregivers, recruited from takiwātanga support groups. Most participants identified as NZ European (80.6%), while 8.7% identified as Māori, 5.2% Asian, 2.9% Pacific Islander and 1.6% "other." In contrast, the New Zealand census (Statistics New Zealand, 2018) reported population figures of 70% New Zealand European, 16.5% Māori, 15.3% Asian, and 9% Pacific Islanders. Eggleston and colleagues make two important observations. Firstly, that parents in their study were highly educated and, secondly, those who belong to support groups are not likely to be representative of all New Zealand parents (Eggleston et al., 2019). So, while a little over half were satisfied with the diagnostic process, and figures were no different for Māori and Pacific Island parents compared with others in their study, the Māori and Pacific Island parents may not have been representative of their wider communities.

It is also important to note that indigenous families might not view their child's behaviours as representations of autism (Bailey & Arciuli, 2020; Bevan-Brown & Moldovanu, 2016). Many "symptoms" of takiwātanga, including lack of eye contact, verbal gesture, and emotional expression, are viewed differently across cultural groups, and might not be noticed because they are considered "normal" in that cultural context (Bailey & Arciuli, 2020; Bevan-Brown & Moldovanu, 2016; Dyches et al., 2004). Further, symptoms may manifest differently because children are exposed to different environments, beliefs, and practices; and in some contexts, they might be ignored because it is believed the child will "grow out of it"; or because they are perceived to be "naughty" (Bevan-Brown & Moldovanu, 2016, pp. 158–159). It is also possible that some indigenous families delay seeking diagnosis and treatment because they experience feelings of whakamā (shame, shyness, and embarrassment) (Bevan-Brown & Moldovanu, 2016). A Sāmoan mum writes of her dilemma about informing her family that her "beautiful boy" had been diagnosed with ASD.

> People who weren't considered "normal" were on the list of things that my Sāmoan parents' generation weren't used to talking about—unless it was to laugh at them and label them as valea (stupid) or leaga le ulu (mental, crazy) [...] After the initial denial and blame, they became staunch advocates and active "trigger monitors" for their grandson, who needed their love and support to cope with the outside world. (Malaeulu, 2020)

Within Māori and Pacifika communities, takiwātanga can be viewed as an individual characteristic which can be supported within the wider community (Bailey & Arciuli, 2020; Bevan-Brown, 2004). Pasifika people often adopt a family or community-based model of care for their children and are likely to try to manage by themselves before seeking professional help outside their community (Bowden et al., 2020). This observation is reinforced by Drysdale et al.'s (2020) findings which suggest while diagnosis for Māori was relatively high in the region of interest the rate for Pasifika people living in the same region was *lower* than the population figure. Moreover, Malaeulu (2020), referenced above, goes on to say, "It takes a village to raise a child and, thankfully, our family village supported us and the changes we had to make to meet (our son's) needs" (no page number). Bevan-Brown (2013) notes that Māori families, too, typically believe their children with disabilities have personal mana (value, power, and prestige) and care for them in genuinely inclusive environments.

Differences in the ways takiwātanga are perceived means that diagnostic tools will not always lead to culturally responsive and respectful assessments. Moreover, assessors do not always have appropriate cultural knowledge and language to facilitate assessment processes. In the New Zealand context, for example, lack of understanding of Māori culture and te reo Māori language has led to the "use of culturally inappropriate assessment questions and content, and the misinterpretation of children's answers and behaviour" (Bevan-Brown & Moldovanu, 2016). Bevan-Brown and Moldovanu (2016) also note that clinic bias (the relationship and attitudes of clinicians towards help-seekers) impacts on both diagnosis and treatment. It is clear then that:

> Interventions developed in Western societies cannot be applied indiscriminately to people with disabilities across the world [...] The expectations, practices and pedagogy involved in certain programs can clash with the family's culture or make members feel 'exposed' or judged. [...] Differing cultural values, attitudes, concepts and manifestations of ASD, educational philosophies, approaches, expectations and child rearing practices can all be problematic. (Bevan-Brown & Moldovanu, 2016, pp. 160–162)

Practitioner understanding of the cultural background of music therapy participants is therefore crucial. Researchers have found that lack of culturally appropriate services, programmes, assessments, and resources has led not only to inadequate provisions for Māori children, but also to their exclusion from schools (Bevan-Brown, 2013). "Positive outcomes are maximised when medical and educational interventions take account of cultural values, attitudes, practices and content, and include culturally appropriate support" (Bevan-Brown & Moldovanu, 2016, p. 163).

Consideration should be given to services that cultivate reciprocity, respect, and collaboration; nurture trust-based relationships in which parents feel safe to talk about their beliefs and the interventions and treatments they are already using; and have the potential to problem solve and resolve conflict (Bevan-Brown & Moldovanu, 2016). Child-centred approaches may be uncomfortable for parents with Asian backgrounds, for example, because they expect programmes to be structured and involve the systematic repetitious practice of skills (Bevan-Brown & Moldovanu, 2016). The concept of "parent as expert" in the lives of their children is highly valued in New Zealand. However, while consulting and involving parents and whānau in assessment, diagnosis, and intervention processes is considered important; the nature and extent of their participation should take account of their comfort levels (Bevan-Brown & Moldovanu, 2016).

References

Alagoz, M., Kherad, N., Gavaz, M., & Yuksel, A. (2019). New genetic approaches for early diagnosis and treatment of autism spectrum disorders. *Review Journal of Autism and Developmental Disorders, 6*(4), 367–380. https://doi.org/10.1007/s40489-019-00167-w

American Psychiatric Association. (2013). *Diagnostic criteria from DSM-V*. American Psychiatric Association.

Ansel, A., Rosenzweig, J. P., Zisman, P. D., Melamed, M., & Gesundheit, B. (2017). Variation in gene express ion in autism spectrum disorders: An extensive review of transcriptomic studies. *Frontiers in Neuroscience, 10*, 601. https://doi.org/10.3389/fnins.2016.00601

Anastasiou, D., & Kauffman, J. M. (2012, May 1). Disability as cultural difference: Implications for special education. *Remedial and Special Education, 33*(3), 139–149. http://dx.doi.org/10.1177/0741932510383163

Antezana, L., Scarpa, A., Valdespino, A., Albright, J., & Richey, J. A. (2017). Rural trends in diagnosis and services for autism spectrum disorder. *Frontiers in Psychology, 8*, 590–590. https://doi.org/10.3389/fpsyg.2017.00590

Bailey, B., & Arciuli, J. (2020). Indigenous Australians with autism: A scoping review. *Autism, 24*(5), 1031–1046. https://doi.org/10.1177/1362361319894829

Bakan, M. B. (2018). *Speaking for ourselves*. Oxford University Press. https://doi.org/10.1093/oso/9780190855833.003.0005

Baron-Cohen, S. (2017). Editorial perspective: Neurodiversity—A revolutionary concept for autism and psychiatry. *Journal of Childhood Psychology and Psychiatry, 58*, 744–747. https://doi-org.helicon.vuw.ac.nz/10.1111/jcpp.12703

Bergmann, T. (2016). Music therapy for people with autism spectrum disorder. In J. Edwards (Ed.), *The Oxford handbook of music therapy*. Oxford University Press. https://doi.org/10.1093/oxfordhb/9780199639755.013.3

Bevan-Brown, J. (2004). *Maori perspectives of autistic spectrum disorder: Report to the Ministry of Education*. Ministry of Education.

Bevan-Brown, J. (2013). Including people with disabilities: An indigenous perspective. *International Journal of Inclusive Education, 17*(6), 571–583. https://doi.org/10.1080/13603116.2012.694483

Bevan-Brown, J., & Moldovanu, A. (2016). The role of culture in the perception, assessment, diagnosis, treatment and education of children and young people with autism spectrum disorder. In J. Bevan-Brown & V. M. Dharan (Eds.), *Autism spectrum disorder in Aotearoa New Zealand: Promising practices and interesting issues* (pp. 155–168). NZCER Press.

Bowden, N., Thabrew, H., Kokaua, J., Audas, R., Milne, B., Smiler, K., Stace, H., Taylor, B., & Gibb, S. (2020). Autism spectrum disorder/Takiwātanga: An integrated data infrastructure-based approach to autism spectrum disorder research in New Zealand. *Autism: the International Journal of Research and Practice, 24*(8), 2213–2227. https://doi.org/10.1177/1362361320939329

Campbell, C. (2008). Further towards an affirmation model. In T. Campbell, F. Fontes, L. Hemingway, A. Soorenian, & C. Till (Eds.), *Disability studies: Emerging insights and perspectives*. The Disability Press.

Chevallier, C., Kohls, G., Troiani, V., Brodkin, E. S., & Schultz, R. T. (2012). The social motivation theory of autism. *Trends in Cognitive Sciences, 16*(4), 231–239. https://doi.org/10.1016/j.tics.2012.02.007

Drysdale, H., & van der Meer, L. (2020). Rates of autism spectrum disorder diagnoses for children and adolescents in the Hutt Valley Region of New Zealand between 2012 and 2016. *Research in Autism Spectrum Disorders, 73*, 101547. https://doi.org/10.1016/j.rasd.2020.101547

Dyches, T. T., Wilder, L. K., Sudweeks, R. R., Obiakor, F. E., & Algozzine, B. (2004). Multicultural issues in autism. *Journal of Autism and Developmental Disorders, 34*(2), 211–222. https://doi.org/10.1023/B:JADD.0000022611.80478.73

Eggleston, M. J. F., Thabrew, H., Frampton, C. M. A., Eggleston, K. H. F., & Hennig, S. C. (2019). Obtaining an autism spectrum disorder diagnosis and supports: New Zealand parents' experiences. *Research in Autism Spectrum Disorders, 62*, 18–25. https://doi.org/10.1016/j.rasd.2019.02.004

Funabiki, Y., Murai, T., & Toichi, M. (2012). Cortical activation during attention to sound in autism spectrum disorders. *Research in Developmental Disabilities, 33*(2), 518–524. https://doi.org/10.1016/j.ridd.2011.10.016

Garcia, E. M. (2020). Covering the politics of neurodiversity: And myself. In S. K. Kapp (Ed.), *Autistic community and the neurodiversity movement: Stories from the frontline* (pp. 233–241). Springer Singapore. https://doi.org/10.1007/978-981-13-8437-0_17

Hemingway, L. (2008). Introduction: Emerging insights and perspectives within disability studies. In T. Campbell, F. Fontes, L. Hemingway, A. Soorenian, & C. Till (Eds.), *Disability studies: Emerging insights and perspectives*. The Disability Press.

Jaarsma, P., & Welin, S. (2012). Autism as a natural human variation: Reflections on the claims of the neurodiversity movement. *Health Care Analysis, 20*(1), 20–30. https://doi.org/10.1007/s10728-011-0169-9

Janzen, T. B., & Thaut, M. H. (2018). Rethinking the role of music in the neurodevelopment of autism spectrum disorder. *Music and Science, 1*, 1–18. https://doi.org/10.1177/2059204318769639

Kapp, S. K., Gillespie-Lynch, K., Sherman, L. E., & Hutman, T. (2013, January). Deficit, difference, or both? Autism and neurodiversity. *Developmental Psychology, 49*(1), 59–71. http://dx.doi.org/10.1037/a0028353

Kapp, S. K. (2020). Introduction. In S. K. Kapp (Ed.), *Autistic community and the neurodiversity movement: Stories from the frontline* (pp. 1–19). Springer Singapore. https://doi.org/10.1007/978-981-13-8437-0_1

Khundrakpam, B. S., Lewis, J. D., Kostopoulos, P., Carbonell, F., & Evans, A. (2017). Cortical thickness abnormalities in autism spectrum disorders through late childhood, adolescence, and adulthood: A large-scale MRI study. *Cerebral Cortex, 27*, 1721–1731. https://doi.org/10.1093/cercor/bhx038

Lai, G., Pantazatos, S. P., Schneider, H., & Hirsch, J. (2012, March). Neural systems for speech and song in autism. *Brain, 135*, 961–975. https://doi.org/10.1093/brain/awr335

Lang, R., Hancock, T. B., & Singh, N. N. (2016). Overview of early intensive behavioral intervention for children with autism. In R. Lang, T. B. Hancock, & N. N. Singh (Eds.), *Early intervention for young children with autism spectrum disorder* (pp. 1–14). Springer International Publishing. https://doi.org/10.1007/978-3-319-30925-5_1

Levitin, D. J. (2013). Neural correlates of musical behaviors a brief overview. *Music Therapy Perspectives, 31*(1), 15–24. https://doi.org/10.1093/mtp/31.1.15

Low, M. Y. (2021). *Experiences of autistic clients in Nordoff-Robbins music therapy: An interpretive phenomenological analysis*. Drexel University.

Malaeulu, D. (2020). We're blessed to have a son with autism. *E-tangata (Web site): A Māori and Pasifika Sunday magazine*. https://e-tangata.co.nz/reflections/were-blessed-to-have-a-son-with-autism/

Marquez-Garcia, A. V., Magnuson, J., Morris, J., Iarocci, G., Doesburg, S., & Moreno, S. (2021). Music therapy in autism spectrum disorder: A systematic review. *Review Journal of Autism and Developmental Disorders*. https://doi.org/10.1007/s40489-021-00246-x

Ministry of Health. (2019). *New Zealand health survey*. Ministry of Health. Retrieved December 9, 2021 from https://www.health.govt.nz/nz-health-statistics/national-collections-and-surveys/surveys/new-zealand-health-survey

Ministry of Education. (2009b). *Special education guidelines*. http://www.minedu.govt.nz/NZEducation/EducationPolicies/SpecialEducation

Molnar-Szakacs, I., & Heaton, P. (2012). Music: A unique window into the world of autism: Molnar-Szakacs & Heaton. *Annals of the New York Academy of Sciences, 1252*(1), 318–324. https://doi.org/10.1111/j.1749-6632.2012.06465.x

Peterson, C. (2014). Theory of mind understanding and empathic behavior in children with autism spectrum disorders. *International Journal of Developmental Neuroscience, 39*, 16–21. https://doi.org/10.1016/j.ijdevneu.2014.05.002

Robertson, C. E., & Baron-Cohen, S. (2017). Sensory perception in autism. *Nature Reviews Neuroscience, 18*(11), 671–684. https://doi.org/10.1038/nrn.2017.112

Ronconi, L., Molteni, M., & Casartelli, L. (2016). Building blocks of others' understanding: A perspective shift in investigating social-communicative deficit in autism. *Frontiers in Human Neuroscience, 10*, 144–144. https://doi.org/10.3389/fnhum.2016.00144

Savarese, E. T., & Savarese, R. J. (2010). "The superior half of speaking": An introduction. *Disability Studies Quarterly, 30*(1), Online. http://dx.doi.org/10.18061/dsq.v30i1

Sharda, M., Midha, R., Malik, S., Mukerji, S., & Singh, N. C. (2015). Fronto-temporal connectivity is preserved during sung but not spoken word listening, across the autism spectrum. *Autism Research, 8*(2), 174–186. https://doi.org/10.1002/aur.1437

Sharda, M., Tuerk, C., Chowdhury, R., Jamey, K., Foster, N., Custo-Blanch, M., Tan, M., Nadig, A., & Hyde, K. (2018). Music improves social communication and auditory-motor connectivity in children with autism. *Translational Psychiatry, 8*(1), 213–231. https://doi.org/10.1038/s41398-018-0287-3

Snyder, S. L., & Mitchell, D. T. (2006). *Cultural locations of disability*. University of Chicago Press. https://doi.org/10.7208/9780226767307

Stanutz, S., Wapnick, J., & Burack, J. A. (2014). Pitch discrimination and melodic memory in children with autism spectrum disorders. *Autism: the International Journal of Research and Practice, 18*(2), 137–147. https://doi.org/10.1177/1362361312462905

Statistics New Zealand. (2018). *2018 census*. https://www.stats.govt.nz/2018-census

Stavropoulos, K. K., & Carver, L. J. (2018). Oscillatory rhythm of reward: Anticipation and processing of rewards in children with and without autism. *Molecular Autism, 9*(4), 1–15. https://doi.org/10.1186/s13229-018-0189-5

Swain, J., & French, S. (2000). Towards an affirmation model of disability. *Disability & Society, 15*(4), 569–582. https://doi.org/10.1080/09687590050058189

Thaut, M., Hoemberg, V., & Abiru, M. (2014). *Handbook of neurologic music therapy* (1st ed.). Oxford University Press.

Trevarthen, C., & Delafield-Butt, J. T. (2013). Autism as a developmental disorder in intentional movement and affective engagement. *Frontiers and Integrative Neuroscience, 7*, 1–16. https://doi.org/10.3389/fnint.2013.00049

Wan, C. Y., Bazen, L., Baars, R., Libenson, A., Zipse, L., Zuk, J., Norton, A., & Schlaug, G. (2011). Auditory-motor mapping training as an intervention to facilitate speech output in non-verbal children with autism: A proof of concept study. *PLoS ONE, 6*(9), e25505. https://doi.org/10.1371/journal.pone.0025505

World Health Organisation, & World Bank. (2011). *World report on disability*. https://www.who.int/publications/i/item/9789241564182

World Health Organisation. (2019). *Autism spectrum disorders*. World Health Organisation. Retrieved August 20, 2020 from https://www.who.int/newsroom/fact-sheets/detail/autism-spectrum-disorders

Yinger, O. S., & Gooding, L. (2014, July). Music therapy and music medicine for children and adolescents. *Child and Adolescent Psychiatric Clinics of North America, 23*(3), 535–553. https://doi.org/10.1016/j.chc.2013.03.003

3

Music Therapy with Tamariki Takiwātanga

Part 1: Music Therapy Research

Therapies that support engagement and creativity are important for children on the autism spectrum (Marquez-Garcia et al., 2021), and music therapy is a popular option (Brondino et al., 2015; Dharan, 2015; Kasilingam et al., 2019). The evidence base comprises many case reports and smaller studies (Accordino et al., 2007; Bergmann, 2016) as well as a growing number of systematic reviews and meta-analyses. With the former, a researcher answers research questions by collecting and summarising all the relevant empirical evidence, and with the latter the researcher uses statistical methods to summarise the results of these studies.

For example, Geretsegger et al.'s (2014) meta-analysis of 10 clinical trials, focusing specifically on research into music therapy for autistic people, found moderate-to-large effects of music therapy on interpersonal skills including social interaction, non-verbal communication, social-emotional reciprocity, and parent–child relationship. These authors were able to conclude that music therapy may help children with ASD to improve skills related to the core of the condition (Geretsegger

D. Rickson, *Music Therapy with Autistic Children in Aotearoa, New Zealand*,
https://doi.org/10.1007/978-3-031-05233-0_3

et al., 2014). Specifically, the analyses suggested music therapy can improve initiating behaviours and verbal communication within sessions, and social interaction within and beyond the therapy context. Similarly, following her meta-analysis, which included 12 studies with a total of 170 participants, Whipple (2018) was able to claim that music therapy is effective for individuals on the autism spectrum across the lifespan, but particularly during early years. Improvements were noted in communication, interpersonal relationships, personal responsibility, and play skills in young children diagnosed with ASD (Whipple, 2018).

Likewise, systematic reviews have suggested music therapy has positive impacts, particularly in supporting social interaction and verbal and non-verbal communication (James et al., 2015; Marquez-Garcia et al., 2021). James et al.'s (2015) review included twelve studies with a total of 147 participants: eight involving preschoolers, three involving older children, and one involving adults. The music therapy approaches included improvisation as well as songs with lyrics to target specific skills, and were focused on decreasing undesirable behaviour, promoting social interaction, improving independent functioning, enhancing understanding of emotions, and increasing communication (p. 39). The authors found positive outcomes in 58% of the studies, mixed outcomes in a further 42%, and no negative outcomes. Similarly, Marquez-Garcia et al. (2021) engaged in a systematic review of 36 articles focusing on improvisation or listening to or singing songs, published between 2008 and 2018. Like James et al., (2015) these authors concluded that the results are encouraging.

Broader reviews also found positive outcomes related to music therapy. For example, Su Maw and Haga (2018) conducted a meta-analysis to determine the effectiveness of a range of cognitive, developmental, and behavioural interventions for preschool children on the autism spectrum. Of fourteen included studies, the three that focused on music therapy (Kim et al., 2008; Lim & Draper, 2011; Thompson et al., 2013) were found to provide the greatest outcome effects—even though one was of short duration and low intensity. While suggesting more evidence-based trials are needed, the authors were able to conclude that music therapy appears to be effective for improving social interaction with young children on the autism spectrum.

Vaiouli and Andreou (2018) identified eleven studies (ten published since 2010), focusing specifically on music to promote language development in young children on the autism spectrum. Six were contextualised as music education interventions, while five were music therapy. These authors concluded that music and music therapy can provide helpful contexts for developing young children's preverbal and verbal communication.

Simpson and Keen (2011) published a narrative review of the literature relating to the use of music as an intervention, or to facilitate an intervention, with children diagnosed with autism. A total of 20 experimental controlled studies were included. Dependent variables were primarily communication, socialisation, and behavioural skills (Kaplan & Steele, 2005; Simpson & Keen, 2011), while independent variables ranged from improvised music to highly structured activities. The researchers found some limited evidence to suggest that music interventions were helpful for developing social, communicative, and behavioural skills in young tamariki takiwātanga although small sample sizes, a wide range of methods and applications, and the use of multiple interventions impacted the review findings (Simpson & Keen, 2011).

Finally, a review of "complementary and alternative medicines" (CAMs), suggests that music therapy represents a popular therapeutic option for this population (Brondino et al., 2015). While they found no conclusive evidence supporting the efficacy of CAM therapies for autism generally, these researchers detected promising results for music therapy primarily based on findings from the Cochrane Review conducted by Geretsegger et al. (2014) described above.

Simpson and Keen (2011) found most studies relating to music interventions with individuals on the spectrum focused on young children (3–11 years), and very few on young people aged between 12 and 18 years. Perhaps this is unsurprising given the generalised belief that early intervention is important whenever a child is experiencing a developmental delay. Lang et al. (2016) note however, that while some studies suggest that outcomes for children on the spectrum tend to be better the earlier an intervention is initiated, others suggest that the child's age may not be of importance. This may be due to the heterogeneity of autism, varieties of research designs, research contexts, and outcome measures used (Lang et al. 2016). With that in mind, even though this book focuses predominantly on older children, the following sections include examples of music therapy research with very young children, as well as adolescents and adults. It is important to note that some of these studies would have been included in the reviews described above, and that only studies published since 2000 have been included here.

Music Therapy Research Focusing on Very Young Children

Studies with very young children have focused on improving peer interactions, the management of activities of daily living and school routines, interpersonal skills, and speech and language. Dependent variables have predominantly included individualised songs with original or familiar tunes. This is possibly because while the way in which songs may be delivered can vary, they are easier to implement consistently than improvised music therapy. However, music therapists have also been able to undertake experimental research involving improvised approaches with mixed results.

The Use of Song with Young Children

Kern and Aldridge (2006) investigated whether music therapy might support four preschool-aged boys diagnosed with autism to improve peer interactions and engage in meaningful play in the playground. An outdoor music centre was created, the therapist composed original songs for each participant, and teachers collaborated in the implementation of the intervention. The combination of environmental adaptations and individualised interventions led to the boys' increased involvement with peers, and teachers were able to successfully facilitate the interventions in the playground.

In another project involving staff collaboration, Kern, Wakeford, and Aldridge (2007) explored whether music therapists, occupational therapists, and classroom teachers could support a three-year-old boy diagnosed with autism to develop independence with basic self-care tasks such as hand washing, toileting, and cleaning up. Spoken words or lyrics sung to familiar or original tunes provided prompts for each step in the tasks, and both strategies were successful in increasing his independence. In a similar study, Kern et al. (2007) were able to demonstrate that therapist composed songs, using lyrics to convey the demands of a morning routine, assisted two boys to enter their classroom, greet their teacher and peers, and to begin engaging in play.

Finnigan and Starr (2010) explored whether music therapy might increase the social responsiveness of a three-year-old girl. The therapist engaged her in turn-taking play with three toys, without and with music. In the music condition the therapist interacted through singing songs accompanied by guitar. Improvements in eye contact, imitation, and turn-taking were noted. Avoidant behaviours became infrequent and only occurred in baseline or no-music conditions. A longer period of music therapy would have been necessary to determine whether the child had maintained her gains.

Lim (2010) investigated the impact of music training, speech training, and no-training on the verbal production of fifty children diagnosed with autism aged between three and five years. Those in the music training group watched a music video which contained songs and pictures of targeted words, while those in the speech training group watched a video with stories and pictures of the targeted words. The children increased their acquisition of target words in both music and speech training conditions, with children considered to have lower abilities making greater gains in the music condition. The authors conclude that children diagnosed with autism gain important linguistic information from patterns embedded in music.

In a further study, Lim and Draper (2011) compared the impact of sung instructions and songs composed by the music therapist with the same texts delivered in spoken form via Applied Behavioural Analysis (ABA). The researchers found that both music and speech training significantly improved the verbal production of children diagnosed with autism compared to control conditions. Janzen & Thaut (2018) argue that singing may provide an important approach to learning for this population because it can be non-reciprocal, structured and ritualized, slower than speech, and lyrics carry associated meaning. In another example, Simpson, Keen, & Lamb, (2013) attempted to improve engagement and learning outcomes for children diagnosed with ASD by focusing on their receptive labelling skills, using a computer-based communication programme. In this study no significant differences were found between infant-directed song interventions or infant-directed speech intervention.

The Use of Music Therapy Improvisation with Young Children

Kim, Wigram, and Gold (2008) conducted a randomised trial to investigate the effects of improvisational music therapy on joint attention, of ten preschool boys on the autism spectrum, by comparing improvisational music therapy and play sessions with toys (30 min per week over 12 weeks). The music therapy and play sessions were carried out by two different therapists, and a semi-flexible treatment manual was used to ensure the intervention was consistent and reliable. In each session the therapist supported and developed the child's play, before gently introducing modelling and turn-taking activities within the child's focus of attention and range of interest.

Music therapy was found to be significantly more effective than play sessions in addressing joint attention skills, with children offering longer periods of eye contact and turn-taking during music therapy than in play. Moreover, participants engaged in longer turn-taking during the more directive second half of the session, in both conditions. The authors suggest turn-taking may occur spontaneously in freer play, but for longer when the therapists were working to direct the children. In summary, this research suggests that child-centred improvised music therapy can promote social engagement and holds important therapeutic potential for children on the autism spectrum.

In a further report on the same study, Kim et al., (2009) argued that when children were engaged in improvisational music therapy, they experienced longer periods of joy and emotional synchronicity, and initiated engagement and responded positively to the therapist's interpersonal demands more readily. The authors were able to produce important evidence that music therapy supports tamariki takiwātanga's social, emotional, and motivational development.

Music Therapy Research Focusing On Children

The relatively recent large-scale international TIME-A study aimed to overcome the methodological limitations of previous studies by using a larger sample size and examining the effects over longer periods of time. Between 2011 and 2015 three hundred and sixty-four children aged between four and seven years, and their parents, were involved in this study. Each family received five months of enhanced standard care (ESC), involving three 60-min sessions of advice and support in addition to usual treatment. In addition, families were randomly assigned to one of three groups to receive 1) one session of improvised music therapy per week, 2) three sessions of improvised music therapy per week, or 3) to receive the enhanced standard care only. No significant differences were found between treatment and usual care groups, on measures of symptom severity, or between low-intensity and high-intensity music therapy treatment groups compared with usual care, according to the Autism Diagnostic Observation Schedule (ADOS) (Bieleninik et al., 2017; Crawford et al., 2017). However, further exploratory post hoc analyses revealed a significant improvement in the music therapy group on the social motivation subscale (SRS) of the ADOS, and improved scores on the social affect subscale.

Bieleninik and colleagues (2017) suggest the inconsistent findings may be explained by variations in local contexts involving just one or few therapists; the implementation of improvisational interventions; the duration of intervention or inconsistent attendance; methodological differences such as the choice of proximal vs distal outcome; and the ADOS as a measurement tool. Nevertheless, improvisational music therapy seemed very "well accepted by parents, children, and staff" (p. 532). In a qualitative study connected to the trial, parents reported that children enjoyed and benefited from the therapy and their own involvement was positive (Bieleninik et al., 2017). These authors note that some commentators are arguing for a shift towards outcomes such as well-being and adaptive functioning and suggest that "being able to engage in learning, participate successfully in school through childhood and adolescence, and work and have meaningful relationships as adults […] may matter more to people with ASD than symptom severity" (Bieleninik et al., 2017, p. 533).

Listening Vs Interactive Music Therapy

Rabeyron and colleagues (2020) conducted a randomised controlled trial comparing music therapy and music listening for thirty-six children on the autism spectrum, aged from 4 to 7 years. The children were randomly assigned to listening or music therapy groups and were involved in 25 sessions over an eight-month period. Changes were measured using the Clinical Global Impression (CGI) scale, the Childhood Autism Rating Scale (CARS) and the Aberrant Behavior Checklist (ABC). The researchers were able to conclude that music therapy results in greater clinical improvement for children on the autism spectrum, than simply listening to music.

Music Therapy to Enhance Social Communication

In Canada, 51 children on the autism spectrum, aged six to twelve years, participated in a study to determine whether improvised music therapy (using song and rhythm) might improve their social communication, family quality of life, and functional brain connectivity (Sharda et al., 2018). Results show that compared to controls, the children in the music therapy group improved their social communication (including semantics, appropriate initiations, social relations, and interests), and family-related quality of life. Moreover, their MRI scans revealed that connectivity increased between auditory and motor regions and decreased between auditory and visual-association regions following music (Sharda et al., 2018).

Gattino et al. (2011) conducted a randomised controlled trial to examine the effects of Relational Music Therapy (RMT) on the verbal, non-verbal, and social communication of children diagnosed with autism, in a hospital setting. Twenty-four boys aged between 7 and 12 years were involved in the study, which compared music therapy (plus clinical routine activities) with standard treatment (clinical routine activities). The 30-min music therapy sessions held over a period of seven months, involved a variety of activities including singing, improvising, composing, and playing musical games. No significant outcomes were found using the "social communication" domain of the Childhood Autism Rating Scale (Brazilian version) (CARS-BR) so results were deemed to be inconclusive.

Joint Attention

LaGasse (2014) compared the developing social skills of 17 children diagnosed with ASD, aged 6–9 years. The children participated in ten 50-min music therapy or social skills group sessions over a period of five weeks. Findings were mixed, including no significant differences between groups in terms of children's initiations or response communications, and/or withdrawals from the interaction. However, children in the music therapy group made greater gains in joint attention with peers, and eye gaze towards others. Results suggest music therapy social groups might support the development of joint attention for children diagnosed with ASD.

Communication and Interaction

Porter et al.'s (2017) randomised controlled trial involving 251 children (aged 8–16), who experienced social, emotional, behavioural and developmental difficulties, included a subgroup of 18 children on the autism spectrum. The researchers found no significant differences between "music therapy plus usual care" groups, or "usual care" groups in terms of the children's communication and interaction skills. It is important to note however, that while children continued to participate in music therapy, there were high rates of dropout from the research. The low numbers of research participants limited the potential to observe significant differences between groups.

Social Stories

Social Stories ™ (Gray & Garand, 1993) are a well established treatment option for children diagnosed with autism or ASD. Carefully crafted stories are used to model and teach the children how to understand and respond to specific social situations, including how to initiate, reciprocate, maintain, and terminate social interactions. Given the attraction that these children have to music, it is not surprising that many practitioners are interested in whether singing social stories may be more helpful than reading them. However, research in this field has brought mixed results.

Brownell (2002) conducted a study with four children on the autism spectrum and found that singing was better than reading in all cases, but differences were only significant in one case. Despite the small sample size, the author concluded that musically adapted social stories are an effective and viable option for children on the autism spectrum. More recent studies have produced mixed results, however. Pasiali (2004) focused on the use of "prescriptive therapeutic songs" to promote the development of social skills in three young children, while Schwartzberg and Silverman (2013) conducted a larger study involving 30 children. Results were inconclusive in both studies. On the other hand, Pasiali (2004) noted that parents of the children in her study were pleased with the results and believed that their child's participation was beneficial; and Schwartzberg and Silverman (2013) argued that children and staff seemed to enjoy the songs and repeated them throughout the day suggesting sung social stories may support the storage and recall of information.

Music Therapy Research Focusing on Adolescents and Adults

Two studies (Boso et al., 2007; Hillier et al., 2011) focus specifically on music therapy with adolescents or young adults diagnosed with autism, while Pasiali, LaGasse & Penn (2014) worked with a group of adolescents who were described as having broader diagnoses of neurodevelopmental delay. In a contrasting study, Low (2021) engaged in participatory action research with four autistic adults to explicate the meaning of their lived experiences in Nordoff-Robbins Music Therapy.

Boso et al. (2007) focused on the effects of long-term music therapy with eight young adults who were described as having severe autism. The young people took part in 52 hour-long interactive music therapy sessions, which included singing, playing piano, and drumming. The study was small, and no control group was used, so it is not possible to generalise findings. Nevertheless, the authors suggest that active music therapy could improve autistic symptoms, as well as personal musical skills in young adults with severe autism.

In contrast, Hillier et al.'s (2011) study involved twenty-two "high functioning" adolescents and young adults on the autism spectrum (aged between 13–29 years). During the music therapy sessions, participants were engaged in a variety of music making activities including listening to and discussing different types of music, exploring, and improvising on various musical instruments, and composing, with a view to producing a short movie and soundtrack using GarageBand. Findings indicate that participants experienced improved self-esteem, reduced anxiety, and an increase in their positive attitudes towards peers.

Pasiali, LaGasse, & Penn (2014) found significant improvements in the selective attention and rapid shifting of attention in adolescents with neurodevelopmental delays, including autism, after eight sessions of Musical Attention Control Training (MACT). Musical Attention Control Training involves "perceptual and structured musical exercises built on rhythmic, melodic and harmonic patterns to train sustained, selective, divided, focused, and shifting attention" (Janzen & Thaut, 2018, p. 9).

To participate in Low's (2021) the autistic adults needed to be able to communicate verbally or with assistive technology, and purposeful sampling was used to recruit participants who could yield the richest data. The four men highlighted the importance of music therapy for the development of their musicianship and personal selves; meaningful relationships with their peers, music therapists, and music; and the valuing of the socio-cultural identities.

Improvisational Music Therapy

Researchers have found improvisational music therapy to be a promising intervention to improve the social communication skills, and the self-awareness, emotional expression, and understanding of children diagnosed with ASD (Geretsegger et al., 2014; James et al., 2015; Janzen & Thaut, 2018; Marquez-Garcia et al., 2021). Kim et al.'s, (2008) investigation of the effects of improvisational music therapy on the joint attention skills of children with ASD found significant improvement in music compared to control conditions. A subsequent microanalysis of the video data from this study (Kim et al., 2009), also suggested that children demonstrated increased emotion in the music condition compared to the toy play. LaGasse's (2014) study, comparing the effects of music therapy and non-musical social skills intervention on the cooperative play and communication of children diagnosed with ASD found significant improvement in joint attention with peers, and eye gaze towards other people, compared to the control group.

On the other hand, the more recent large-scale multicentre randomised clinical trial (RCT) described above, involving 364 children aged between 4 and 7 years, did not support these results (Bieleninik et al., 2017). Moreover, Gattino et al., (2011) found no significant differences between improvisational music therapy and standard care in improving the verbal, non-verbal, and social communication skills of children diagnosed with autism, PDDNOS, and Asperger's Syndrome; although a subgroup analysis suggested that for those diagnosed with autism only there was a significant increase in non-verbal communication following the music condition.

It is important to examine the reasons behind contradictory results because RCTs and meta-analyses are considered the most rigorous forms of positivist research (Broder-Fingert et al., 2017). Variations in local contexts; the ways interventions are implemented; inconsistent attendance of participants; and the measurement tools that are used can all have an impact on results (Bieleninik et al., 2017; Marquez-Garcia et al., 2021). When flexible improvisational approaches are used, and results are averaged across heterogeneous populations, the potential to demonstrate differences is reduced. Diagnostic measures such as the Autism Diagnostic Observation Schedule (ADOS) do not appear to be sensitive enough to capture the change that occurs in music therapy (Bieleninik et al., 2017; Marquez-Garcia et al., 2021). A combination of assessment methods, such as parent/self-reports, psychometric measures, coded analysis of video recordings, and before and after neurophysiological measures might be needed.

Following their systematic review of music therapy involving improvisation or listening to or singing songs (Marquez-Garcia et al., 2021) agreed that "studying music therapy through a scientific lens can be problematic due to the multiple theoretical approaches and techniques employed and individual differences in patient populations and cultures" (Marquez-Garcia et al., 2021). Building on Sharda et al.'s (2018) finding that music therapy may be able to improve brain function in children on the autism spectrum, Marquez-Garcia et al. (2021) recommend music therapy researchers include neuroimaging techniques to gain a more objective understanding of the effect of music therapy on individuals with the diagnosis of ASD.

Part 2: Music Therapy Practice

Music therapists have been working with children on the autism spectrum for many decades, and practice in this field is now well established (Bergmann, 2016; Janzen & Thaut, 2018; Oldfield et al., 2019; Reschke-Hernandez, 2011). Recent workforce surveys have revealed that 44% of music therapists worldwide (Kern & Tague, 2017) and 48% of Australian music therapists (Jack et al., 2016) work with people on the autism spectrum. A New Zealand survey published in 2015 (Rickson et al. 2015) indicated almost 50% of NZ RMThs (29) were working with an estimated 150 children and 30 adults on the spectrum in this country. These high percentages are perhaps not surprising given that takiwātanga often have an affinity for music and may exhibit special musical abilities (Bergmann, 2016; Heaton, 2004; Janzen & Thaut, 2018). Music is a non-verbal form of communication and play which can be powerful in addressing the core features of autism (Bergmann, 2016) and music therapy is considered to have high potential as a therapeutic option (Bergmann, 2016; Wigram & Gold, 2006).

Theoretical Underpinnings

Music therapy approaches used with people diagnosed with autism or ASD have been grounded in various behavioural, developmental, educational, relational, creative, psychoanalytic, and neurological theories (Bergmann, 2016; Carpente & LaGasse, 2015; Geretsegger et al., 2015; Wigram & Gold, 2006) and have become well established (Bergman, 2016).

Berger (2002), for example, argues that difficulties with sensory integration play a prominent role in autistic processing and therefore in the way children respond to environmental stimuli. She promotes a multi-dimensional physiologic perspective of music therapy which focuses on ways music can interact with and alter sensory responses in children diagnosed with autism. She describes how fun and creative musical activities can support children's internal rhythmic organisation, and the ways in which playing instruments and moving to music can improve sensory integration and coordination. Ultimately these outcomes are assumed to transfer to other areas of learning.

Other neurological approaches also focus on rhythmic organisation, or "entrainment". For example, a neurological approach which aims to support a child diagnosed with ASD to develop speech might involve the introduction of rhythmic exercises to stimulate initiation, gradually moving to rhythmic tapping on their body, or rhythmic body movement (Carpente & LaGasse, 2015). Music therapists using a Neurologic Music

Therapy technique called "Developmental Speech and Language training through Music (DSLM)" (Thaut et al., 2014) would engage children in activities involving singing, chanting, playing musical instruments, and a combination of music, speech, and movement (Janzen & Thaut, 2018).

It seems that the relationship difficulties that children on the autism spectrum may experience, including difficulties with facial expressions, gesture, prosody, and turn-taking, might also be explained by challenges with timing, or temporal synchrony (Wimpory & Gwilym, 2019). Situating the origins of autism in systems that programme time, serial coordination, and prospective control of movements, as well as regulate affective evaluations of experiences, might explain why improvisational music therapy seems to be effective with this population (Trevarthen & Delafield-Butt, 2013). Improvisational music therapy (IMT) involves therapist and participants using the spontaneous creation of music as a primary therapeutic experience for social engagement and expression of emotions (Bruscia, 2014; Geretsegger et al., 2015). Therapists respond to the child's impulses or motivations, consciously and sensitively attuning to their movements, feelings, and intentions (Geretsegger et al., 2015). In this way, just as sensitive carers do, they support the child's communication attempts, and co-regulate arousal (Hardy & Lagasse, 2013).

Improvisational music therapy can be incorporated into other music-centred, child-centred, and psychodynamic approaches. The music- and child-centred "Creative Music Therapy" approach (Nordoff & Robbins, 1971) is one such example. Creative Music Therapists believe that all human beings are musical, and that music can therefore reach and affect all children, including those who experience severe developmental challenges. Their ideas have been reinforced by more recent "communicative musicality" theories (Malloch & Trevarthen, 2009; Trevarthen, 2002; Trevarthen & Malloch, 2017; Trevarthen & Malloch, 2000) which demonstrate how the "natural growth of a musical self in relationship" begins with intimate imitative dialogues and proto conversations (sensitively timed conversational turn-taking) between infants and carers (Trevarthan & Malloch, 2017, p. 2). Using vocalising or movement, new-born babies can synchronise precisely with their carer's communicative gestures (Trevarthen & Aitken, 2001).

Similarly, relationship-based approaches to music therapy assessment and intervention are grounded in the child's ability to attend, adapt, and engage with their own and others' musical play (Carpente & LaGasse, 2015). The core features of autism spectrum disorder, relating and communicating, can be managed through a collaborative music making process. Fundamental elements of the Creative Music Therapy approach have continued to underpin the work of many contemporary music therapists, including practitioners in New Zealand.

Methods and Goals

Previous paragraphs summarising music therapy research, demonstrate that music therapists employ a wide range of methods and techniques in their work with children on the autism spectrum including interactive playing or learning of instruments; vocalisation and singing; song writing and composition; movement and dance; and improvisation. Education tools such as the SCERTS (Prizant et al., 2006), Social Stories™ (Gray & Garand, 1993); and Floortime (Greenspan & Wieder, 2006) models, have been employed by music therapists working within interdisciplinary and multimodal approaches.

Most music therapy practices primarily focus on supporting children to improve their communication, social interaction, emotional skills (Bergmann, 2016; Carpente & LaGasse, 2015; Geretsegger et al., 2015; Janzen & Thaut, 2018; Kern et al., 2013; Wigram & Gold, 2006)motor functioning, and cognitive functioning (Carpente & LaGasse, 2015). In addition to rehabilitative goals, music therapy has also been used to support children's well-being, self-expression, creativity, and "psychological enrichment" (Reschke-Hernandez, 2011); and might focus on music-centred goals such as musical relatedness or musical interrelatedness (Aigen, 2014a). Music therapists might also support parents to create music experiences that enhance their interaction with the child (Thompson et al., 2013), or support other professionals to use music with clinical intent and purpose within their scope of practice (Carpente & LaGasse, 2015; Rickson, 2012).Early intervention can lead to better outcomes for children, so it is natural that music therapists would put significant focus on music therapy for young children and their families (Kern & Humpal, 2012; Nugent, 2019; Thompson, 2012, 2017; Thompson & McFerran, 2015).

With some exceptions, early pioneers of music therapy tended to utilise the predictability inherent in music, by engaging children in structured activities such as singing groups, folk dancing, and rhythm activities (Reschke-Hernandez, 2011). However, following the leads of Alvin (1978) and Nordoff & Robbins' (Nordoff & Robbins, 1971) child-centred improvisational music therapy has become the primary means to promote expression, communication, and interaction(Geretsegger et al., 2015; Janzen & Thaut, 2018; Kim et al., 2009; Wigram & Gold, 2006; Wigram et al., 2002). Receptive, precomposed music, and/or song-writing methods are still used (Carpente & LaGasse, 2015; Oldfield et al., 2019) with music therapy practitioners working in the USA utilising singing, vocalising, instrument play, and dance more frequently than child-centred improvisation (Kern, 2018). Kern (2018) also reports that practitioners in the USA are more likely to employ behavioural approaches in their work.

Nevertheless, the utilisation of improvisation techniques in the large multicentre randomised clinical trial (RCT) TIME-A study with children aged 4–7 years, reinforces the suggestion that improvisation is widely used internationally. In improvisational music therapy music therapists establish a meaningful relationship with a child through a shared music making process (Kim et al., 2009). They create unique opportunities for children to engage in safe musical encounters, leading to relationships of trust. Some children diagnosed with ASD might find it easier, initially at least, to respond to "music" or "instruments" rather than to people. The music therapist follows the child, creating empathic and supportive musical structures that respond to their emotional state and synchronise with their sounds and movement, while also introducing elements of anticipation and surprise. As the dyad becomes attuned, a sense of togetherness is created, the child's communication increases and becomes more flexible, and social reciprocity develops (Carpente, 2017; Geretsegger et al., 2015; Kim et al., 2009; Simpson & Keen, 2011; Wigram, 1992, 1993, 2004; Wigram & Elefant, 2009).

Music therapy therefore offers a unique interaction setting for children diagnosed with ASD to develop communication skills (Walworth, 2007). For example, the utilisation of "babbling" vocal exchanges which typically occur between carers and infants, and the incorporation of children's vocalisations and musical sounds into interactive improvised musical exchanges, can lead to speech development (Oldfield, 2020, p. 110). Drawing on decades of experience working with this population, Oldfield (2006) suggests that music therapy is powerful because it is motivating; children are supported by the structure inherent in music making as well as in the music therapy sessions; it provides opportunities for following and initiating; involves basic non-verbal exchanges; and enables children to be in control in a constructive way. It combines movement with music; can involve integration of playfulness, drama, and music; and can include joint work with parents (Oldfield, 2006, p. 90).

Epstein, Elefant & Thompson (2020) suggest music therapists working with verbal children might be more likely to utilise their intellectual and language skills by focusing on vocalisation and songs, to develop mutual play and expand play routines. Thompson (2018) for example, describes a process of building on a young child's actions and verbal stories, making meaning of their contributions, and interpreting and representing the communication musically. This process relied on Thompson attuning to the child, as well as enhancing the emotional content of the story. The work supported the child to spontaneously share real-life events within their storytelling, rather than repeating scripts learnt from movies and television programmes. Songs can be improvised in response to the children's spontaneous verbal expressions; precomposed songs or adapted songs might be used to facilitate further improvisation; and/or children's stories or non-verbal gestures might be incorporated into an improvised story or song (Baker et al., 2009).

Music therapy practice has become increasingly diverse as music therapists have begun to view autism through the socio-cultural lens. Many people who live with autism would prefer to receive support to manage or remove the challenges they face in their everyday lives rather than looking for treatment or a "cure" for their autistic symptoms (Bakan, 2018). It is in this context that Music-centred (Aigen,

2014a, 2014b), Resource-oriented (Rolvsjord, 2010), and Community Music Therapy (Stige & Aaro, 2012) approaches that focus on providing access to musicking and turn the lens towards maximising health and well-being through the mobilisation of the children's strengths and resources, become highly relevant. Music therapists recognise that within an autism-friendly environment, such as a music space, children can sometimes function at a higher level than their neurotypical peers (Baron-Cohen, 2017). Yet they, and their communities, often continue to need support beyond the music therapy room to ensure they can comfortably engage in musicking in other contexts.

Specific information about the practice of New Zealand music therapists is provided in the introduction to the case studies, in Chapter 5.

References

Accordino, R., Comer, R., & Heller, W. B. (2007, January–March). Searching for music's potential: A critical examination of research on music therapy with individuals with autism. *Research in Autism Spectrum Disorders, 1*(1), 101–115. https://doi.org/10.1016/j.rasd.2006.08.002

Aigen, K. (2014a). Music-centered dimensions of Nordoff-Robbins music therapy. *Music Therapy Perspectives, 32*(1), 18–29. https://doi.org/10.1093/mtp/miu006

Aigen, K. (2014b). *The study of music therapy: Current issues and concepts.* Taylor and Francis.

Alvin, J. (1978). *Music therapy for the autistic child.* Oxford University Press.

Bakan, M. B. (2018). *Speaking for ourselves.* Oxford University Press. https://doi.org/10.1093/oso/9780190855833.003.0005

Baker, F., Wigram, T., Stott, D., & McFerran, K. S. (2009). Therapeutic songwriting in music therapy, Part II: Comparing the literature with practice across diverse clinical populations. *Nordic Journal of Music Therapy, 18*(1), 32–56. https://doi.org/10.1080/08098130802496373

Baron-Cohen, S. (2017). Editorial perspective: Neurodiversity—A revolutionary concept for autism and psychiatry. *Journal of Childhood Psychology and Psychiatry, 58*, 744–747. https://doi-org.helicon.vuw.ac.nz/10.1111/jcpp.12703

Berger, D. S. (2002). *Music therapy, sensory integration and the autistic child*. Jessica Kingsley.

Bergmann, T. (2016). Music therapy for people with autism spectrum disorder. In J. Edwards (Ed.), *The Oxford handbook of music therapy*. Oxford University Press. https://doi.org/10.1093/oxfordhb/9780199639755.013.3

Bieleninik, L., Geretsegger, M., Mossler, K., Drusmus, J. A., Thompson, G., Gattino, G., Elefant, C., Gottfried, T., Igliozzi, R., Muratori, F., Suvini, F., Kim, J., Crawford, M. J., Odell Miller, H., Oldfield, A., Casey, O., Finnemann, J., Carpente, J. A., Park, A.-L., … Gold, C. (2017). Effects of improvisational music therapy vs enhances standard care on symptom severity amount children with autism spectrum disorder. The TIME-A randomized clinical trial. *Journal of the American Medical Association, 318*(6), 525–535. https://doi.org/10.1001/jama.2017.9478

Boso, M., Emanuele, E., Minazzi, V., Abbamonte, M., & Politi, P. (2007, September). Effect of long-term interactive music therapy on behavior profile and musical skills in young adults with severe autism. *Journal of Alternative & Complementary Medicine, 13*(7), 709–712.

Broder-Fingert, S., Feinberg, E., & Silverstein, M. (2017). Music therapy for children with autism spectrum disorder. *Journal of the American Medical Association, 318*(6), 523–524. https://doi.org/10.1001/jama.2017.9477

Brondino, N., Fusar-Poli, L., Rocchetti, M., Provenzani, U., Barale, F., & Politi, P. (2015). Complementary and alternative therapies for autism spectrum disorder. *Evidence-Based Complementary and Alternative Medicine, 2015*, 258531–258589. https://doi.org/10.1155/2015/258589

Brownell, M. D. (2002, Sum). Musically adapted social stories to modify behaviors in students with autism: Four case studies. *Journal of Music Therapy, 39*(2), 117–144. https://doi.org/10.1093/jmt/39.2.117

Bruscia, K. (2014). *Defining music therapy*. Barcelona.

Carpente, J. A., & LaGasse, A. B. (2015). Music therapy for children with autism spectrum disorder. In B. L. Wheeler (Ed.), *Music therapy handbook* (pp. 290–301). The Guilford Press.

Carpente, J. A. (2017). Investigating the effectiveness of a developmental, individual difference, relationship-based (DIR) improvisational music therapy program on social communication for children with autism spectrum disorder. *Music Therapy Perspectives, 35* (2), 160–174. https://doi.org/10.1093/mtp/miw013

Crawford, M. J., Gold, C., Odell-Miller, H., Thana, L., Faber, S., Assmus, J., Bieleninik, Ł, Geretsegger, M., Grant, C., Maratos, A., Sandford, S., Claringbold, A., McConachie, H., Maskey, M., Mössler, K. A., Ramchandani,

P., & Hassiotis, A. (2017). International multicentre randomised controlled trial of improvisational music therapy for children with autism spectrum disorder: TIME-A study. *Health Technology Assessment (winchester, England), 21*(59), 1–40. https://doi.org/10.3310/hta21590

Dharan, V. (2015, July 22–23). *Hearing from the experts: Parents' knowledge of what works for their children*. Altogether Autism Conference, Auckland, New Zealand.

Epstein, S., Elefant, C., & Thompson, G. (2020). Music therapists' perceptions of the therapeutic potentials using music when working with verbal children on the autism spectrum: A qualitative analysis. *The Journal of Music Therapy, 57*(1), 66–90. https://doi.org/10.1093/jmt/thz017

Finnigan, E., & Starr, E. (2010). Increasing social responsiveness in a child with autism. *Autism, 14*(4), 321–348. https://doi.org/10.1177/1362361309357747

Gattino, G. S., Riesgoa, R. D. S, Longo, D., Leite, J. C. L., & Faccini, L. S. (2011). Effects of relational music therapy on communication of children with autism: A randomized controlled study. *Nordic Journal of Music Therapy, 20*(2), 142–154. https://doi.org/10.1080/08098131.2011.566933

Gray, C. A., & Garand, J. D. (1993). Social stories: Improving responses of students with autism with accurate social information. *Focus on Autistic Behavior, 8*(1), 1–10. https://doi.org/10.1177/108835769300800101

Geretsegger, M., Elefant, C., Mössler, K. A., & Gold, C. (2014). Music therapy for people with autism spectrum disorder. *The Cochrane Database of Systematic Reviews*. https://doi.org/10.1002/14651858.CD004381.pub3.

Geretsegger, M., Holck, U., Carpente, J. A., Elefant, C., Kim, J., & Gold, C. (2015). Common characteristics of improvisational approaches in music therapy for children with autism spectrum disorder: Developing treatment guidelines. *Journal of Music Therapy, 52*(2), 258–281. https://doi.org/10.1093/jmt/thv005

Greenspan, S. I., & Wieder, S. (2006). *Engaging autism: The floortime approach to helping children relate*. Da Capo Press.

Hardy, M. W., & Lagasse, A. B. (2013). Rhythm, movement, and autism: Using rhythmic rehabilitation research as a model for autism. *Frontiers in Integrative Neuroscience, 7*, 19–19. https://doi.org/10.3389/fnint.2013.00019

Heaton, P. (2004). Interval and contour processing in autism. *Journal of Autism and Developmental Disorders, 35*(6), 787–793. https://doi.org/10.1007/s10803-005-0024-7

Hillier, A., Greher, G., Poto, N., & Dougherty, M. (2011, March 1, 2012). Positive outcomes following participation in a music intervention for adolescents and young adults on the autism spectrum. *Psychology of Music, 40*(2), 201–215. https://doi.org/10.1177/0305735610386837

Jack, N., Thompson, G., Hogan, B., Tamplin, J., Eager, R., & Arns, B. (2016). *My profession, my voice: Results of the Australian Music Therapy Association's 2016 workforce census.* https://www.austmta.org.au/resources

James, R., Sigafoos, J., Green, V., Lancioni, G., O'Reilly, M., Lang, R., Davis, T., Carnett, A., Achmadi, D., Gevarter, C., & Marschik, P. (2015). Music therapy for individuals with autism spectrum disorder: A systematic review. *Review Journal of Autism and Developmental Disorders, 2*(1), 39–54. https://doi.org/10.1007/s40489-014-0035-4

Janzen, T. B., & Thaut, M. H. (2018). Rethinking the role of music in the neurodevelopment of autism spectrum disorder. *Music and Science, 1,* 1–18. https://doi.org/10.1177/2059204318769639

Kasilingam, N., Waddington, H., & Van Der Meer, L. (2019). Early intervention for children with autism spectrum disorder in New Zealand: What children get and what parents want. *International Journal of Disability, Development, and Education, 68*(4), 521–537. https://doi.org/10.1080/1034912X.2019.1696949

Kaplan, R. S., & Steele, A. L. (2005). An analysis of music therapy programme Goals and outcomes for clients with diagnoses on the autism spectrum. *Journal of Music Therapy, 42*(1), 2–19. https://doi.org/10.1093/jmt/42.1.2

Kern, P., Rivera, N. R., Chandler, A., & Humpal, M. (2013, Win). Music Therapy services for individuals with autism spectrum disorder: A survey of clinical practices and training needs. *Journal of Music Therapy, 50*(4), 274–303. https://doi.org/10.1093/jmt/50.4.274

Kern, P., & Tague, D. (2017). Music therapy practice status and trends worldwide: An international survey study. *Music Therapy Perspectives, 54*(3), 255–286. https://doi.org/10.1093/jmt/thx011

Kern, P., & Aldridge, D. (2006). Using embedded music therapy interventions to support outdoor play of young children with autism in an inclusive community-based child care program. *Journal of Music Therapy, 43*(4), U1-294. https://doi.org/10.1093/jmt/43.4.270

Kern, P., Wakeford, L., & Aldridge, D. (2007). Improving the performance of a young child with autism during self-care tasks using embedded song interventions: A case study. *Music Therapy Perspectives, 25*(1), 43–51. https://doi.org/10.1093/mtp/25.1.43

Kern, P., Wolery, M., & Aldridge, D. (2007). Use of songs to promote independence in morning greeting routines for young children with autism. *Journal of Autism & Developmental Disorders, 37*(7), 1264–1271. https://doi.org/10.1007/s10803-006-0272-1

Kern, P., & Humpal, M. E. (2012). *Early childhood music therapy and autism spectrum disorders: Developing potential in young children and their families* (edited by Petra Kern and Marcia Humpal; foreword by David Aldridge). Jessica Kingsley.

Kern, P. (2018). Evidence-based practice in music therapy: Identifying effective interventions for children with Autism Spectrum Disorder. In P. Kern & M. Humpal (Eds.), *Early childhood music therapy and autism spectrum disorder: Supporting children and their families* (2nd ed., pp. 35–49). Jessica Kingsley.

Kim, J., Wigram, T., & Gold, C. (2008). The effects of improvisational music therapy on joint attention behaviors in autistic children: A randomized controlled study. *Journal of Autism and Developmental Disorders, 38*(9), 1758–1766. https://doi.org/10.1007/s10803-008-0566-6

Kim, J., Wigram, T., & Gold, C. (2009). Emotional, motivational and interpersonal responsiveness of children with autism in improvisational music therapy. *Autism, 13*(4), 389–409. https://doi.org/10.1177/1362361309105660

LaGasse, A. B. (2014). Effects of a music therapy group intervention on enhancing social skills in children with autism. *The Journal of Music Therapy, 51*(3), 250–275. https://doi.org/10.1093/jmt/thu012

Lang, R., Hancock, T. B., & Singh, N. N. (2016). Overview of early intensive behavioral intervention for children with autism. In R. Lang, T. B. Hancock, & N. N. Singh (Eds.), *Early intervention for young children with autism spectrum disorder* (pp. 1–14). Springer International Publishing. https://doi.org/10.1007/978-3-319-30925-5_1

Lim, H. A. (2010). Effect of "developmental speech and language training through music" on speech production in children with autism spectrum disorders. *Journal of Music Therapy, 47*(1), 2–26. https://doi.org/10.1093/jmt/47.1.2

Lim, H. A., & Draper, E. (2011, Win). The effects of music therapy incorporated with applied behavior analysis verbal behavior approach for children with autism spectrum disorders. *Journal of Music Therapy, 48*(4), 532–550. https://doi.org/10.1093/jmt/48.4.532

Low, M. Y. (2021). *Experiences of autistic clients in Nordoff-Robbins music therapy: An interpretive phenomenological analysis*. Drexel University.

Malloch, S., & Trevarthen, C. (2009). *Communicative musicality: Exploring the basis of human companionship.* Oxford University Press.

Marquez-Garcia, A. V., Magnuson, J., Morris, J., Iarocci, G., Doesburg, S., & Moreno, S. (2021). Music therapy in autism spectrum disorder: A systematic review. *Review Journal of Autism and Developmental Disorders.* https://doi.org/10.1007/s40489-021-00246-x

Nordoff, P., & Robbins, C. (1971). *Therapy in music for handicapped children.* St. Martin's Press.

Nugent, J. (2019). Music therapy with children with autistic spectrum conditions and their families. In H. Dunn, E. Coombes, E. Maclean, H. Mottram, & J. Nugent (Eds.), *Music therapy and autism across the lifespan: A spectrum of approaches* (pp. 179–196). Jessica Kingsley.

Oldfield, A. (2006). *Interactive music therapy: A positive approach.* Jessica Kingsley.

Oldfield, A., Blauth, L., Finnemann, J., & Casey, O. (2019). Clinical trials: Are music therapists deluding themselves? In H. Dunn, E. Coombes, E. Maclean, H. Mottram, & J. Nugent (Eds.), *Music therapy and autism across the lifespan: A spectrum of approaches* (pp. 35–56). Jessica Kingsley.

Oldfield, A. (2020). Book Review. In P. Kern & M. Humpal (Eds.), Early childhood music therapy and autism spectrum disorder. *British Journal of Music Therapy, 34*(2), 108–120.

Pasiali, V. (2004). The use of prescriptive therapeutic songs in a home-based environment to promote social skills acquisition by children with autism: Three case studies. *Music Therapy Perspectives, 22*(1), 11–20. https://doi.org/10.1093/mtp/22.1.11

Pasiali, V., LaGasse, A. B., & Penn, S. L. (2014). The effect of musical attention control training (MACT) on attention skills of adolescents with neurodevelopmental delays: A pilot study. *The Journal of Music Therapy, 51*(4), 333–354. https://doi.org/10.1093/jmt/thu030

Porter, S., McConnell, T., McLaughlin, K., Lynn, F., Cardwell, C., Braiden, H. J., Boylan, J., Holmes, V., Rogan, S., Clinician, L., Diamond, K., Allen, J., Reilly, C., Davidson, F., McDowell, C., Boyd, R., Oldfield, A., Mullowney, M., Downes, C., … Heale, A. (2017). Music therapy for children and adolescents with behavioural and emotional problems: A randomised controlled trial. *Journal of Child Psychology and Psychiatry, 58*(5), 586–594. https://doi.org/10.1111/jcpp.12656

Prizant, B. M., Wetherby, A. M., Rubin, E., Laurent, A. C., & Rydell, P. J. (2006, November 3, 2007). *The SCERTS model in practice: Program planning and intervention*. Retrieved November 3, 2007 from http://www.scerts.com/frequently_asked_questions.htm.

Rabeyron, T., Robledo del Canto, J.-P., Carasco, E., Bisson, V., Bodeau, N., Vrait, F.-X., Berna, F., & Bonnot, O. (2020). A randomized controlled trial of 25 sessions comparing music therapy and music listening for children with autism spectrum disorder. *Psychiatry Research, 293*, 113377. https://doi.org/10.1016/j.psychres.2020.113377

Reschke-Hernandez, A. E. (2011). History of music therapy treatment interventions for children with autism. *Journal of Music Therapy, 48*(2), 169–207. https://doi.org/10.1093/jmt/48.2.169

Rickson, D. J. (2012). Music therapy school consultation: A unique practice. *Nordic Journal of Music Therapy, 21*(3), 268–285. https://doi.org/10.1080/08098131.2012.654474

Rickson, D. J., Molyneux, C., Ridley, H., Castelino, A., & Upjohn-Beatson, E. (2015a). *Music therapy for children who have autism spectrum disorder ASD: Exploring the potential for research in New Zealand using a mixed methods design*. Victoria University of Wellington.

Rolvsjord, R. (2010). *Resource-oriented music therapy in mental health care*. Barcelona.

Sharda, M., Tuerk, C., Chowdhury, R., Jamey, K., Foster, N., Custo-Blanch, M., Tan, M., Nadig, A., & Hyde, K. (2018). Music improves social communication and auditory-motor connectivity in children with autism. *Translational Psychiatry, 8*(1), 213–231. https://doi.org/10.1038/s41398-018-0287-3

Su Maw, S., & Haga, C. (2018). Effectiveness of cognitive, developmental, and behavioural interventions for autism spectrum disorder in preschool-aged children: A systematic review and meta-analysis. *Heliyon, 4*(9), e00763. https://doi.org/10.1016/j.heliyon.2018.e00763

Schwartzberg, E. T., & Silverman, M. J. (2013). Effects of music-based social stories on comprehension and generalization of social skills in children with autism spectrum disorders: A randomized effectiveness study. *The Arts in Psychotherapy, 40*(3), 331–337. https://doi.org/10.1016/j.aip.2013.06.001

Simpson, K., & Keen, D. (2011). Music interventions for children with autism: Narrative review of the literature. *Journal of Autism and Developmental Disorders, 41*, 1507–1514. https://doi.org/10.1007/s10803-010-1172-y

Simpson, K., Keen, D., & Lamb, J. (2013). The use of music to engage children with autism in a receptive labelling task. *Research in Autism Spectrum Disorders, 7*(12), 1489–1496. https://doi.org/10.1016/j.rasd.2013.08.013

Stige, B., & Aaro, L. E. (2012). *Invitation to community music therapy.* Routledge.

Thaut, M., Hoemberg, V., & Abiru, M. (2014). *Handbook of neurologic music therapy* (1st ed.). Oxford University Press.

Thompson, G. A. (2012). Family-centered music therapy in the home environment: Promoting interpersonal engagement between children with autism spectrum disorder and their parents. *Music Therapy Perspectives, 30*(2), 109–116. http://ezproxy.massey.ac.nz/login?url=http://search.ebscohost.com/login.aspx?direct=true&db=ccm&AN=2012088717&site=eds-live&scope=site

Thompson, G. A., McFerran, K. S., & Gold, C. (2013). Family-centred music therapy to promote social engagement in young children with severe autism spectrum disorder: A randomized controlled study. *Child: Care, Health And Development, 40*(6), 840–852. https://doi.org/10.1111/cch.12121

Thompson, G. A., & McFerran, K. S. (2015a). Music therapy with young people who have profound intellectual and developmental disability: Four case studies exploring communication and engagement within musical interactions. *Journal of Intellectual & Developmental Disability, 40*(1), 1–11. https://doi.org/10.3109/13668250.2014.965668

Thompson, G. (2017b). Long-term perspectives of family quality of life following music therapy with young children on the autism spectrum: A phenomenological study. *Journal of Music Therapy, 54*(4), 432–459. https://doi.org/10.1093/jmt/thx013

Thompson, G. A. (2018). Dramatic role play within improvisational music therapy: Joey's story. In A. Oldfield & M. Carr (Eds.), *Collaborations within and between dramatherapy and music therapy* (pp. 31–51). Jessica Kingsley.

Trevarthen, C., & Malloch, S. N. (2000). The dance of wellbeing: Defining the musical therapeutic effect. *Nordic Journal of Music Therapy, 9*(2), 3–17.

Trevarthen, C., & Aitken, K. J. (2001). Infant intersubjectivity: Research, theory, and clinical applications. *Journal of Child Psychology and Psychiatry, 42*(1), 3–48. https://doi.org/10.1111/1469-7610.00701

Trevarthen, C. (2002). Origins of musical identity. In R. A. R. MacDonald, D. J. Hargreaves, & D. Miell (Eds.), *Musical identities.* Oxford University Press.

Trevarthen, C., & Delafield-Butt, J. T. (2013). Autism as a developmental disorder in intentional movement and affective engagement. *Frontiers and Integrative Neuroscience, 7*, 1–16. https://doi.org/10.3389/fnint.2013.00049

Trevarthen, C., & Malloch, S. (2017). The musical self. In R. A. R. MacDonald, D. J. Hargreaves, & D. Miell (Eds.), *Handbook of musical identities* (1st ed.). Oxford University Press.

Vaiouli, P., & Andreou, G. (2018). Communication and language development of young children with autism: A review of research in music. *Communication Disorders Quarterly, 39*(2), 323–329. https://doi.org/10.1177/1525740117705117

Walworth, D. D. (2007, Spr). The use of music therapy within the SCERTS model for children with autism spectrum disorder. *Journal of Music Therapy, 44*(1), 2–22.

Whipple, J. (2018). Music therapy research: Effective interventions for young children with autism spectrum disorder. In P. Kern & M. Humpal (Eds.), *Early childhood music therapy and autism spectrum disorder: Supporting children and their families* (2nd ed., pp. 49–69). Jessical Kingsley.

Wigram, T. (1992). Differential diagnosis of autism and other types of disability. *Australian Journal of Music Therapy, 3*, 16–26.

Wigram, T. (1993). Music therapy research to meet the demands of health and educational services. In M. Heal & T. Wigram (Eds.), *Music therapy in health and education.* Jessica Kingsley.

Wigram, T. (2002). Indications in music therapy. Evidence from assessment that can identify the expectations of music therapy as a treatment for autistic spectrum disorder (ASD): Meeting the challenge of evidence based practice. *British Journal of Music Therapy, 16*(1), 11–28.

Wigram, T., & Gold, C. (2006). Music therapy in the assessment and treatment of autistic spectrum disorder: Clinical application and research evidence. *Child: Care, Health And Development, 32*(5), 535–542.

Wigram, T., & Elefant, C. (2009). Therapeutic dialogues in music: Nurturing musicality of communication in children with autistic spectrum disorder and Rett syndrome. In S. Malloch & C. Trevarthen (Eds.), *Communicative musicality: Exploring the basis of human companionship* (pp. 423–445). Oxford University Press.

Wimpory, D., & Gwilym, E. (2019). Musical interaction therapy (MIT) for children with autistic spectrum conditions (ASCs): Underlying rationale, clinical practice and research evidence. In H. Dunn, E. Coombes, E. Maclean, H. Mottram, & J. Nugent (Eds.), *Music therapy and autism across the lifespan: A spectrum of approaches* (pp. 97–136). Jessica Kingsley.

4

An Innovative Research Design

Research Questions

How is music therapy with autistic children (tamariki takiwātanga) in New Zealand (Aotearoa) perceived by family members and other autism experts?

1. How do commentators perceive music therapy in each case?
2. How do they perceive the potential of music therapy for tamariki takiwātanga overall?
3. In what ways is music therapy perceived similarly or differently according to the position/lens of the observer (i.e., people who know the child, their music therapists, and people who don't know the child)?

D. Rickson, *Music Therapy with Autistic Children in Aotearoa, New Zealand*,
https://doi.org/10.1007/978-3-031-05233-0_4

The Context

In 2018, research funding enabled ten music therapists to offer sessions to tamariki takiwātanga who had no previous experience of music therapy. The funding would allow for weekly sessions, for up to twelve months, but could be used flexibly according to tamariki takiwātanga needs. All New Zealand Registered Music Therapists (85) were invited to express interest. A list of those who were available, and their geographical locations, was compiled. Then an email was sent to Autism New Zealand, requesting expressions of interest from families who might want to be involved in the project. Respondents were provided with the list of available therapists in their local area and were asked to contact a therapist directly.

Music therapists were encouraged to give the families an information sheet and consent form but to ensure that they understood this did not necessarily mean they would be included in the project (see discussion of "Ethical Considerations"). Music therapists were also asked to let me know that they had given families the information, so I could record the incoming expressions of interest in chronological order. It was anticipated that the families would be able to digest the research information while simultaneously going through a music therapy referral process. The first ten dyads who had completed their referral process, and agreed to work together, would be included in the project.

The therapists and children would be encouraged to work in the ways that suited them best, and not to alter any aspect of their practice for the research. However, at the end of the year, or end of their programme, whichever came first, the music therapists would provide me (the researcher) with case materials in "Narrative Assessment" form (see below) with video examples where possible. Informed consent was obtained from music therapists, as well as children and their families, for this clinical data to be reused for research purposes. The case materials were not treated as data to be "analysed"; but as artefacts to be read, viewed, and critiqued by a team of commentators. The purpose of the research was to learn how music therapy might be understood by these commentators, people who were experts in the field of autism. Twenty-six of the commentators were family members, teachers, or other professionals who knew one of the children, and interpreted their case. Six other autism experts who did not know the children, interpreted all ten cases. The "other" autism experts had various and multiple expertise as parents, teachers of typical and diverse populations, a member of ASD disability action group, an education lecturer, a psychologist, an autism advisor, a policy analyst, an autistic adult, and a cultural advisor.

Narrative Assessment

New Zealand music therapists working with tamariki takiwātanga predominantly evaluate the music therapy process using descriptive assessment methods (Rickson et al., 2016) which are a good match with Narrative Assessment as it is outlined by the Ministry of Education. The research protocol maximised this congruence by asking the music therapists involved in the project to present case reports of their work with the tamariki takiwātanga, in Narrative Assessment form (Ministry of Education, 2009). Narrative Assessments involve observing children as they engage in purposeful and meaningful activity and documenting authentic accounts of their learning and development to make their learning visible to the writer, as well as others who are interested. They are "designed to combine observation, interpretation, analysis, and possible responses" (Ministry of Education, 2009, p. 28).

A key feature of the approach is that it details the progress of an individual rather than comparing them to other learners. Moreover, it goes further than simple description, to identify *how* the therapy and other environmental factors contributed to the child's learning and development.

> Narrative Assessment provides a rich picture of students' skills, strengths, and learning support needs. It uses learning stories to capture progress in students' learning and records the often-subtle interactions between the student, their learning environments, their peers, their learning support team, and their learning activities. (p. 1)

The music therapists were therefore enabled to engage in child-centred practice, which is a preferred approach in New Zealand (Rickson, Molyneux, Ridley, Castelino, & Upjohn Beatson, 2015). They were able to collaborate with the child, parents, and other professionals to ensure goals, plans, and evaluation procedures were suitable for individual children. During sessions they could respond to the child in the moment, focusing on their strengths, allowing them to lead the therapy process, and giving them time to demonstrate learning.

> Learning stories capture a sense of progress in learning, and of the impacts of that learning on important life outcomes, that is sometimes missing from IEP's. (Ministry of Education, 2009, p. 13)

The therapists would document sessions in ways that felt comfortable for them. Towards the end of the therapy process they would reflect on their documentation to uncover meaningful examples in the child's learning and development and write a short story (Learning Story) about why the moment was considered meaningful. They were encouraged to keep the stories brief but evocative—the kind of stories they might tell their colleagues. For example, they might describe the child developing a sense of agency, purposefully doing something, and "owning" the skill, or using a skill in different ways, in different circumstances, in different contexts, or in more complex situations. Enough detailed description of key interactions would need to be included to give a rich context to the learning being described, and audio and/or video examples would complement the stories and clarify details not readily revealed in the text. The perspectives or voices of the children and/or their family or whānau could be included in the story.

Narrative Assessment enabled the focus to remain on actions and relationships. It was acknowledged that children's learning and development are not necessarily predictable. When learning stories were strung together, they would capture individual progress and achievement as well as the facilitative factors. Importantly, a series of learning stories can demonstrate progress towards goals that have not been previously identified. In this way, the children's learning or development could be evaluated with the benefit of hindsight.

The Narrative Assessment also included music therapists' personal perspectives and interpretations. However, for the purposes of the research project, these were presented to the researcher in a separate document that was not provided to commentators. Instead, the commentators were asked to give their own summary of whether learning and development had been demonstrated; what the stories told them about music therapy for this child; the potential for music therapy to help other children; and what might have been done differently.

Data Gathering

Qualitative Descriptions

Commentators were asked to read the case carefully and listen to and/or view any accompanying audio or audio-visual material, several times; and to write and/or record their responses on a secure website. They were advised that they could respond in any way they felt appropriate, and there were no limits on how much they could write or say about the case; but that it was anticipated that they might write around one A4 page of typed responses or record 15–20 min of spoken response. The following questions were offered as a prompt:

- What learning and/or development, if any, has been demonstrated?
- What does this tell us about music therapy for this child?
- What personal reactions and feelings are you having to this story?
- What does this tell us about the potential for music therapy to help other children?
- What might have been done differently?

Commentators who looked at all ten cases were also asked to write (or speak and record) a summary of what they believed the stories demonstrated overall.

Questionnaires

Using a Likert scale questionnaire each commentator was asked to note whether they "Strongly Agreed" (6), "Agreed" (5), "Somewhat Agreed" (4), "Somewhat Disagreed" (3), "Disagreed" (2), or "Strongly Disagreed" (1) to a list of statements including:

- The child made progress towards their stated individual goal.
- The child is clearly developing skills that will help them learn (Key Competencies) [For information on "Key Competencies"]
- In the light of the background provided, music therapy is important for this child
- In the light of the background provided, the interaction would be meaningful for the child
- The child seemed to enjoy music therapy sessions overall
- In the light of the background provided, the child appeared positively engaged
- The music was important in these interactions
- The way the therapist facilitated this interaction was important
- In the light of the background provided, the child made timely progress towards their individualised goal
- The stated goal seemed appropriate for this child

After scrutinising the case materials, the 32 commentators completed a total of 85 Likert questionnaires. They also produced a total of 86 qualitative descriptions to communicate whether, how, and why they believed music therapy was helpful for the children they observed, and their personal reactions to the story. In each case, findings from the questionnaires were examined to see whether they confirmed or contradicted the narrative accounts. Where there was contradiction, I searched for an explanation by reanalysing the descriptive data (see "Mixed Methods Research"). When all cases had been analysed, I engaged in cross-case analysis (see "Data Analysis").

Ethical Considerations

Music therapists would engage tamariki and their whānau (family and community) in a process of "typical music therapy practice." The music therapists and families would not be "primary participants" in the research, but "secondary participants" (Given, 2008) who would give informed consent for data from the music therapy practice to be used for research. Only New Zealand Registered Music Therapists (NZ RMTh) with current practising certificates would be involved to ensure safe, valid, and supervised practice. Ongoing supervision is a requirement for Registered Music Therapists in this country so it was also anticipated that they would discuss issues related to their practice with the tamariki takiwātanga during their professional supervision sessions, as needed. In addition, the ten music therapists were encouraged to develop a community of practice, or a peer supervision group, where they could provide confidential support to each other and develop their practices, without any involvement from me, the researcher.

It would be usual to encourage potential research participants, including those who might be described as "secondary participants," to take at least two weeks to consider whether they want to be involved in a research project. Information sheets are always complex and potential participants need time to read, discuss, and digest the content, before deciding to participate. Similarly, music therapists would typically engage thoroughly with families who are referred to music therapy, to determine whether a programme is likely to be beneficial for the child, whether this music therapist is best to deliver the service and, if so, how, and when the therapy might take place. They would find out what parents wanted for their children, who would be involved in the process, and so on. Information might be shared verbally and/or via a referral form, and they would get to know families and help families to know them before they made the decision to work together. The referral and/or assessment process can therefore take some time.

As noted earlier, the inclusion criteria stated that the first ten dyads who had completed their referral process, and agreed to work together, would be included in the project. There was therefore a risk that some families who expressed interest in being involved in this project would go through the referral and/or assessment process yet not be accepted. While they would still be able to have music therapy if they could afford to pay for it in the usual way, there may have been some who would be unable self-fund it. Expressions of interest were received from thirty-five different families and were prioritised according to the day/time their expression of interest was first received. However, several parents wrote to me first, and some contacted more than one therapist, seemingly excited about their potential involvement. Some consented to be involved in the research unreasonably quickly, and one family who contacted two therapists even gave consent twice.

In the circumstances, it was necessary for me to initially "receive" but not "accept" consent forms. Music therapists were asked to reinforce with families the importance of taking time to decide whether music therapy would be right for their child and only then to consider whether they would like to be involved in the project. Consent forms would only be accepted when the referral and/or assessment process was complete. Caution was needed to ensure that everyone had all the information they need to make a good decision about this significant commitment to work together.

Further, while there would be no research protocol for the music therapy practice, and the work would not be monitored by the researcher at all, there were two particularly important issues for music therapists to consider together with families; specifically, how they might gather video material of sessions for their case reports, and the importance of nominating people who might be willing to comment on their child's case at the end of the year. Families were asked whether they would be able to name up to five people to be commentators, but their names would not be required and informed consent would not be obtained until towards the end of the period of work.

When the research commenced, ten music therapists were working with one child each, and some had other children on a waiting list. As usual, music therapists would keep family information confidential. The research data would come from commentators and was therefore one step removed from direct practice. The real names of families, commentators, and music therapists have not been used in this book, or any other research publications. Nevertheless, all parties have been informed that in such a small field as music therapy with tamariki takiwātanga, there is a risk that they might be identified.

Theoretical Underpinnings

Critical Realism

The aim of this project was to learn about the ways family members and other experts might understand music therapy with tamariki takiwātanga. As is seen in the chapters ahead, the commentators were able to observe and explicate some of the complexities of music therapy interaction, in which child and therapist mutually influence each other. Critical realism is a theory that acknowledges the mutual influence humans have on each other, the ways our actions shape society, and the need we have for explanations. It is used in research relating to a range of disciplines, particularly those which focus on real problems situated in a complex social world (Williams et al., 2017). In the context of this research, the theory provided support for an examination of music therapy processes that would help us understand what music therapy might mean for a child or group of children, in a particular location and time. The purpose of this project is to explain the complex process of music therapy, rather than "prove" that it is effective. On the other hand, in asking experts to comment on whether learning or development occurred, I was seeking information that might help us understand whether certain conditions can lead to observable patterns of change in particular contexts (Bhaskar, 1989). While multiple descriptions of the same phenomenon can be valid, critical realists are interested to find out what works for whom and in what circumstances. Williams et al., (2017, p. 6) explain that *people* determine whether programmes are successful or not. "In essence, we are interested in identifying and understanding people's responses to different resources offered within complex social programmes or interventions."

A Multiple Case Study Design

Bhaskar (1989), who is considered the initiator of critical realism, believed it is important to explain behaviours, such as the relationships between structures and values, and to describe phenomena in an understandable way. I aimed for the research to be transparent, accurate, ethical, and accessible to practitioners, families and other professionals, and the multiple mixed method case study approach seemed to be the most appropriate way to do this. Case studies include a great deal of information about music therapy participants, therapists, and the context of the therapy, and afford researchers and readers opportunities to make connections between pre-existing theories and practices, ultimately to enhance understanding and generate new and/or improved practices (McLeod, 2010). It is not possible however to determine causation from case study material, i.e., to claim that any improvement in tamariki takiwātanga well-being was due to music therapy. It is also not possible, especially from a single case, to generalise findings, or to say that music therapy practised in the same way with similar children will have similar outcomes.

On the other hand, by integrating findings from several interrelated qualitative studies researchers can provide comprehensive coverage, both in-depth and broad, of a topic (Kinn et al., 2013) and it is possible to make tentative generalisations when trends are strongly supported across cases (McLeod, 2010; Pilkington, 2018; Solesbury, 2002). Multiple case study research enables researchers not only to study the situational uniqueness of each case, but also to uncover common characteristics across cases, and to understand the phenomenon under study as applicable to the whole bounded group rather than just each individual case (Stake, 2006). That is, the current project aimed to understand not only what music therapy processes might mean for the individual children, but to understand music therapy with tamariki takiwātanga in New Zealand more broadly. Stake (2006) identified that a multiple case study ideally consists of between four to ten cases. Four or more cases are needed to show enough of interactivity between the programmes and their situations, and more than ten can result in the data providing more uniqueness of activity than can be usually analysed by a research team.

This study also contains elements of the hermeneutic single case efficacy design (HSCED) (Elliott, 2002; McLeod, 2010), which uses case material to determine whether clients may have improved because of the therapy they have received. In HSCED, individual researchers or a research team systematically examine clinical data to determine whether the outcome is good, whether it can be attributable to therapy or has been brought about by some other means, and what elements in the therapy process might have influenced the changes (McLeod, 2010, p. 26). McLeod goes on to argue that HSCED answers important questions around the effectiveness of therapy, and thus contributes to debates around evidence-based practice. However, the main weakness of the approach is that it "involves the assembly of a rich data set, and then proceeds to reduce this complexity to answer a single question: can this therapy be shown to have been effective?" (McLeod, 2010, p. 26). As noted above, this study was less focused on causality, but aimed to understand what music therapy processes might mean for individual children and, more broadly, for tamariki takiwātanga in New Zealand.

Mixed Methods Research

While there are many definitions of mixed methods research the broad purpose is to generate breadth and depth of understanding, and corroboration (Johnson et al., 2007). It allows for "multiple ways of seeing the social world" and the integration of multiple ways of knowing (Creswell et al., 2011). Moreover, the researcher is a critical component of the research process, and their reflexivity guides the project (Timans et al., 2019). I wanted to understand how individual commentators perceive the practice of music therapy with tamariki takiwātanga (having viewed individual and/or multiple cases), and whether examining the perceptions of multiple commentators might highlight common understandings. I was able to obtain this information from their written descriptions of witnessing music therapy (open-ended information) . Commentators also completed Likert questionnaires indicating how strongly they might agree or disagree to predetermined questions about music therapy processes (closed-ended information). Data was analysed separately and, for each of the ten in cases, I examined the ways in which the findings from the descriptions and Likert questionnaires related to each other and converged or diverged. Where there was divergence, particularly in James' case, I searched for an explanation by reanalysing the data. Overall, there were high levels of corroboration between data sets.

Reflexivity

> An Israeli Saying is 'things that You See from Here, You can't See from There' (Berger, 2015, p. 230).

In chapter 1 I wrote that, as a qualitative researcher, I have tried to be "reflexive," to be critically aware of the ways in which my experiences and beliefs have been influencing my research, and the ways the research processes have been influencing me, through each and all its stages. Research is a performance, with researchers as central protagonists, implicated in every aspect of the research process, in the choice of questions, design of the project, data collection process, and most importantly in the analysis and final account.

Reflexivity is important to "minimise projecting our own experiences and using them as the lens to view and understand participants' experience" (Berger, 2015, p. 230) and to expose unexpected possibilities (Porter, 2007). It involves researchers actively acknowledging that their actions and decisions will inevitably impact on the meaning and context of the experience they are investigating. Scrutinising the lens through which they view the phenomenon is an important way for researchers to generate credible, trustworthy, and nonexploitative research (Berger, 2015, p. 229).

However, reflexivity does not avoid the problem of speaking for others, and I am aware "the intellectual conviction that self-awareness is important may not be sufficient to expose masks and blind spots to self-scrutiny" (Probst, 2015, p. 38). Nevertheless, I am hopeful that my extensive experience as an action researcher, which includes initiating participatory action research with a team of young people with intellectual disabilities, has made me alert to my mistakes, limitations, and vulnerabilities. I am used to closely scrutinising my own thoughts and actions (an internal process), by engaging in external activities (Probst & Berenson, 2014) which includes processing ideas through journaling and arts-based activities. For example, during this project I kept a diary in which I grappled with questions such as:

- What am I imagining I will find? For instance, as a music therapist, and music therapy lecturer, I was tired of being asked to "prove" that music therapy was effective. I *did* want to demonstrate that it was helpful. Was my desire for "positive results" influencing how I collect and analyse my data?
- How are the music therapists and commentators viewing me? What power dynamics are at play? Will the commentators say what they think I want to hear?
- In what ways are my own experiences as 1) aunt of Tim (who was takiwātanga), 2) a music therapist who has worked extensively with tamariki takiwātanga, and 3) a music therapy teacher, influencing my thoughts, feelings, and actions?

Having autism in my family, and my experience of working with autistic communities, may have given me *some* helpful insight into the experiences of autistic people. Being a music therapy clinician gave me *some* understanding and connection with the music therapists who facilitated the sessions. I was also a music therapy lecturer, who had taught some of the music therapists, and a researcher who was interested in developing a genuine understanding of how their work might be viewed by others. These experiences would all influence the way I engaged with this research.

My experiences indicate that, like many researchers, I was positioned to take both "insider" and "outsider" perspectives. While I could bring some knowledge and experience to help me understand what was being said, my interpretations were also "coloured." Even reflexive researchers cannot truly understand and convey participants' experiences when they are not shared (Berger, 2015). When writing our reports, we determine how stories will be told, and make decisions about what to leave in and what to take out. The stories of our participants intermesh with our own—and we can only aspire to faithfully represent the views of others.

My data analysis process therefore involved debriefing with others, writing analytic memos, constantly checking for statements that contradicted positive findings, letting the analysis sit and coming back to it, and consulting a colleague who confirmed that the data analysis seemed a trustworthy representation of the themes in the narratives rather than reflection of my biases (Berger, 2015). Most importantly, I have made a concerted effort to highlight participants' own words in the research findings.

It is important to notice that "commentators" too, held various positions. Parents who chose music therapy for their children clearly believed, at least initially, that it would be valuable for the children. Others who knew them, such as extended family or educators, may have been less invested in the process, and some of the commentators who did not know the children may even have been sceptics. In all cases, their "positions," or the lens through which they viewed the work, would have had an impact on what they noticed and commented on.

Data Analysis

A convergent parallel mixed methods design was employed to determine whether descriptive statistics drawn from questionnaires affirmed the themes that emerged from qualitative descriptions (Bradt et al., 2013). The questionnaires and descriptive data were analysed separately, and, in each case, as qualitative themes emerged, findings from the questionnaires were examined to see whether they confirmed or contradicted the narrative accounts. Where there was contradiction, I searched for an explanation by reanalysing the descriptive data.

Descriptive Text

Participants' transcripts and survey responses were accepted as accurate representations of their understandings and beliefs regarding the phenomenon they had observed, and thematic analysis was applied to the data sets. Thematic analysis is a flexible process of identifying patterns or themes within qualitative data and interpreting those themes to make sense of them in the light of the research question (Clarke & Braun, 2013). The aim of the analysis was to generate a comprehensive thematic summary, "moving beyond what individual participants report, clustering together common ideas from multiple individuals to re-present the data" (Willis et al., 2016, p. 1193). The analysis interprets and explains commentator's views, rather than just describing what they shared. My process was grounded in six steps outlined by Braun and Clarke (2006).

1. Familiarisation: Each document was read thoroughly several times, to ensure I was familiar with the data set before it was carefully and consistently named according to "case," "author," "relationship" (e.g., Liam, Familiar, Mother) and uploaded to NVivo software. I reread the data in NVivo and made annotations to mark specific points of interest.
2. Initial "open" coding
    (a) Each document was coded to a "case" and assigned an "attribute" ("Familiar Expert"; "Other Expert"; or "Music Therapist").
    (b) Each document was examined individually and chunks of data describing specific aspects of the music therapy process were labelled according to concepts and meaning in the context of the research question. These data were organised into "Nodes" in NVivo. Throughout the process I modified my codes many times, moving back and forward, recoding, deleting codes, renaming, and/or adding new codes. At the end of this step the codes had been organised into broad themes.
3. Search for themes: At this point I transferred the data from each Node into Word documents. Using the "cut and paste" function I moved the data around searching for coherent and meaningful patterns in

relation to the research question, and constructed themes. During this phase, I was still occasionally returning to NVivo and moving data to other nodes until I was confident that I had collated all the relevant data to each theme. I used the "node properties" function in NVivo to describe my themes and was constantly revising the ways in which these themes were worded and/or positioned.

4. Reviewing themes: I reread the data to make sure the themes were supported; and reviewed, modified, and developed the themes to ensure they were coherent and distinct, and relevant to the research question. A colleague also reviewed the data and the themes to ensure the findings were valid and credible. A "case report" describing how commentators perceived the impact of music therapy was developed for each child, and returned to music therapists and their families, asking for feedback, to ensure descriptive and interpretive validity. Positive feedback was received, and minor changes were incorporated into the data.
5. Refining and defining themes: I refined the themes to identify the essence of what each theme is about, and. I revised the descriptions of my themes to ensure they encapsulated the essence of the theme; that the subthemes were relevant to the overarching theme; and that the themes were convincing and relevant to the research question. I constructed an informative name for each theme.
6. Writing Up: I created an analytic narrative and illustrated it with excerpts from the raw data and contextualised my findings in the literature.

Questionnaires

Commentators also completed Likert questionnaires indicating how strongly they might agree or disagree to predetermined questions about music therapy processes. As noted earlier, this data was analysed separately and, for each of the ten in cases, I examined the ways in which the qualitative findings and Likert questionnaires related to each other and converged or diverged. Where there was divergence, I searched for an explanation by reanalysing the data.

References

Berger, R. (2015). Now I see it, now I don't: Researcher's position and reflexivity in qualitative research. *Qualitative Research, 15*(2), 219–234. https://doi.org/10.1177/1468794112468475

Bhaskar, R. (1989). *Reclaiming reality: A critical introduction to contemporary philosophy*. Verso.

Bradt, J., Burns, D. S., & Creswell, J. W. (2013, June 20). Mixed methods research in music therapy research. *Journal of Music Therapy, 50*(2), 123–148. https://doi.org/10.1093/jmt/50.2.123

Braun, V., & Clarke, V. (2006, April). Using thematic analysis in psychology. *Qualitative Research in Psychology, 3*(2), 77–101. http://dx.doi.org/10.1191/1478088706qp063oa

Clarke, V., & Braun, V. (2013). *Successful qualitative research: A practical guide for beginners*. Sage.

Creswell, J. W., Klassen, A. C., Plano Clark, V. L., & Clegg Smith, K. (2011). *Best practices for mixed methods research in the health sciences*. Office of Behavioral and Social Sciences Research, National Institute of Health.

Elliott, R. (2002). Hermeneutic single-case efficacy design. *Psychotherapy Research, 12*(1), 1–21. https://doi.org/10.1080/713869614

Given, L. M. (2008). Secondary participants. In L. M. Given (Ed.), *The Sage encyclopedia of qualitative research methods* (pp. 805–809). Sage. https://dx.doi.org/10.4135/9781412963909

Johnson, R. B., Onwuegbuzie, A. J., & Turner, L. A. (2007). Toward a definition of mixed methods research. *Journal of Mixed Methods Research, 1*(2), 112–133. https://doi.org/10.1177/1558689806298224

Kinn, L. G., Holgersen, H., Ekeland, T. J., & Davidson, L. (2013). Metasynthesis and bricolage: An artistic exercise of creating a collage of meaning. *Qualitative Health Research, 23*, 1285–1292. https://doi.org/10.1177/1049732313502127

McLeod, J. (2010). *Case study research in counselling and psychotherapy*. Sage.

Ministry of Education. (2009a). *Narrative assessment: A guide for teachers*. Learning Media. http://www.throughdifferenteyes.org.nz/a_guide_for_teachers

Pilkington, H. (2018). Employing meta-ethnography in the analysis of qualitative data sets on youth activism: A new tool for transnational research projects? *Qualitative Research, 18*(1), 108–130. https://doi.org/10.1177/1468794117707805

Porter, S. (2007). Validity, trustworthiness and rigour: Reasserting realism in qualitative research. *Journal of Advanced Nursing, 60*(1), 79–86. https://doi.org/10.1111/j.1365-2648.2007.04360.x

Probst, B. (2015). The eye regards itself: Benefits and challenges of reflexivity in qualitative social work research. *Social Work Research, 39*(1), 37–48. https://doi.org/10.1093/swr/svu028

Rickson, D. J., Castelino, A., Molyneux, C., Ridley, H., & Upjohn-Beatson, E. (2016). What evidence? Designing a mixed methods study to investigate music therapy with children who have autism spectrum disorder (ASD), in New Zealand Contexts. *The Arts in Psychotherapy, 50*, 119–125. https://doi.org/10.1016/j.aip.2016.07.002

Rickson, D. J., Molyneux, C., Ridley, H., Castelino, A., & Upjohn Beatson, E. B. (2015b). Music therapy with people who have autism spectrum disorder—Current practice in New Zealand. *New Zealand Journal of Music Therapy, 13*, 8–32. https://www-proquest-com.helicon.vuw.ac.nz/docview/1897698669?accountid=14782

Solesbury, W. (2002). The ascendancy of evidence. *Planning Theory & Practice, 3*(1), 90–96. https://doi.org/10.1080/14649350220117834

Stake, R. E. (2006). *Multiple case study analysis*. The Guilford Press.

Timans, R., Wouters, P., & Heilbron, J. (2019). Mixed methods research: What it is and what it could be. *Theory and Society, 48*(2), 193–216. https://doi.org/10.1007/s11186-019-09345-5

Williams, L., Rycroft-Malone, J., & Burton, C. R. (2017). Bringing critical realism to nursing practice: Roy Bhaskar's contribution. *Nursing Philosophy, 18*(2), e12130-n/a. https://doi.org/10.1111/nup.12130

Willis, D. G., Sullivan-Bolyai, S., Knafl, K., & Cohen, M. Z. (2016). Distinguishing features and similarities between descriptive phenomenological and qualitative description research. *Western Journal of Nursing Research, 38*(9), 1185–1204. https://doi.org/10.1177/0193945916645499

5

Introduction to the Case Studies

Music Therapy Practice with Tamariki Takiwātanga in New Zealand (Aotearoa)

The following information utilises findings from the exploratory research undertaken with New Zealand colleagues in 2015 (Rickson et al., 2015a,b). Data describing music therapy practice was drawn from focus groups, individual interviews, and questionnaires completed by/with New Zealand Registered Music Therapists.

Stages

Music therapy processes typically include stages of referral, assessment, programme planning, and evaluation (Hardy & LaGasse, 2018). We found that tamariki takiwātanga in New Zealand are often referred to music therapy because they have an interest in music, and need help to manage their behaviour, anxiety, or other emotions; to develop attention and/or other communication skills; to increase curiosity and motivation, improve social interaction and/or develop relationships; or to have fun.

D. Rickson, *Music Therapy with Autistic Children in Aotearoa, New Zealand*, https://doi.org/10.1007/978-3-031-05233-0_5

An assessment process determines whether music therapy is likely to be helpful for the child and, if so, what the focus of the music therapy programme might be, and how and where it might be implemented (individual, group, or family sessions; at home, in a private room, or in the classroom). In addition to music making with the child, therapists are likely to collaborate with other team members and to draw on existing documentation such as the child's Individual Education Plan (IEP), and the New Zealand Curriculum Key Competencies (Ministry of Education, 2014).

Key Competencies

The New Zealand Curriculum is underpinned by a vision of "young people as lifelong learners who are confident and creative, connected, and actively involved" in daily life with peers, families, and communities. It defines five key competencies that are considered "critical to sustained learning and effective participation in society" (Ministry of Education, 2014). These include "thinking," "using language, symbols, and texts," "managing self," "relating to others," and "participating and contributing." The development of these competencies can be considered an achievement, but they are also the means to succeeding in other areas. The ministry recognises that children develop the competencies in social contexts, that the competencies develop over time and are "shaped by interactions with people, places, ideas, and things" and that students need to be "challenged and supported to develop them in contexts that are increasingly wide-ranging and complex." They are therefore useful constructs for music therapists who are working in school settings in this country.

Context

Most New Zealand music therapists provide individual therapy, especially when the child experiences auditory sensitivity, has extreme difficulty paying attention, or needs to develop more awareness of self and others. However, many also work with children in group settings involving typically developing children, family members, or children who have another diagnosis, particularly when social skills are a focus. Family or other team members are also often present as observers or supporters of therapy.

The Therapeutic Relationship

The importance of the therapeutic relationship was highlighted in our earlier study with some of the therapists resisting the temptation to focus on specific goals, until a relationship had been established. Their primary emphasis seemed to be on developing "a caring, respectful, intimate and creative environment in which people can share meaningful experiences and grow" (Rickson et al. 2015a,b, p. 46). They argued when children feel understood, they are more likely to "open up" and demonstrate their abilities and potential. Further, they suggested that "music therapy often allows families and others to see the person in a new light, and to celebrate their strengths," and that "this can be extremely valuable for families who are often confronted with lists of things that their child is unable to do" (p. 49).

Goals and Outcomes

Communication and socialisation seemed to be the most common areas of focus for the music therapy programmes (Rickson et al. 2015). However, these are broad concepts that encompass many subskills. A focus on communication for example might include receptive skills such as listening, attending, concentrating, and engaging; and expressive skills such as vocalisation and creative musical expression, or speech and language development. Similarly, a focus on socialisation might include developing awareness of others and their needs, listening, engaging, participating, sharing, turn-taking, cooperating, and developing confidence.

We also found that the development of relationships is a frequently cited goal. Sometimes the focus is on developing the child–therapist relationship; sometimes it is on engaging children in meaningful activity with others, making or maintaining relationships with peers, or developing wider social networks. Tamariki takiwātanga often need support to interact, to participate, to express themselves in socially acceptable ways, and to develop independence. New Zealand RMTh therefore suggested they sometimes focus on "music therapy to support well-being or quality of life", or engagement in "meaningful activity", and highlight the inclusion of children with their peers, particularly within school communities, as an important goal. Finally, music therapists are also concerned to support children to manage sensory difficulties, particularly auditory sensitivity, and sensory integration. They suggest that child-centred music therapy, which enables children to be in control of sound-making, seems to support increased tolerance for sounds—particularly when they may occur unexpectedly.

Overall, then, while the music therapists valued diversity, acknowledged individual difficulties and strengths as part of the human condition, and argued that tamariki takiwātanga might be allowed to do things differently, or to "be" different people, they also suggested that tamariki takiwātanga might need support to engage in typical activities. That is, in some circumstances it would be enough for a child just to be happy during a music therapy session. In other circumstances it would be considered beneficial to challenge them to develop new skills so they might be able to engage more readily with neurotypical peers and others.

Approaches

In terms of approach, music therapy practice with tamariki takiwātanga in New Zealand is predominantly informed by creative, psychodynamic, improvisational music therapy theory. Practice is "child-centred", or community-oriented, although music therapists do engage with medical, behavioural, creative, relationship-based, and music-centred approaches in certain contexts.

For example, some described engaging in "improvisatory" or "music-centred" approaches, suggesting the primary outcome of music therapy might be for children to have opportunities to engage and to communicate with others through music making. Others suggested music and/or the elements of music can be used as a "tool" for therapy; or argued that skill development can be embedded in "musical play" or "drama" experiences. For some, psychodynamic thinking was important to their work, as they reflected "on all aspects of the music therapy process, including that external to the session itself," and used their reflections to guide the sessions. Some described helping children to settle in the classroom and working with staff to encourage the use of music therapy strategies across contexts, an approach which aligns with community music therapy. A few of the therapists indicated they would at times reflect on behavioural antecedents and consequences and introduce specific strategies to help children manage their behaviour. Interestingly, it seemed that a more "behavioural" approach was also expected and/or desired to a certain extent by some parent interviewees involved in the study. Finally, we found that some music therapists align their work with specific non-music therapy approaches such as intensive interaction.

It was clear that the music therapists held the therapeutic relationship central to the work, and that they aimed to develop caring, respectful, intimate, and creative environments in which children can grow. Flexibility within sessions, and within music, was considered crucial to enable participants to "'open up' and to show their abilities and potential within the context of the therapeutic relationship" (Rickson et al. 2015a,b, p. 21). The music therapists sought to construct the music therapy process *with* the children; accepting them as they are; responding to them in the moment with adapted, composed, or improvised music; drawing on their interests and strengths; and providing stimulation, comfort, and security according to the children's needs. The child-centred (or person-centred) approach involves "seeing beyond autism, meeting participants 'where they are,' and being committed to an approach that starts with what participants bring, valuing and developing authentic relationships them" (Rickson et al. 2015a,b p. 46).

However, despite strongly advocating for child-centred approaches with tamariki takiwātanga overall, the music therapists described varying their practices according to their personal situations and/or the context in which they were working. The approach that they would take would be influenced by a variety of factors including "the unique skills and knowledge they bring to music therapy from other fields, other countries, and previous music therapy experiences; the context in which they are working; and their knowledge of, and/or the needs of the participant/s they are working with" (Rickson et al. 2015a,b, p. 43). For example, one practitioner suggested their sessions became less structured, more child-led, and increasingly improvisational as they gained more experience as a music therapist. Another suggested that a change in living circumstances for the child they were working with led to a change in behaviour that signalled the need for more structure and containment.

Freedom and Structure Within Sessions

Despite advocating for flexible, child-led, approaches, the music therapists also suggested that sessions are typically carefully structured, particularly at the beginning of the music therapy process, with children being encouraged to take more of a lead as they feel ready to do so. Importantly, they argued that the structure of and repetition within the *music* provides a sense of safety, supports the child's engagement, or contains their expressive communication. "It is the way the music and its elements are used in relation to vitality affects and attunement that makes music therapy unique" (Rickson et al. 2015a,b, p. 50). Music is the "bridge" that connects child and therapist. Nevertheless, "while structure and routine can be important, 'rigid' expectations that people with ASD will be able to adhere to typical social norms can be unrealistic" (p. 40).

Methods

Many New Zealand music therapists use improvisation in their work. They believe that the potential to adapt, compose, and improvise in the moment is crucial to both attune and add vitality to the children's actions, and thus to promote interaction. However, most use a range of methods which might include, for example, listening to familiar music, which might reduce anxiety; playing instruments, which can promote reciprocal interaction and provide opportunities for expressive communication; or singing, which can be an engaging, expressive, and inclusive medium, to support vocalisation and speech development. Sessions might involve vocal or instrumental improvisations, rhythm activities (such as drumming), or improvised songs.

For example, they might sing improvised or adapted songs to describe what tamariki takiwātanga are doing, thus making their activity meaningful or purposeful, providing language for what they are doing, and/or songs might be used to help them to transition from one activity to another. They might provide musical structure and repetition to give tamariki takiwātanga important non-verbal cues about when and how they might contribute to an interaction, thus supporting their turn-taking and other social skills. One music therapist described tamariki takiwātanga playing wind instruments to promote oro-motor development, and another reported that audio recording one child's singing motivated further vocalisations.

Layout of the Case Studies

All the work undertaken for the current study involved music therapists working with individual children rather than with groups. This is perhaps unsurprising since the research funding was offered to individual children. Ethical complications can arise when music therapists are paid to work with individuals, and other children are involved in the interactions. As noted above, music therapists in New Zealand do, of course, facilitate group programmes which include or are specifically for takiwātanga, in classrooms or community settings. However, in these instances, the music therapist is more likely to be employed by or contracted to a facility or community group to work somewhat flexibly within their wider population, rather than being employed to work with an individual child.

In the chapters that follow, each case study begins with a brief description of the child, and their music therapist (the background). The music therapists have been classified as "beginning" (those who have worked with less than eight tamariki takiwātanga); "established" (those who have worked for less than five years as a registered music therapist but have already worked with over 25 tamariki takiwātanga); "experienced" (those who have worked for more than five years with over 25 tamariki takiwātanga); and "highly experienced" (those who have worked for over ten years with more than 30 tamariki takiwātanga).

The brief description of the child and therapist is followed by a narrative of the music therapy process based on the written descriptions provided by the music therapists. The descriptions have been edited for publication while keeping the primary content intact. This is important because the descriptions were part of the package of raw data, i.e., the Learning Stories / Narrative Assessments (see Sect. "Narrative Assessment") that the experts were commentating on. Each case differs in terms of the amount as well as the type of information that the music therapists chose to include. For example, Liam's music therapist offered minimal written description, relying instead on the video data to "tell the story." In contrast, in Sophia and Oliver's cases video data was not submitted, but the written description was accompanied by photographs.

Music therapists also submitted summaries of the music therapy process which were *not* made available to commentators. This was to increase the potential for commentators to make their own minds up about what was happening in/through the music therapy. In the following chapters I have included the music therapists' summary statements in italics, within boxed borders.

The central focus of each case study is the rich feedback provided by family members and other experts. However, I have also provided brief personal reflections on each case. With ten case studies available to me, I have had the privilege to be able to reflect on the individual and collective cases, and, drawing on the literature as well as my own experience as a clinician and teacher, to consider the way an aspect/s of the work might align with current theories and practices. My approach to this has been instinctive. That is, I have simply chosen to focus on one or two characteristics of the work that intrigued me personally, in terms of the way the music therapist carried out and/or described the work, and/or the interpretations of the commentators. My intention is not to judge, but to add another perspective having had the opportunity to read the case notes as well as the commentators' opinions of the cases. Music therapists, students, and other readers are likely to think of other, perhaps contrasting, questions, ideas, and ways of conceptualising the work.

The music therapy approach is the lens that guides and justifies the music therapist's choice of methods and techniques (Pasiali, 2018) and influences the ways they explain "the role of music, the role of the therapist, and the processes (they employ)" (Edwards, 2016, p. 418). Music therapists in New Zealand tend to draw on a variety of approaches in their work (Rickson et al. 2015a,b) and this seemed to be the case for many of the music therapists whose work is described in this book. Edwards (2016) suggests the delivery of various music therapy methods (activities) can look similar across various approaches, while the way in which the music therapists explain their work may be different. It can be difficult therefore to interpret other music therapists' work and I therefore feel it is important to reiterate that the reflective musings following each case are my own. They are not necessarily the opinions of the practitioners, and they are not the only way to think about the work.

In the chapters that follow, to protect the anonymity of participants, commentators who knew a child have been identified by their relationship to the child (e.g., mother, teacher, aunt) while the six autism experts who commented on all ten cases have been given nom-de-plumes (Hilda, Freya, Ruella, Vivian, Dana, and Mike). The children and their music therapists have also been given nom-de-plumes.

References

Edwards, J. (2016). Approaches and models of music therapy. In J. Edwards (Ed.), *The Oxford handbook of music therapy* (1st ed., pp. 418–427). Oxford University Press. https://doi.org/10.1093/oxfordhb/9780199639755.001.0001

Hardy, M., & LaGasse, A. B. (2018). Music therapy for persons with autism spectrum disorder. In A. Knight, A. B. LaGasse, & A. A. Clair (Eds.), *Music therapy: An introduction to the profession* (pp. 185–202). The American Music Therapy Association Inc.

Ministry of Education. (2014). *Key competencies*. Te Kete Ipurangi, Ministry of Eudcation. Retrieved August 25, 2020 from https://nzcurriculum.tki.org.nz/Key-competencies

Rickson, D. J., Molyneux, C., Ridley, H., Castelino, A., & Upjohn-Beatson, E. (2015a). *Music therapy for children who have autism spectrum disorder ASD: Exploring the potential for research in New Zealand using a mixed methods design.* Victoria University of Wellington.

Rickson, D. J., Molyneux, C., Ridley, H., Castelino, A., & Upjohn Beatson, E. B. (2015b). Music therapy with people who have autism spectrum disorder—Current practice in New Zealand. *New Zealand Journal of Music Therapy, 13*, 8–32. https://www-proquest-com.helicon.vuw.ac.nz/docview/1897698669?accountid=14782

Pasiali, V. (2018). Approaches to music therapy. In A. Knight, B. LaGasse, & A. A. Clair (Eds.), *Music therapy: An introduction to the profession* (pp. 139–159). The American Music Therapy Association Inc.

6

LIAM—"It Made Me Laugh Out Loud!"

Background

Liam was an 8-year-old boy who loved music. His family actively engaged in musicking, and he knew the words of many songs which he sang well. He was generally talkative, and was progressing well academically, although he frequently had difficulty concentrating and was often described as being "in his own world." Liam also had difficulty engaging with and relating to his peers, and therefore in developing friendships. He needed support with listening, interacting, making choices, and taking turns.

His music therapist, Jodie, was highly experienced in this context. She employed a child-centred approach, in which "the child's preferences and responses to the music shaped the music therapy planning and intervention." Music therapy was typically provided weekly, for five months, and a total of 14 sessions took place, in Jodie's studio. The work ended abruptly due to changes in family circumstances. The broad, initial, music therapy goal was for Liam to develop peer friendships.

D. Rickson, *Music Therapy with Autistic Children in Aotearoa, New Zealand*,
https://doi.org/10.1007/978-3-031-05233-0_6

The Music Therapy Process

In the first example Liam arrived at music visibly upset. Although he was quiet and tearful, he was able to sit at the keyboard, and became interested when Jodie showed him how a note could be "bent" by swivelling a knob on the panel. From there he moved with her to the drum and cymbal where they took turns to make rhythm patterns for each other to copy. Quite suddenly, he smiled and said "we need something else" indicating towards the guitar. Jodie began to sing a song, accompanying herself on the guitar, before pretending to go to sleep. When Liam woke her with a "boo!" Jodie immediately instigated a song about him waking her up, and he began to laugh and dance happily around the room, pleading to repeat the game "because it (was) so funny".

> Jodie surmised that allowing Liam time to be upset, while demonstrating empathy, enabled a 'shift' from his watching her, to mutual understanding and interaction. Prior to this session his interactions had appeared 'mechanical', and now they seemed more genuine.

While Jodie had established that he loved singing, Liam did not want "to sing in front of everyone." In the second example from session eight, Jodie is focusing on supporting Liam to participate in the making of his own CD. Having this tangible product would enable him to share his music with peers and others, without singing in front of them, should he choose to. In this session, with his cousin present, Liam was able to assert himself more readily and to communicate his choice of musical material, pictures, font colour and cover layout, for his CD.

> Jodie felt Liam had improved in his ability to listen and to interact, and that he demonstrated increased confidence in choice making, and 'performing' with voice for the recording.

The third example, from session ten, focused on Liam's ability to engage in shared musical interaction. While he enjoyed playing the keyboard, he would play in a solitary way preferring to use the automated rhythms on the keyboard than to share his music with Jodie. In this session, for the first time, he was able to wait while Jodie played, and to engage in several exchanges of turn-taking.

Jodie noted that Liam's developing awareness of others, increase in concentration, and the emergence of turn-taking was important. He was interacting in more natural ways. A longer term of music therapy might include peer or small group music therapy sessions to promote his ability to develop friendships.

Commentators' Interpretations of Liam's Case

Commentators observed that Liam's enjoyment of the music therapy sessions ensured that he had a context in which he could gradually develop his cognitive abilities. When playing the piano Liam paid keen attention to the notes (Vivian), appeared to be planning (Hilda), "tried to keep in time with the beat by the end [...] (and) although it took him a while, he did eventually pick up on the tempo" (Aunt Amanda). He was participating with enthusiasm (Freyer) and, according to his grandmother, achieved well considering he had no musical training. His Aunt Rachelle suggested he developed an understanding that it was important to wait patiently, "for it not to be all about him and his wants and needs." He began "watching," "taking an interest" (Aunt Rachelle), "paying attention," and "concentrating hard" (Aunt Rachelle; grandmother). At one point Liam was "eagerly waiting for his turn to play the piano" (grandmother) with "his hands poised ready [...] - but he was able to exercise restraint and wait until he was told it was his turn to play" (Ruella).

> Children with ASD often have difficulty waiting their turn and while they can be rule driven, it is not unusual for them to become frustrated. It was good to see that the turns were of different durations and at some points Liam clearly thought it was his turn and was about to jump in and then held himself back. He had great concentration. (Freyer)

It is likely that Liam's auditory sensitivities contributed to his initial cautious approach to shared music making, and that opportunities to "experiment" and to control sound, gave him increasing confidence to engage in music making with others. As a small child Liam was always disturbed by loud noises (Aunt Amanda; Liam's grandmother). His auditory sensitivity continued to be evident in music therapy (Aunt Amanda; Liam's grandmother; Mike), but he seemed to "have conditioned himself to get used to the noise" (Aunt Rachelle) and was able to manage it well. Family members were surprised for example that he seemed to be "enjoying" and "at ease" playing the cymbal (Aunt Amanda; Aunt Rachelle; Liam's grandmother). Aunt Amanda noticed "I could see a definite progress in the sessions, in his confidence in his ability to play the instruments and to hit the cymbal or piano keys without flinching" (Aunt Amanda). Liam's Aunt Rachelle suggested he was "quite shy" when he initially started playing the piano but hit more notes and "played quite vigorously and loudly [...] as he builds up this confidence". In turn, Liam's music became more creative or, in his grandmother's words, "experimental."

> Although at the start Liam played some quite basic notes on the piano, as he progressed and gained more confidence it sounded more tuneful and expressive. I thought it interesting that he tried to play a melody rather than crashing on the keyboard. I loved the very confident improvised scale at the end. (Liam's grandmother)

> I can honestly say I've never heard Liam play on a piano before and it sounded like his confidence grew the more he interacted with the keys. He repeated some of the sounds near the end. [...] It sounded like he was enjoying the freedom to play as he liked without judgement. (Aunt Amanda)

The child-centred music therapy approach afforded Liam opportunities to employ adaptive strategies to reduce his own anxieties. For example, he may have introduced the "Boo" game because it was familiar and comforting for him. His Aunt explained, "Liam loves playing the Boo game with his family; this is something he seems to do when we first arrive at our family gatherings and (it) acts as an ice breaker" (Aunt Amanda). He also employed humour by, for example, saying "boo" to the "audience," through the camera (Freyer). Aunt Amanda suggested he also used the music as a cue to allow him to keep moving around the room, which in turn helped him to remain calm. Liam was able to move as he needed to, while being contained by the structure of the music. Hilda observed:

> Liam is twirling in space – a favourite of autistic kids as it can be soothing – but when the music stops, he joins in the game of waking up Jodie by saying 'boo'. Playing such an interactive game requires imagination and suggests to me that Liam is enjoying the learning that is taking place. (Hilda)

Several commentators noted Liam's increasing ability to manage his anxiety when being filmed (Freyer; Hilda: Aunt Amanda). Given his reluctance to share his music making with others it was notable that he continued to participate with enthusiasm when he was aware of the camera (Hilda; Vivian). "Playing to the video camera" seemed like an important adaptive strategy in which the camera itself served as an intermediary object through which Liam could share his music.

> (At home) he can quite happily sing if he thinks no one is listening but then gets all shy when he realises that we are listening to him. [...] (Here) he started to play to the camera which I thought was great! It shows that he can interact with others [...] (he) is aware that other people will also be watching him. (Aunt Rachelle)

> Liam sings quite faintly at the beginning but by the end he is very clear and confident. It is one of his favourite songs and he seemed to enjoy belting out the song despite an audience which usually makes him quite shy. (Aunt Amanda)

Commentators argued that Liam developed a strong connection with Jodie over the course of the therapy, and that "it was a pleasure to be able to see the connection between him and his therapist" (Freyer). He was "at ease with her" (Liam's grandmother), and trust developed at least in part because of her respect for his sensory needs (Hilda). This led to an increase in genuine engagement and allowed him to try "something new" (Freyer). He wanted to work collaboratively with her to develop his interests in music (Freyer) and in doing so his "social skills developed as much as could reasonably be expected for an eight-year-old in this short but sustained period" (Mike).

> I loved it! Jodie created an environment where it was 'ok' for Liam to be himself. There was no pressure placed upon him to do as he was told rather, she created a space for Liam to learn by experimenting. He was able to take the lead. (Dana)

Neurotypical people and takiwātanga often have difficulty understanding each other's non-verbal communication. For example, Mike was uncomfortable with the description of Liam being "in his own world." He argued that takiwātanga ways of being can draw too much or too strong scrutiny, leading to inaccurate assumptions. Freyer too was keen to have "evidence of when Liam was in another world or lacking in concentration to illustrate the contrast when he was engaged." Family members, who understood Liam's non-verbal communications well, were more confident in drawing conclusions. Aunt Rachelle shared that "Liam can appear standoffish at times and as if he isn't listening, but I don't believe this to always be true," while Aunt Amanda said, "He can also tend to get wrapped up in his own thoughts at times and zone out, but this never seemed to be the case in the videos."

However, Mike and Aunt Amanda both suggested that Liam may have lacked genuine engagement at times. Mike wrote "when Jodie talked about smiling at the same time [as Liam], and a positive shift in the therapist relationship" he may have been "just humouring her […] and complying" because he views her as an authority figure. Similarly, Aunt Amanda shared:

> I have to say it made me smile how serious Liam looked throughout this clip. It was like he wanted to get it right and please Jodie. He understood by the end that turn taking was the rule and waited patiently for his turn on the keys. (Aunt Amanda)

Jodie was disappointed that the sessions ended abruptly due to changes in family circumstances, suggesting there was considerable potential for more learning and development to take place, particularly regarding friendship development. While the experience of music therapy may have provided a positive basis for the goal of making friends (Hilda), in this case Liam was only able to demonstrate the ability to build a positive relationship with Jodie (Vivian). While "the sessions were well planned, engaging and offered a range of learning opportunities to stimulate Liam's body and mind" (Dana), "there was no peer engagement in the therapy" (Mike). Vivian, similarly, noted:

> What was unclear was that one of the goals in the intervention plan as noted by Jodie was for Liam to begin generalising his responses from music to social play at school. This aspect was somehow not pursued or not reported […] Nevertheless, the brief preview of what is possible in a term of therapy is indeed promising. (Vivian)

Moreover, the inclusion of his cousin in one of the sessions provided an opportunity for Liam to watch and learn from a peer (Ruella) and he improved in his choice making following this modelling (Freyer). The way that this supported Liam to make decisions provides a good case for involving a peer/s in subsequent sessions to provide opportunities for developing social skills with his peers (Ruella). The recording project was particularly helpful for Liam because it gave him opportunities to make choices (Ruella) and engaged his logic (Mike).

> Overall, I think (the music therapy) was great and used an interest of Liam's (music), to help build his confidence around people he doesn't know well and enable him to be patient and wait his turn when he needs to. I can see how music therapy could possibly help Liam with his confidence over time and in turn with his social relationships with people that he doesn't know well. (Aunt Rachelle)

Liam was responsive because the therapist worked with his skills and interests (Hilda). He was passionate about music, and "Jodie did a wonderful job creating a repertoire of musical opportunities which appealed to (him) and kept him engaged" (Dana). He was variously observed to have "natural musicality," "interest," appreciation," "passion," and "love" for music, and to have "expressed himself well through the arts" (Dana). He created an "interesting rhythmic composition" (Freyer) and did some "amazing singing" (Dana). He "obviously enjoyed the sensory experiences and learning challenges provided by music, which indicates it is important for his wellbeing" (Hilda). Ongoing "therapy through music would enable him to develop confidence in other areas of his life including at school [and] with friendships" (Aunt Rachelle).

> Listening to the Audio clip (of 'Can't Stop the Feeling') reminded me how much Liam loves to sing along to this song. It is one of his favourite songs and he knows the words very well. He usually dances along as he sings. Liam has a lovely voice and was chosen to sing a solo piece at his school at the end of last year. I was amazed at how in tune he was and surprised he had the courage to stand in front of so many people and sing. In the past he has always hovered in the background and kept well out of the limelight. I felt very tearful but proud watching him. To me this is a great example of how music therapy has really helped Liam gain confidence. (Liam's grandmother)

Liam's case highlights the positive cycle of success leading to further successes. As his confidence increased, he was naturally more able to participate, and this in turn supported his abilities to manage sensory and cognitive stimuli. Commentators could see opportunities for further developing Liam's interest in singing (Mike) and in guitar (Hilda). "Skills with, and enjoyment of music, are a good way to develop relationships with others throughout life who share these skills" (Hilda).

> This case demonstrates that for those children with autism who have a natural flair for music in combination with an intuitive therapist, can be a win-win combination for increasing specific competencies that can be generalised by students to their learning and social settings. (Vivian)

Commentators described their experience of watching the clips as enjoyable, exciting, delightful and a pleasure, and at times it not only made them smile but also laugh out loud. Family members felt proud of Liam. Other commentators summarised that the learning Liam demonstrated shows that music therapy has been a valuable and successful intervention (Freyer; Hilda; Ruella) which should continue (Dana; Hilda).

> Music Therapy has been very good for Liam helping him to express himself, gain confidence and to be more aware of others around him. He has always loved music, so it has been a great way to grab his interest. There has been quite a noticeable change in him this year and I believe the music therapy course has helped to minimise his autistic traits enabling him to start to develop some friendships at school. (Liam's grandmother)

Integration of Findings from Descriptions and Liam's Questionnaires

The findings from questionnaires were predominantly in line with qualitative findings. Commentators agreed that music therapy was meaningful and important for Liam; that he was positively engaged, seemed to enjoy music therapy sessions overall, and that he made timely progress towards his individualised goal. They also agreed that music was an important aspect of the therapeutic interaction, and most agreed that the way Jodie facilitated the interaction was also important. However overall results (from all ten cases) suggest the latter question was unclear and therefore difficult to answer.

An important finding from Liam's case is that one commentator (Dana) strongly *disagreed* with the statements that Liam made progress towards his stated individual goal (Q1) and that he was clearly developing skills that would help him learn (Q4). Yet her qualitative report was very positive and included the statement "The sessions were well planned, engaging and offered a range of learning opportunities to stimulate Liam's body and mind" (Dana). It is therefore likely that the commentators who strongly disagreed or somewhat disagreed that he made progress towards his goals were focusing on the broad goal of "developing friendships." This goal was not directly addressed in the programme of therapy, although some of the skills that underpin the development of friendships were being addressed.

Music Therapist's Summary

Jodie reported that the music therapy process held Liam's interest. He was encouraged to listen, to participate, and to take turns. His concentration increased, and the production of a CD gave him something he could share with others. She argued that while the changes he made were small, Liam moved from being self-absorbed, resistant to making decisions, and lacking in concentration, to interacting with her, and after some encouragement, making his own decisions. She anticipated he would continue to develop skills if he had more time in therapy.

My Reflections on Liam's Case

Despite the acceptance that tamariki takiwātanga prefer their "own time and space" the notion that they are living "in their own worlds" is contentious. Autistic people are "push(ing) back against the damaging and pervasive stereotypes that have historically cast them as people in their own world" (Bakan, 2015, p. 117) so it is not surprising that Mike challenged this description of Liam. Under responsivity to auditory stimuli, can lead to the perception that takiwātanga are inattentive, "living in their own world," or even deaf (Tomchek & Dunn, 2007). Similarly, if they have difficulties with auditory-visual integration, i.e., looking and listening at the same time, they are often perceived to be not concentrating. While attending and concentrating, by definition, rely on children being able to focus on specific stimuli while putting other stimuli aside until a task is completed, tamariki takiwātanga may be concentrating keenly on auditory stimuli while keeping their eyes averted. So, lack of eye contact does not necessarily imply lack of engagement.

Moreover, Liam seemed to be working hard to learn the rules that would enable him to live up to the expectations of neurotypical people. Jodie initially experienced him as "mechanical," going through the motions, while others suggested he was "complying" or "just humouring (her)." That is, he appeared to be performing, rather than being performative. Yet as their relationship developed, and his anxiety decreased, he was observed to be more genuinely engaged. His initial desire to "get it right" *may* have been to please Jodie, as Aunt Amanda suggested, and/or he may have been working hard to create a particular musical aesthetic. Liam loved singing, sang many songs, and could play keyboard, yet was not keen "to sing in front of everyone." Performance anxiety is common even for very young children, and this can have both innate and developed components (Boucher & Ryan, 2011). That is, some children may be innately performance anxious while others might be wary or anxious about performing because they feel unable to meet the expectations and responses of peers, siblings, teachers, and parents in performance situations.

It was therefore noteworthy that Liam was gradually more able to cope with performing through an intermediary object, the video camera, which served as a communication bridge (Rojas-Bermúdez & Moyano, 2020). While he found it difficult to sing in front of people, he was able to "belt out a song" in front of the video camera even when he knew there would be an "audience" behind it. Further, when he was working on his CD project the focus shifted from performing works for others and trying to act in ways that others would appreciate, to taking part in music therapy activities that afforded him opportunities to be himself. He was able to be "performative", genuinely engaged in a musical collaboration with Jodie, which in turn enabled him to produce a musical work that *could* be performed (Small, 1998).

> The performance of identity is a way that we (takiwātanga) can reclaim our agency and autonomy from a system which would try to tell us who we are allowed to be, and what aspects of the self we are able to express. At the same time, there are real consequences for violating social norms,

> or deviating from the scripts that our culture gives us which define the roles we are allowed to take. (Sayre, 2020, no page number)

Liam and Jodie's collaborative CD project seems to sit comfortably within the theoretical frame of Resource-Oriented Music Therapy. Resource-Oriented music therapy (Rolvsjord, 2010) emphasises children's strengths and potentials and focuses on developing collaborative projects that lead to positive experiences, skill development, and strategies for managing, rather than on difficult emotions, conflict, and problems. When takiwātanga are listening to and discussing music while creating music artefacts they can experience reduced anxiety, and an increase in self-esteem and positive attitudes towards peers (Hillier et al., 2011). Resource-oriented approaches in turn sit comfortably within a cultural neurodiversity framework, which,

> ...privileges autistic ability over disability and draws on the creative initiatives and impulses of children with autism rather than trying to restrain, retrain, or redirect them" [...] Musical cultures, social norms, and priorities can grow directly from the preferences, directives, and agency of autistic children who are making music together. (Bakan, 2014, no page number)

Jodie did not describe her work as resource-oriented, instead suggesting she employed a child-centred approach in her work, in which "the child's preferences and responses to the music shaped the music therapy planning and intervention." Her playful improvisation with the Boo game, which supported Liam to move from a distressed to a joyful mood, could readily be situated within the child-centred Creative Music Therapy frame in which the therapist spontaneously plays, moves, and vocalises with the child to establish and support developing reciprocal communication patterns (Nordoff & Robbins, 2007; Pasiali, 2018).

However, Jodie also seemed to provide overt direction to ensure that Liam knew when "it was his turn to play" which, according to his Aunt Rachael meant that he ultimately learnt that life is "not to be all about him and his wants and needs." A structured approach in which music is used as "a cue for facilitating responses, as a way to structure responses, as a reward, and as a way to structure attention to task" (Madsen, 1999, in Pasiali, 2018, p. 7) aligns with behavioural music therapy. However, the language Jodie uses to describe her work, in this context at least, does not include words familiar to behavioural approaches such as "problem behaviours," "treatment," "contingencies," or "reinforcing stimulus." While she describes using the structure of songs and musical elements to invite Liam's participation, she does not appear to adhere to a highly structured programme of repetitive activities with the aim of observing behavioural responses that can be readily replicated (Knight et al., 2018, p. 7). Instead, she followed his lead, and by celebrating his natural musicality and passion for singing she was able to open possibilities for him to develop relationships with others who share his interests and skills (Hilda).

References

Bakan, M. B. (2014). Ethnomusicological perspectives on autism, neurodiversity, and music therapy. *Voices: A world forum for music therapy, 14*(3). https://doi.org/10.15845/voices.v14i3.799

Bakan, M. B. (2015). "Don't go changing to try and please me": Combating essentialism through ethnography in the ethnomusicology of autism. *Ethnomusicology, 59*(1), 116–144. https://doi.org/10.5406/ethnomusicology.59.1.0116

Boucher, H., & Ryan, C. A. (2011). Performance stress and the very young musician. *Journal of Research in Music Education, 58*(4), 329–345. https://doi.org/10.1177/0022429410386965

Hillier, A., Greher, G., Poto, N., & Dougherty, M. (2011, March 1, 2012). Positive outcomes following participation in a music intervention for adolescents and young adults on the autism spectrum. *Psychology of Music, 40*(2), 201–215. https://doi.org/10.1177/0305735610386837

Knight, A., LaGasse, B., & Clair, A.-A. (Eds.). (2018). *Music therapy: An introduction to the profession.* American Music Therapy Association.

Nordoff, P., & Robbins, C. (2007). *Creative music therapy* (2nd ed.). John Day.

Pasiali, V. (2018). Approaches to music therapy. In A. Knight, B. LaGasse, & A. A. Clair (Eds.), *Music therapy: An introduction to the profession* (pp. 139–159). The American Music Therapy Association Inc.

Rojas-Bermúdez, J., & Moyano, G. (2020). Puppets as psychotherapeutic instrument: Intermediary and intra-intermediary object in psychodrama. *Journal of Applied Arts & Health, 11*(1), 135–141. https://doi.org/10.1386/jaah_00025_7

Rolvsjord, R. (2010). *Resource-oriented music therapy in mental health care.* Barcelona.

Sayre, D. N. (2020). What does it really mean to talk about "performative" activism? *All the World's a Stage.* https://www.danasayre.com/what-does-it-really-mean-to-talk-about-performative-activism/

Small, C. (1998). *Musicking: The meanings of performing and listening.* University Press of New England.

Tomchek, S. D., & Dunn, W. (2007). Sensory processing in children with and without autism: A comparative study using the short sensory profile. *The American Journal of Occupational Therapy, 61*(2), 190–200. https://doi.org/10.5014/ajot.61.2.190

7

AVA—"Lots of Reasons to Smile"

Background

Ava was an 8-year-old NZ European girl who was verbal, and her communication could be expressive when she was talking about topics of interest but rigid and repetitive when she was anxious. She attended a regular school. Ava has three siblings, one of whom was just six months old when music therapy sessions began. Bonding had been difficult because she found his crying hard to tolerate. Ava's other brothers and father played musical instruments, and she also had regular experiences of music at church.

Ava's music therapist, Pamela, was highly experienced in this context. She practiced in a child-centred way drawing on psychotherapeutic principles in this piece of work. Music therapy was typically provided weekly, for 10 months, and a total of 34 sessions took place. The sessions were held in Ava's family home, after school. The broad, initial, music therapy goals were to extend Ava's interpersonal skills and interest in music, increase her adaptable vocal self-expression, and decrease her feelings of anxiety when exposed to unexpected change.

D. Rickson, *Music Therapy with Autistic Children in Aotearoa, New Zealand*,
https://doi.org/10.1007/978-3-031-05233-0_7

The Music Therapy Process

In the first vignette Ava is excited because Pamela has brought an additional red guitar to the session. Even while Pamela is tuning it, Ava is eagerly leaning over it asking "Can I have it? I have a guitar just like my Daddy?" When Ava has the guitar on her lap Pamela introduces a song developed in the previous session, which involves improvising lyrics according to what Ava is playing or talking about. Pamela accompanies herself on her own guitar, while Ava holds "her" red guitar flat on her knees, plucking, strumming, and tapping intermittently, and interjecting with questions and observations about the guitar. She looks around and comments that there are three guitars in the room, and one is her daddy's. When the lyrics of the song include her observation, she smiles and imitates, adding the words "beautiful music." Towards the end of the activity, she calls her mum to take notice of what she is doing.

> Pamela surmised this was a significant moment because Ava had not wanted to share instruments, and now they were mutually engaged with the same type of instrument.

In the second description Pamela is focusing on a song, "M is for Music," which was originally improvised, but was becoming familiar through repetition over time. As Pamela sang it, she would leave a space at the end of each of the four phrases, thus inviting Ava to add the last word of each phrase. Ava now recognised the structure of the music and began anticipating her turn. In this example, at first Ava sang the word quietly while watching Pamela carefully. During the second playing of the song, Ava began to explore the harmonica she had in her hands and started to play, while Pamela accompanied her. Ava then noticed an underwater scene on the ocean drum, verbalising "Mr Crab." As Pamela began to sing about "Mr Crab," Ava's playing became more sustained. She looked at Pamela as she played and moved her body to the music.

> Pamela surmised this was an important moment because Ava had begun to use her voice and to breathe in new ways. She seemed more relaxed and was not using rigid speech or focusing on other people while she was immersed in this experience.

In the third description Ava does not want to play any instruments, including the ocean drum that she had enjoyed previously, declaring them "too loud". As she focused on eating her afternoon tea, Pamela found some paper and wrote the word "tui" on it. Ava was immediately interested in what she was doing, smiled when she read the word, and moved to sit next to Pamela on the sofa. Pamela asked, "What colour is the tui?" After a brief pause Ava replied "Bluey-black with white under its chin." Pamela continued to question her carefully about where the tui lives, and what it eats. Ava watched closely and repeated her words as Pamela wrote them down. She nodded and smiled when Pamela suggested they could write a song about other birds too. From pictures of native birds, she chose the fantail (piwakawaka) and the wood pigeon (kereru) before suggesting "[…] chickens?" She remained focused for a long time as they sang the song that emerged (see section "Ava's Song"). Pamela accompanied the song with her guitar, and Ava contributed the last line of each verse and the occasional last word of a phrase.

> Pamela noted that this was the first time that songwriting had been introduced, and Ava easily adapted to and accepted the new experience. She was relaxed and did not use any rigid speech patterns. This level of collaboration had not been observed before.

Pamela wrote that after the songwriting session described above, Ava had been enjoying singing vocal sounds, making "silly sound combinations" involving pitch and rhythm (vocables). Pamela had introduced "Love to Play Music," a song which encouraged Ava to contribute her vocables. In the fourth description Pamela reintroduced this song and Ava began to play her red "flute" (recorder). Her playing sometimes matched the rhythm of the music and in the vocables sections she imitated Pamela's sounds with her voice. Her vocalisations were strong and clear, and she matched pitch and rhythm sounds accurately and expressively, in a sustained manner.

> Pamela noted that Ava remained engaged and flexible, adapting to changing sounds, and was spontaneous, organised, and purposeful in her play, overall.

Commentators' Interpretations of Ava's Case

Commentators observed that in early music therapy sessions Ava appeared very chatty, excited, and somewhat distracted (Dana) and that her comments were observational in their nature (Freyer). However, in subsequent sessions significant improvements were noticed, and it became clear that music therapy would be an appropriate way to help Ava gain confidence in using her voice expressively (Ruella; Freyer).

> The video for story four was my favourite to watch, there was such good eye contact and genuine smiles and sense of fun between them. Ava's vocalisations were adaptable as well as being purposeful and responsive. She had the agency to choose how she wanted to express herself and did so in a fluid and fun way which shows she was relaxed enough to let go of some of her earlier more rigid ways of responding. (Freyer)

There was clear improvement in Ava's interpersonal skills (Freyer; Ruella). As she became increasingly relaxed (Hilda; Teacher) and confident (Freyer; Dana) she gave more eye contact (Freyer; Ruella) and her use of rigid speech decreased (Ruella). She demonstrated improved listening, attention, and concentration (Freyer; Ruella; Teacher) became more focused and engaged (Dana; Hilda; Ruella; Ava's grandmother), was able to participate in more interaction and musical collaboration while developing skills with turn taking (Freyer; Hilda; Ruella). Moreover, despite family reporting that sensory issues impacted on Ava's ability to manage daily life, they did not appear to impact significantly on her ability to engage in music therapy. Freyer noted for example:

> In some sessions when she became engaged with the task she was not distracted or bothered by noise that was coming from another room [...] it is possible with further interventions Ava could develop tools to distract herself from unpleasant auditory stimuli. (Freyer)

> The main development I observed from the four learning stories over the course of therapy was the increase in Ava's engagement. In the first learning story, her attention appeared to wane quickly, and she would focus on other things (e.g., who made the guitar). Changes were evident even by the second story, where she was able to re-engage much more readily. In the third and fourth learning stories, Ava seemed to be fully immersed in the activity and did not require any redirection. (Ruella)

On the other hand, while Mike could see from the learning stories that Ava had developed strongly in several areas, he was less convinced that she experienced a decrease in her anxiety. His caution was reinforced by Ava's grandmother who suggested the reduction in anxiety could be brief. However, they agreed that Pamela's careful planning to produce the red guitar, an instrument that was meaningful to Ava, contributed significantly to keeping her calm and engaged.

> As soon as Ava had the guitar in her hands her excitement level rose, and she became extremely fixated on holding it and working out how she could play it. Her Daddy's guitar sat behind the sofa in the room where the session was taking place and she began to compare the red guitar with that of her fathers. [...] As she strums the guitar, she keeps making comparisons between her guitar and that of her daddy's which seems to make her relax and makes it familiar to her, lowering anxiety. (Ava's grandmother)

However, in this example it was not just the object—the red guitar—that held Ava. Rather, as Ava's grandmother argued, Pamela worked hard to provide steady, consistent, gentle music which eventually contained Ava and enabled her to engage with the music, rather than just the instrument. The structure and repetition in Pamela's music generated "familiarity."

> Ava has referred to the similarities (between the guitars) many times (and) she constantly draws Pamela to these facts thus gaining a common ground between Pamela, Daddy, and herself. Her body is slightly stiff, and her focus becomes about the instrument and less about what Pamela is doing. She constantly interrupts about "who made the guitar, who made the guitar" [but] Pamela […] continues singing and strumming. I notice that she will not give up this questioning until Pamela manages to engage her focus on playing the guitar and singing. (Ava's grandmother)

> Ava relaxes more when she feels she is familiar with her surroundings. [As she] senses she's leading the music, and relaxes into having control over what's sung, she joins in more. This introduces another level of engagement – [when] Ava is introduced to new things normally she would have a meltdown. (Ava's grandmother)

Freyer also noted that the wind instruments used in music therapy potentially helped Ava manage her anxieties, because they encouraged mindful breathing which in turn can have a calming effect. She also argued that the mouth organ and flute could both be used in other settings to "help her cope with situations she feels stressed by" (Freyer). Similarly, Ava's teacher observed how the playing of musical instruments could both energise and relax.

> When playing the harmonica, Ava is sitting upright - arms up and elbows out and putting good energy into playing. While in full swing she moves her body into Pamela […] (and) when fully 'in the moment' she is relaxed. […] I certainly see the value of music therapy in helping children such as Ava (and all children) in reducing anxiety to reach calmness so they can connect with others by responding to and making music. From this, a possibility that the children may recognise the difference they feel from other experiences so they can reflect and develop self-awareness. (Teacher)

Commentators also highlighted the positive relationship Ava had with Pamela which supported her interest and motivation to engage. As Freyer observed, her enthusiasm and willingness to participate in all sessions, was a strong indication that she valued her time with Pamela. Interestingly commentators noted that predictability and familiarity were not only important features of the music, but of Pamela's presence as well.

> Ava is probably familiar with and feeling safe with Pamela who comes to the house regularly and does predictable things. Once they get to know and trust them, autistic children often enjoy the one-to-one attention of an empathetic adult as illustrated with this relationship. (Hilda)

Freyer summarised that Ava's case study demonstrates the potential of music therapy to support takiwātanga to improve interpersonal skills. The repetition of familiar musical patterns and routines allowed her to become more relaxed in her interactions (Freyer) and the "safe boundaries allowed her to let another person to enter her guarded world" (Ava's grandmother). Music gave her opportunities to explore, be creative, and to communicate with another person in a different medium (Ava's Teacher).

> (Ava's responsivity) clearly shows not only her enjoyment of what she hears, plays, sings and vocalises, but also a genuine interest in exploring what she can do with music. [...] (She) extends her imitation to spontaneously creating her own music to join in. I have only seen her do this during our folkdance lessons [...] when she physically linked hands to the shoulders of another child, unprompted, to join in a dance complete with rhythm, movement and big smiles. (Teacher)

> She began to use her voice more in the shared interaction, particularly when she could anticipate what was coming. She filled in gaps at the end of phrases, suggested lyrics for a song writing activity, and imitated vocables - matching rhythm and following pitch contours. (Ruella)

The medium of music enabled Ava to connect with Pamela, and to demonstrate the key competency of relating to others (Ava's Teacher). Further, the music therapy sessions were able to provide a special and personal experience for Ava and, as her mother noted, it can be difficult to create experiences that are just for her. Ava enjoyed sharing her achievements with her family.

> A number of times she encouraged us to listen to her. Her love language is words of encouragement, so she wanted assurance from us that we were proud of her. I think she also just really loved it that the afternoon was largely all about her which to be honest isn't often the case in a busy family. (Ava's mother)

Commentators argued that it was a "privilege to witness a small part of Ava's musical journey [...] her excitement and enthusiasm" (Dana); the story gave them "lots of reasons to smile" (Freyer) and it was "delightful to see Emma's confidence and sense of humour shine through as the sessions progressed" (Freyer); "lovely to see how she engaged in music therapy" (Ruella) and "wonderful to see her... interested, engaged and curious" (Ava's teacher). Ava's grandmother felt "happy to see Ava less vulnerable."

> In the first story it was lovely to see the connection she made to the guitar and her father and the genuine excitement she wanted to share with her mother. While she may seek her parents out for affirmation, especially when anxious, as an outside observer this also looked as if she was sharing her joy. I was also encouraged to hear her describe her feelings 'I was happy playing music' which shows the potential music therapy has to help her articulate her emotions. (Freyer)

Integration of Findings from Descriptions and Ava's Questionnaires

The findings from the questionnaires support the highly positive comments made about this case, with two exceptions. Ava's grandmother "somewhat disagreed" that Ava made progress towards her goals. As noted above she observed the temporary nature of Ava's calm periods, and therefore could not agree that there was a decrease in her feelings of anxiety. Ruella disagreed with the statement "the way Pamela facilitated this interaction was important." However, she was positive about Ava's developing interpersonal skills, and thought that music therapy could help Ava continue to gain vocal confidence saying, "It was personally very rewarding to see her using her voice so playfully in the final video, and to read about the way she contributed lyrics for the songwriting activity" (Ruella).

Ruella did note that one of the therapy goals was to "decrease anxiety when exposed to unexpected change" and, while acknowledging the importance of structure and predictability initially, wondered whether Pamela might have introduced more "surprise" in the music to challenge Ava in this area. She also noted that Ava called out to her mother for affirmation during sessions and wondered whether it might have been helpful to include family in the music making. However, none of this information points to dissatisfaction with the way Pamela facilitated the interaction, so I proffer two further explanations. Specifically, it is possible that (1) the meaning behind the statement is unclear, and/or (2) the answer was entered in error. The latter seems possible as a visual scan of the raw data shows that the previous question was unanswered which in turn suggests Ruella's process of completing the questionnaire may have been disrupted.

Music Therapist's Summary

As her anxiety reduced Ava was more able to tolerate loud sounds. She learnt to initiate and share ideas in music, to be expressive and creative. In her musical interactions she demonstrated the ability to take turns, imitate and initiate, and to remain engaged for extended periods. Through the physical act of playing wind instruments her breathing became more controlled, she was soothed and more relaxed. Over time she learnt to increase and vary her vocal expression (melodic and pitch range expanded; phrase length extended) and her music skills improved (she could match pitches and melodic phrases). Songs appeared to offer Ava a structure she could anticipate, and she was able to both contribute (in a song writing activity) and remember, lyrics. Her vocalisations and singing became more flexible, spontaneous, adaptable, and at times playful, and supported her developing relationship with me.

My Reflections on Ava's Case

Ava was demonstrating a genuine interest in exploring what she could do with music and desired to be a "musician" like other family members. However, despite her interest in music, her anxiety, and the demands of neurotypical musical cultures and social norms, restricted her opportunities to communicate and share music freely with others.

Pamela therefore created a range of musical opportunities for Ava to engage with. She trusted that the music, carefully presented in the moment and in response to Ava's presentation, would motivate her to respond and be rewarded for her efforts. She aimed to help Ava to extend her interpersonal skills and interest in music. However, the focus was not on "changing" Ava but on pooling child and therapist resources to maximise the potential for growth and development.

Pamela began her work with Ava using improvised play songs focusing on what Ava was interested in, with the aim of getting to know her and developing the therapeutic relationship through interactive play. She recognised the importance of "musically attuning to a child's emotional, physiological, creative, and playful qualities, even when the child has verbal skills," and of introducing play songs in dynamic ways to support children to regulate their arousal, attention, and emotions (Epstein et al., 2020, pp. 66–67). By taking time to come to know Ava first, Pamela was able to engage her in a meaningful, productive, collaborative music project (composing a song) which she could share with others. As Michael Bakan, an autistic ethnomusicologist explains,

> We will never go wrong by making it a priority to first listen closely, attentively, and with deep engagement, flexibility, and creativity to what Autistic people have to say and the ways they choose to play, whether

via verbal conversations, shared musical experiences, or any other means. (Bakan, 2014, no page number)

Pamela described practising in a child-centred way, but suggested she also employed psychotherapeutic principles in her work with Ava. Her description of the "M is for Music" activity, and the introduction of song frameworks which invited Ava to contribute vocables and to blow her "flute," seem well aligned with Creative Music Therapy which involves promoting learning and development within playful musical interaction. The purposeful introduction of the red guitar "just like daddy's," however, exemplifies Pamela's psychodynamic thinking, as the guitar seemed to serve as a transitional object, a physical object that safely connected Ava's love of music, family, and the music therapist. A psychodynamic approach considers ways children's behaviours, thoughts, and emotions are influenced by unconscious motivations; and "transitional objects [...] aid the process of keeping inner and outer reality 'separated yet interrelated'" (Winnicott, 2008, p. 3).

Ongoing engagement in music has the potential to enrich Ava's life. Nurturing her abilities to music with her family and others opens opportunities for connection, and joy. Drawing on the words of his musical collaborators, Bakan (2018) notes that music can create for takiwātanga "a welcome refuge from the interpersonal engagements of the outside world" (p. 45) or, alternatively, an essential bridge to social relationship.

Ava's Song

BIRDS IN THE FOREST

There are chickens at home, chickens at home
Making lots of noise
They are laying some eggs, laying some eggs
Yum that means scrambled eggs for tea

There's a tui at school, a tui at school
Bluey, black with white under its chin

Tui sings a song so beautiful, so beautiful
And loves to eat red berries

There are fantails in the forest, fantails in the forest
Tails spread out for us to see
Singing and flying through the trees, through the trees
And loves to eat orange berries

The kereru are wood pigeons, kereru are wood pigeons
Swooping as they fly
Hanging out in the forest, in the forest
And loves to eat brown berries

References

Bakan, M. B. (2014). Ethnomusicological perspectives on autism, neurodiversity, and music therapy. *Voices: A world forum for music therapy, 14*(3). https://doi.org/10.15845/voices.v14i3.799

Bakan, M. B. (2018). *Speaking for ourselves.* Oxford University Press. https://doi.org/10.1093/oso/9780190855833.003.0005

Epstein, S., Elefant, C., & Thompson, G. (2020). Music therapists' perceptions of the therapeutic potentials using music when working with verbal children on the autism spectrum: A qualitative analysis. *The Journal of Music Therapy, 57*(1), 66–90. https://doi.org/10.1093/jmt/thz017

Winnicott, D. W. (2008). *Playing and reality.* Routledge.

8

"NOAH"—Developing Friendships

Background

Noah was a 6-year-old boy who loved music, soccer, and maths and aspired to be a rock star. He struggled to concentrate on subjects he was not strong in, including reading and writing, especially when he was experiencing sensory overload. While he was able to communicate verbally, Noah did not understand neurotypical social norms and found it difficult to interact with his peers. As a result, he sometimes displayed emotional volatility. He reportedly needed support to develop fine motor skills. In addition to his diagnoses of ASD, Noah was labelled with Attention Deficit Hyperactivity Disorder (ADHD) and Sensory Processing Disorder (SPD).

His music therapist, Amy, was highly experienced in this context. She suggested she employed a humanistic approach which integrated strengths-based, music-centred, and child-centred principles of active participation and collaboration. She worked with Noah for 27 weekly sessions, in a small private room at his primary school. At school he was working to develop the key competencies (Ministry of Education, 2014) of "managing self" and "using language, symbols and text". The broad

D. Rickson, *Music Therapy with Autistic Children in Aotearoa, New Zealand*,
https://doi.org/10.1007/978-3-031-05233-0_8

initial goals for music therapy were to help Noah regulate his emotions, improve his concentration, and develop interpersonal skills, ultimately to support him to find ways to adapt to the world and the social needs placed on him. Noah initially attended individual sessions during which he would eventually gain the motivation and skills to work with a peer.

The Music Therapy Process

In the first description, from the second session they attended together, Noah and his peer are playing musical instruments. Noah explored the instruments freely, whereas his peer was more focussed on playing a familiar tune. While their music did not always connect, they were able to play alongside one another, and Noah was able to tolerate the sound of several instruments played simultaneously. Later in the session, Noah took a toy plane out of the drawer and wanted to play with it. Amy reminded him that this was music time, and this toy was for another time. He reacted by kicking some of the instruments, shouting and declining to participate further. His peer seemed surprised and said that she had enjoyed the music making earlier in the session, when "Noah was more kind."

> Amy surmised that Noah's preoccupation with the toy plane was a request for a break. She felt that it would be important to continue to work with peers, and to focus on increasing Noah's active participation and positive behaviour.

The second description is of the first session with a different peer, approximately one month later. When they arrived, the children were chatting excitedly about his recent birthday party. Amy encouraged them to unpack the instruments, curious to see how they would interact. As they spread out the percussion instruments on the mat, Noah began to introduce the instruments to his peer, describing them verbally and modelling their use. They began a spontaneous improvisation, which sounded a little chaotic as they became engrossed in exploring the drums, before moving to the tuned percussion. When Noah's attention waned, he tried to engage his peer in a game of musical statues but when this was rejected, he was able to continue improvising. He used quiet self-talk to direct his own play, particularly when he was rearranging the order of the chime bars and checking their letter names with Amy.

> Amy noted that Noah had showed renewed interest in playing a wide range of instruments, sustained attention, and willingness to postpone a preferred activity [musical statues], and that this seemed to be motivated by the presence of his peer. Peer work would therefore continue with a focus on developing shared music-making and continued positive behaviour.

The third description is of a session which took place approximately one month later, with a third peer. After unpacking the instruments and some initial free play, the children and music therapist agreed to play a "Copy Me" game, with self-chosen instruments. Noah had often preferred to take the lead, but in this session, he was willing to follow instructions and to wait for his turn to lead. When he took his turn as leader, he chose an instrument and allowed others to choose their own. He was tolerant when they produced loud sounds and was able to play his own music quietly, self-regulating while encouraging others to listen to him.

The fourth description is of the final session, which took place one week later. Noah took the lead in suggesting activities, but he looked at his peer each time to seek his agreement. His peer accepted his suggestions, and the two children negotiated instrument choices. Amy introduced a visual timer, to help them agree on and manage the amount of time each activity would run. In the first activity, "musical statues," a familiar children's game, the three moved or danced until the music stopped, then froze. Typically, anyone who moves in the silence would be "out" but, as there were only three people, Noah suggested they have two dancers and one musician, and that the dancer who was "out" would swap places with the musician. The musician was free to choose any available instrument. The trio played this game for about ten minutes, with several changes of role.

A period of drumming also took place in this session. There was a clear start to the activity, with Noah waiting until Amy and his peer signalled that they were ready. A period of energetic free improvisation followed. At times, the children's music became synchronised, and they occasionally glanced at one another. The improvisation ended with Noah lifting his arms up suddenly, surprising his peer in so doing, pausing, and verbally confirming the ending as his arms came down.

> Amy surmised, in both activities Noah was able to negotiate the rules, participate actively and cooperate well. His drumming was lively and loud, and he was able to tolerate more than one instrument being played simultaneously, something that he has previously identified as "too loud". After an initial gentle protest, he accepted that he was "out" in musical statues. His choice to play quietly seemed to sometimes be a means of avoiding being overwhelmed by sounds. She concluded that Noah experienced a positive ending to his music therapy programme, as he demonstrated his preference for partner work and a growing capacity to manage himself and cooperate well.

Commentator's Interpretations of Noah's Case

Noah demonstrated clear improvement in his ability to self-regulate, i.e., to calm when things did not go as he expected (Dana, Freyer, Mike, Noah's mother, Ruella, Vivian), to consider the perspectives of others and to negotiate with them (Freyer, Ruella), and to engage in meaningful social interaction (Dana, Freyer, Mike). He became more "at ease with himself" (Vivian). His learning and development were "very strong," particularly in terms of emotional regulation and social skills, "especially for takiwātanga who was six […] a tremendous amount seemed to happen in the sessions I saw" (Mike). Several commentators noticed improvement in Noah's ability to cope with the rules of games, to tolerate mistakes, to go "out" without becoming frustrated (Freyer, Ruella, Dana, Vivian), and to negotiate and cooperate with others (Noah's teacher and mother). "Turn taking, sharing, and listening skills were being put into practice" (Noah's teacher).

> (The later examples) of Noah negotiating his environment in the session to best meet his needs (provided) such a strong contrast to his initial way of responding when things did not go his way [...] and shows the success that this child led intervention has had for him. (Freyer)

> The final session was one that both boys clearly enjoyed. It showcased how far Noah had come with his social interaction and managing his frustrations. I loved watching the game of musical statues between the boys and the way Noah asked, 'when are you going to stop' rather than letting his frustration show in his body language. (Freyer)

Noah was able to focus on the music therapy activities, to respect his peers' personal space, and to tolerate their proximity (Dana). Those who knew him emphasised his increasing confidence and excitement about being familiar with "rules" and being able to share these with others (Noah's teacher and mother). His mother noted that Noah had tended to follow the instructions of certain dominant peers in the playground and therefore valued his increasing ability to take the lead in music therapy sessions. Dana observed a moment when Amy appeared to speak on Noah's behalf and suggested that it would be important for adults to take a step back to allow his relationships with his peers to develop and prosper.

> The initial individual sessions enabled Noah to first become familiar with the therapist and what was involved in the sessions, and this gave him confidence in sharing the sessions with peers. [...] He enjoyed involving peers in the music therapy sessions interacting positively with several partners in this setting. He began to progress from playing in parallel to playing together with his peers. (Ruella)

> (Music therapy) has given Noah some confidence to be able to show his friends how things work, in a non-pushy way, and you can hear (it) in his tone of voice. He does tend to try to tell people/kids what to do when he is feeling anxious about something. [...] I can see that he has learnt to observe and adjust what he is doing to include others in an invitational way rather than feeling the need to dominate and instruct others what they must do. While he does tend to be decisive and directional in these sessions, he doesn't control it the way I have heard and seen (before). (Noah's mother)

Dana felt that Noah would have benefited from more direct guidance regarding "rules of behaviour." However, while Hilda also highlighted Noah's need for rules, and his desire to make the music therapy games and activities more predictable and therefore less stressful and anxiety-inducing, she valued the child-led nature of the sessions. She commented on the way Noah liked to make up rules, expecting others to follow them, often with little explanation, and appreciated the ways these "typical autistic characteristics" were able to be accommodated in music therapy. She, like Noah's teacher, felt it was important for Noah to have opportunities to keep moving when he needed to. The incorporation of movement in sessions allowed Noah to expend his energy in a fun and engaging way. "(Music therapy) seems to encourage a range of positive social interactions using music and movement that are helpful for children like Noah, in everyday life" (Noah's Teacher).

Amy provided "a safe environment for Noah without the pressures of a classroom learning environment [...] She developed a positive relationship with Noah over the course of the year and he obviously felt very comfortable with her" (Noah's teacher). At music therapy he experienced being accepted, and "the realisation that he (would) not 'get into trouble' would have been reassuring for him and would have helped him build trust in his relationship with her" (Freyer).

> He had the agency to decide how he wanted to engage with music therapy. His opinions were taken into consideration and the sessions were adapted to accommodate his wishes and make them partner sessions. The

> decision to do this allowed Noah to develop his interactive communication as well as engage in reciprocal play with increasing confidence. (Freyer)

Having control within his environment gave Noah opportunities to develop appropriate strategies to regulate his sensory input and develop his self-regulation (Freyer, Ruella, and Vivian). The music therapy environment was observed to be a place where he could manage his own comfort levels (Ruella, Freyer), and "although the music room was quite a small space" (Freyer), Noah tolerated a variety of noises (Vivian), and noise levels (Freyer) without becoming overloaded. Noah's mother also noticed he had developed a better tolerance for noise and "for understanding that you cannot always tell people not to speak." She argued that while he still struggles when he is trying to concentrate and there is too much talking around him, or when there are sounds that can't be controlled, the sessions helped him build up a little tolerance especially to "discordant sound" (Noah's mother). Moreover, some children, perhaps many, are immediately "held" by music and can express their emotions musically without becoming overwhelmed. For example, when she read the first description of his music therapy, Noah's teacher wrote:

> I remember this day. Noah was not having the best day before going to music therapy [...] seeing him in this video I can tell that he is a bit emotional and frustrated and on the verge of becoming upset or angry; he looks quite tense. I am impressed that he managed to keep up the playing of instruments so long. (Noah's teacher)

Hilda and Freyer argued that towards the end of the therapy programme Noah and his peers "were managing themselves and using language—(just like) regular 6-year-olds" (Hilda). Freyer wrote that it was very telling that "the first time I viewed the musical statues clip I needed to go back and check which child was Noah as it was not immediately clear who of the two of them was takiwātanga" (Freyer). And, in her final statements, Noah's mother confirmed her perception not only of his developing sensory and emotional regulation and social skills but also transferability of skills to wider contexts.

> Since these sessions he has gone to birthday parties of both boys who participated (in music therapy) and had a great time. Each time he did have a moment where he got overwhelmed (once upset at not being able to do something well, and once because the noise level in the room of very loud kids was too much for him) but was able to take himself away from the others, give himself some time, […] and then return to participate when he felt ready. (Noah's mother)

> At neither party did he ask to leave early, and he definitely wanted to be there for his friends. This is an improvement in his understanding of others socially and willingness to try to work through feeling a little uncomfortable in order not to miss out on the rest of the fun and time with his friends. Before (his experience of) music therapy he would have probably insisted on leaving and that would be it, repeating himself until we left, he wouldn't care about how the other child might feel about him wanting to leave so quickly. The fact that he had friends who wanted to invite him to his birthday party this year was a big step from last year where he felt he had friends in his class but was never invited for playdates or to go to their birthdays even though quite a few came to his. The friendship seemed all one sided from his side and not theirs. So, he is now socially connecting at a better level […] His friends think of him and want to have him around. (Noah's mother)

Integration of Findings from Descriptions and Noah's Questionnaires

The eight commentators who reviewed Noah's case reinforced their positive statements when completing the Likert Questionnaires. All agreed that music therapy was important and meaningful for him and that he appeared to enjoy sessions overall. All also agreed that he was clearly developing skills that would support his learning, and most agreed that he was making timely progress towards appropriate specified goals. Commentators unanimously agreed that the music, as well as the way the therapist facilitated the sessions, was important in promoting his interactions.

Dana, however, "somewhat disagreed" that he made progress towards his specified goals and did not agree that progress towards these goals was timely. She also "somewhat disagreed" that he was positively engaged. She felt the sessions were a little chaotic because of "the high intensity of the drum playing and the excitement this created for Noah." She had a sense that Amy struggled to manage Noah's behaviour and argued that for sessions to be successful the therapist would need to establish clearer guidelines around what was acceptable and unacceptable behaviour. To do this, she recommended that there be more communication with parents and classroom staff who can provide important information regarding behaviour management strategies and give insight into the "real child." Interestingly, when Noah's mother responded to the case study, she expressed strong appreciation for the child-centred approach which gave him opportunities to "show his friends how things work, in a non-pushy way," that he learnt to "observe and adjust what he is doing to include others" without "controlling" them, and that he was able to develop genuine friendships as a result.

Music Therapist's Summary

Amy recorded: Music therapy has provided opportunities for Noah to relate to others (me, and his peers) in a different setting. Noah demonstrated improvements in self-management and cooperative play with me and a classmate. Therapy focused on his ability to attend, cooperate, negotiate, accept rules, and to remain calm. He has become more flexible in his shared play, more accepting of others' opinions, and better able to talk about experiences and perceptions, rather than reacting defensively or angrily. He is more able to manage his sensory processing issues—particularly his auditory sensitivity. The next step would be small group work.

My Reflections on Noah's Case

As Thompson and Elefant (2019) note, the diagnosis of ASD provides little information about the ways an individual may be impacted in daily life. While Noah was verbal, he still needed significant support in managing his emotions, and communicating and socialising with others (Thompson & Elefant, 2019).

Amy enabled Noah to engage in games of his choice (e.g., the game of "Musical Statues") by maintaining high levels of structure within sessions, supporting him to concentrate and to regulate his emotions, even to the extent of redirecting him when he tried to bring a toy plane into the music therapy session. She seemed to want to keep him focussed on the musical instruments, presumably to maximise opportunities for him to freely express himself within improvised music making. Noah had already had some sessions of individual music therapy prior to the three described here and had developed a positive relationship with Amy through improvised music making. So, it seems likely she was interested to see whether he could continue to improvise with peers, thus generalising his goal of "relating to others."

Many music therapists favour non-verbal, music-centred, relational approaches (Thompson & Elefant, 2019) because music making experiences are valued forms of human expression and connection and a unique means for therapeutic change (Aigen, 2014). However, Amy does not describe her role in the music making with Noah and his peers, as a music-centred music therapist would. It is possible that with the focus being on Noah's ability to negotiate and collaborate with peers, Amy has deliberately distanced herself from the musical interaction. The brief description of Noah's drum improvisation with his peer appears to reinforce her decision to allow the pair to play freely and independently, since it seems they valued the opportunity to work things out together and were able to express emotions safely. Being afforded agency to express anger and frustration, without rules, in a musical context can be highly valued.

> It's the fact that I'm allowed to bang on drums for a while—and (on) any instrument I want (as long as I don't break it or it's not meant to be

> banged)—without anybody telling me I'm supposed to do it this way, or I'm supposed to do it that way, or I'm supposed to put this there or that THERE, or I'm doing it wrong. (Bakan, 2014, no page number)

In contrast, Amy refers on at least two occasions to the need for Noah to develop the "positive behaviours" that might be anticipated in a school setting. The importance of differentiating the therapy process from educational processes is also highlighted in Dana's reaction to the "chaotic" nature of music therapy. The emergence of "order" over "chaos" is clearly desirable when music therapists are supporting tamariki takiwātanga to regulate their moods and manage their frustrations in ways that will enable them to interact successfully with others. However, as Oosthuizen (2019) suggests, a therapists' perception of chaos can significantly influence how this is approached. She argues that while chaos might be seen to hinder the therapy process and need to be avoided or controlled, it can also be viewed as a representation of participants' complex lives, and ways of constructing and expressing meaning, as they strive to make music with others (Oosthuizen, 2019). Oosthuizen goes on to suggest the goal of "emotional release" might be a more helpful term for music therapists than "emotional expression" because it allows for resistance and destructiveness. She also prefers "enhancing relationships" over the development of "healthy relationships" because it allows tamariki to participate actively in the complexity of human relationships that involve conflicts and challenges alongside connectedness. Thus, she argues, chaos can be conceptualised as a resource, especially when working with groups.

The music therapy process gave Noah opportunities to be himself while learning other ways of being with people that enabled him to develop genuine friendships. Amy provided structures (such as specifying the use of instruments; encouraging games with "rules"; and providing a visual timer) to encourage order within the sessions. As the commentators suggested, while it was important for Noah to be able to move and/or to play freely within each activity, the "rules" were helpful in reducing his anxiety. And, drawing on his experience of improvising with Amy, Noah was not only able to manage with less support from her but also to provide some supportive musical structures for his peers by, for example, (1) making a sudden physical gesture, lifting his arms up, and surprising his peer; (2) pausing; and (3) verbally confirming the ending of their improvisation.

Thompson and Elefant (2019) suggest that when working with verbal takiwātanga "it sometimes feels like musical interactions are secondary to verbal interactions, and the music therapist is working hard to find ways to engage the child in musical play" (p. 349). In Noah's case the hard work to engage Noah and his peers in musical play seemed to pay off, as he began to develop relational awareness and understanding through seeing and experiencing the reactions of others (Thompson & Elefant, 2019, p. 355) and to develop friendships beyond the therapy room.

References

Aigen, K. (2014). Music-centered dimensions of Nordoff-Robbins music therapy. *Music Therapy Perspectives, 32*(1), 18–29. https://doi.org/10.1093/mtp/miu006

Bakan, M. B. (2014). Ethnomusicological perspectives on autism, neurodiversity, and music therapy. *Voices: A world forum for music therapy, 14*(3). https://doi.org/10.15845/voices.v14i3.799

Ministry of Education. (2014). *Key competencies*. Te Kete Ipurangi, Ministry of Eudcation. Retrieved August 25, 2020, from https://nzcurriculum.tki.org.nz/Key-competencies

Oosthuizen, H. (2019). The potential of paradox: Chaos and order and interdependent resources within short-term music therapy groups with young offenders in South Africa. *Qualitative Inquiries in Music Therapy, 14*(1), 1–39.

Thompson, G. A., & Elefant, C. (2019). "But I want to talk to you!" Perspectives on music therapy practice with highly verbal children on the autism spectrum. *Nordic Journal of Music Therapy, 28*(4), 347–359. https://doi.org/10.1080/08098131.2019.1605616

9

"OLIVER"—As Busy as a Bee

Background

Oliver was a 7-year-old boy of Māori, Japanese, and Pakeha descent, who was homeschooled. He was described as lively, nimble, and entertaining; expressive in his body, often moving with delight, or with frustration: He had a bright intelligent personality, gentle caring nature, and a good sense of humour. He was constantly seeking information, seemed quick to absorb new knowledge, and used verbal communication.

Oliver's desire to seek new knowledge and his quick movements impacted both positively and negatively on his ability to focus and socially engage. He showed sensitivity to perceived approval or disapproval, and with positivity, he seemed to blossom. Yet he often appeared distressed, expressed frustration, was rough with objects, and moved away from people. Calm, comforting, small sounds, and the act of redirection, helped him to refocus and engage. Oliver often sought touch and particularly enjoyed being under a blanket. He preferred to be alongside rather than opposite people.

Oliver was exposed to music in his home—his mother was a dance teacher, and her new partner a musician. However, during the period of

D. Rickson, *Music Therapy with Autistic Children in Aotearoa, New Zealand*,
https://doi.org/10.1007/978-3-031-05233-0_9

the music therapy programme, Oliver had to manage significant family changes, in his parents' relationships, accommodation, and with his younger sister starting preschool, which were mitigated to a degree by his supportive extended family network.

His music therapist, Karen, was an "established therapist" in this context. Karen's approach was child-centred, and she employed a lot of imaginative play in her sessions. The music therapy took place in the lounge of Oliver's home, where Karen used a floor rug to define the therapeutic space. The goal of the music therapy was to support Oliver to develop his ability to regulate his emotions, i.e., to promote self-calming, and reduce anxiety and destructive behaviours.

The Music Therapy Process

In the first description, Oliver looked in the music bag, selected a castanet, and asked, "What is this?" He was sitting on his knees moving a little from side to side. He played with the castanet, snapped it together, and repeated the sound while bouncing his knees up and down on the carpet. Karen took another castanet and began singing a variation of La Cucaracha (The Cockroach, traditional Mexican folk song of unknown origin). She varied the tempo and pace, adding surprise to the song. Oliver found this very funny; he was smiling and giggling and copying her words and actions. He moved his whole body to the music sometimes getting up and moving away but maintaining eye contact while singing and moving. He was animated and excited as he and Karen added original lyrics, in dialogue form and with humour, to the song. After about 10 minutes, when he slowed in his vocalising and movement, Karen redirected him to the mat.

> Karen summarised that it seemed helpful to include both newness/surprise and simple repetitive songs that would enable Oliver to easily improvise new words.

The second description began with Oliver spilling the small percussion instruments out of the bag in a rough manner. He picked several up and threw them down again, ran around the mat, and when he returned, fell on his knees, intentionally, quite hard. During the greeting song, when the therapist asked, "how are you today?" he replied "Bad"—and threw an instrument. He ran to his mother who was sitting across the room and asked for something, using a whining tone. Mum redirected him to Karen who sat on the music mat, hunched up as if hiding something in her hand. As Oliver came close, she began to chant about bees in a hive using a quiet, slow, mysterious voice. Bringing each "hiding" finger out, she slowly circled each in front of him returning her hands together again and counting…1, 2, 3, 4, 5 until on "five" she brought out her hand and buzzed the "bees" around. Oliver was still, watching her hand.

She repeated the rhyme and observed that Oliver was still focussed on her hand, seeming to like the anticipation. Karen continued to repeat the rhyme, becoming increasingly animated as she varied her dynamics. Oliver began to use his hand as well, buzzing with her at the end of the verse. Then he hopped up from the mat and, using his whole body as if he was the bee buzzing around, began skipping, jumping, and running around the room. He returned and remained by therapist for the quiet part of the verse. However, as the chant progressed, he increasingly widened his movements until he was running out of the room, round the house, and re-entering by another door. He was laughing as he was running and buzzing around. Karen sang "Come back bees, come back to your hive." However, when she reduced the volume of her chant, he moved close to her and became quiet and attentive.

> Karen surmised Oliver was able to be calmed and engaged. The rhythm contained him, and the playful interaction was supporting their developing relationship.

On the day of the third description, Karen had brought two kazoos to the session. Oliver blew through them, persevering as he strived to make a sound. Karen demonstrated, and he began to hum into the kazoo, to enjoy the sounds he was making and to follow her lead as she made long sounds of varying loudness. Oliver sat close to her on the mat, giving eye contact. He began to "perform," improvising sounds and movement. He seemed to enjoy the attention as Karen and his mother watched him, his mother laughing as she filmed him. Oliver said "It sounds like bee" before running to the kitchen to fetch a pot and a comb. When he returned, he made the kazoo and comb vibrate on the pot as Karen improvised a song "There's a bee and it's buzzing all around …" A creative and excited dialogue ensued. Oliver got up from the mat, and "flew" around the room, moving his body to the rhythm and making bee sounds. Eventually, he said "Oh, no, we have to save the bee, and let it out." He walked slowly towards the window, opened it, shook his hand, and put the "bee" out of the window. He returned to the music mat looking proud.

> Karen surmised this was a rare moment of quiet focussed attention within creative play. She noted Oliver seemed to enjoy this activity and was fully involved in the story which suggested he might benefit from opportunities to perform.

The fourth description begins with Oliver very animated. He had jumped and climbed and was sitting on the back of the couch. Although he was looking at Karen, and humming, he was finding it difficult to remain in one place. However, when she reached for a blanket and held it up, Oliver moved quickly underneath it. Karen began to sing, beating rhythmically on the floor, "the ants came marching two by two […] to get out of the rain…" She gently tapped on Oliver's feet, then his back as if the rain was falling on him, maintaining a steady rhythm as he stayed hiding under the blanket. This was followed by another song about a baby bird, hiding in its shell and slowly coming out. Oliver seemed to like the anticipation of acting out the words where the "baby bird" slowly came out, flew around the room, and came back down to the nest. After two repetitions, he began to talk about a dog. "I like Milo, because he is kind to me." Karen talked with him about being kind and looking after animals. Oliver had some soft toys nearby; he lined them up and said, "I love my friends."

> Karen surmised when Oliver feels safe, he is more likely to be able to build relationships.

On the day of the fifth description Oliver seemed irritated and unhappy. He had been half-hearted about the music Karen played, pushed his sister, banged on the floor, and thrown an instrument. Karen brought her guitar, which was in a large hard case, to the centre of the mat and asked, "I wonder how this opens?" Oliver approached, found the latches, and lifted each one carefully, opening the case. As he began to pluck the strings Karen said "We need to tune the guitar. Can you please play each string very carefully, just once?" Oliver became engrossed in the sound and sight of the single strings vibrating. He was using his fine motor skills to pluck the strings and listening sensitively to the slight changes in tone as Karen turned the tuning pegs. Listening to his own playing, he was focussed on the present moment. When the guitar was tuned, Karen began to finger some chords, directing Oliver to strum the strings. He watched carefully as her fingers moved, and he played the strings in different ways, sometimes strumming all strings, sometimes plucking one or more.

> Karen noted that Oliver was clearly intrigued by the music, and how he was influencing the sounds. From the tuning to the more formal music making, it seemed as if they were working as a team on a meaningful task. Oliver was listening intently, focused, and relaxed. Karen noted that tuning the guitar seemed to engage his whole being, cognition, vision, and hearing; and he seemed content as he carefully plucked the strings. She surmised that this activity was meaningful and would support his learning.

The sixth description begins with Karen shaking the bag of percussion instruments to encourage Oliver to come back to the mat. She picked through the many small instruments, naming the songs he associated with each one. She asked him to choose three instruments and line them up in order of their next three music activities. He chose four—castanets, maracas, drumsticks, and egg shakers. With the egg shakers, Karen sang "Morningtown Ride" (Reynolds, 1957). Oliver had a shaker in each hand, was weighing them up, listening to the sounds, and keeping the beat. She extended the song, pretending the train was far away and quiet, then coming near and very loud, then modulating back to quiet. Oliver listened to this three times. As Karen was leaving this session Oliver said, "I love you." She replied, "I love you too, Oliver."

> Karen thought Oliver was very engaged with the rhythm, and that he seemed to enjoy listening to sounds fading away. She surmised that music therapy was continuing to provide learning opportunities for Oliver.

In the seventh description Karen arrives to find Oliver climbing on the bookcase, protesting, and ignoring his mother when she asked him not to climb. When Karen began their welcome song, asking how he was today…Oliver replied "bad!" and threw an instrument. The family was preparing to move and there was a large empty cardboard box near the music space. Oliver climbed inside and looked at his mother, as if he were challenging her. Karen said "I like boxes" as she began to improvise a song about being inside, where it is dark and safe. Oliver watched her before joining in the song, repeating her words. She rocked the box from side to side, gently at first, and then making bigger and bigger movements, before tipping the box on its side. Oliver crawled out onto the mat towards her, seeming sad and flat. He picked up the wooden frog instrument, and she sang "there's a little brown frog…." Oliver stroked the beater across the frog's back, which made a croaking sound. "The frog is hurt" he said. She continued singing, and added, "Let's look after the frog." Oliver cradled the frog in his hand, and was quiet and focussed, while she continued to sing. "Look after the frog" he said. "Yes, we will. I like the way you look after the frog" she replied.

Karen surmised music might help him understand and manage feelings.

Commentators' Interpretations of Oliver's Case

> The learning stories presented in this case study demonstrated three main things: Oliver becoming engaged in the music therapy sessions, focusing his attention, and calming through music therapy activities. These three things fit well with the stated goal, which was to "reduce distress and promote self-calming, so that he could learn, interact and play." (Ruella)

Mike argued that Oliver clearly demonstrated increased engagement within the sessions, as well as along the course of the therapy. Four commentators who did not know Oliver (Dana, Freyer, Mike, and Ruella) all drew attention to the positive therapeutic relationship that developed between Oliver and Karen, while Ruella noted that it was clear that Karen had formed a lovely relationship not only with Oliver but also his family.

> For the most part Oliver loved participating in music therapy and could hardly contain his excitement when the music therapist would arrive. He would willingly participate in the activities set out for him and loved taking a leading role in some sessions. (Dana)

> I loved the way Oliver developed his trust in Karen and the increased confidence he showed in their relationship to want discuss things that were important to him that were not directly related to activities in the sessions, such as his dog and stuffed animals. (Freyer)

Two of the commentators who did not know Oliver also drew attention to his spontaneous comment, "I love you" (in the sixth description), but in differing ways. Mike was "uncomfortable" with Karen's response. He reasoned that "children on the spectrum can be very bright (as Oliver appears to be) and we can have an abstract understanding of emotions [...] for a bright seven-year-old that could be challenging to process" (Mike). In contrast, Freyer was "very moved" by the event, especially since it occurred in a session in which Karen had been quite strict with him. Commentators suggested Oliver's case study highlights his empathy, which bodes well for his relationships with others. One of Freyer's "favourite moments was when Oliver put the 'bee' out of the window; it showcased how much empathy Oliver can feel for others as well as his capacity for imaginative play" (Freyer).

Oliver had several sensory challenges, and his anxiety and destructive behaviours had been identified as areas of concern. Music was used in engaging ways to connect with Oliver, support him regulate his emotions and behaviour and in turn to interact (Mike, Freyer, Ruella).

> I was struck by how motivated Oliver was by sensory input and how he would both seek it, for example by getting the pot to feel the vibrations of the kazoo and comb and remove himself from it by seeking security under his blanket. The kazoo could be an effective calming tool for Oliver as he responds to the sensation and sound of it, but also needs to control his breathing when using it which can have a similar regulatory effect as other breathing tools such as blowing bubbles [...] (Further) the music provided familiar patterns and repetitions that can be comforting to children with ASD. The repetition of songs and activities from earlier sessions appeared to help Oliver feel safe, especially under his blanket where he could shut out other sensory information and focus on the music and his responses to it. (Freyer)

On the other hand, Dana observed that Oliver struggled to stay on task for prolonged periods and had a sense that it was difficult for Karen to gauge his mood on any given day. While she agreed that music therapy gave Oliver the opportunity to release anxiety through musical expression, she felt that the implementation of a behaviour management plan would have increased potential for positive change. And yet, as Ruella observed, "(Oliver's) mother almost cancelled a session because he was having a 'bad' day, but the music therapy session helped him become calm."

> Oliver's mood was often unpredictable across the sessions and this showcased how music therapy was able to be adapted to help him redirect his energies when frustrated and help support him to engage in a positive way, often with a combination of music and imaginative play [...] The music and activities associated with it would often excite Oliver and by changing the tone and pace of the songs and their actions he was able to bring himself back from an excited state [...] He was able to be guided to calm down [...] and this was achieved by auditory input and physical items that helped promote his sense of safety and need for sensory support. (Freyer)

Integration of Findings from Descriptions and Oliver's Questionnaires

In this case qualitative feedback from commentators was rather brief, and findings from the questionnaires were mixed. For example, all seven commentators (six "other commentators" and Oliver's mother) "agreed" or "somewhat agreed" that the goals set for Oliver were appropriate and that he was developing skills that would help him learn. However, only three were able to completely agree that he was able to meet his goals and only two were able to completely agree that this happened in a timely manner. Freyer suggested a lack of progress would not be surprising given the significant changes that Oliver was managing over the period of the music therapy programme, whereas for Mike it seemed that the case study did not have the information he needed to make that judgement.

> The way the narrative was written, the learning and development was unclear. At times I felt like I was reading more about the therapist than I was about the child [...] Clear goals and links to the curriculum are extremely important for clarity of understanding whether an intervention has been of full assistance or not. (Mike)

> Change can cause escalated anxiety in many children, but this can be particularly heightened for children with ASD. As the changes taking place for Oliver were ongoing throughout the therapy including an unintended final session it was harder to see the progression for Oliver over the sessions. (Freyer)

Commentators were therefore also generally unsure about whether the music therapy interaction was meaningful and important for Oliver. Nevertheless, there was relatively strong agreement that he enjoyed music therapy overall, that he was positively engaged, and that the way Karen facilitated the interaction was important. Oliver was reportedly going through a particularly difficult period in his life, and the therapist was able to provide moments of positivity which would likely contribute to his developing resilience and overall well-being.

> It was special to read about (Oliver's) engagement during what was a time of upheaval in his life... this was a moving account of a young man who has so much potential. Karen accomplished some important breakthroughs with (him). (Freyer)

Music Therapist's Summary

Karen recorded: Oliver demonstrated improvement in his abilities to self-manage, particularly with emotion regulation. He learnt how to withdraw when overwhelmed, to self-calm, and return to social engagement; and accept direction from me. He was gradually more readily drawn into play, and he was able to offer joint attention for longer periods. He developed an ability to engage in creative spontaneous storytelling.

My Reflections on Oliver's Case

Karen focussed on engaging Oliver in imaginative play: using her body and hands to indicate she had a "secret", using her hands to create a hive while singing about bees, and in a subsequent session introducing a kazoo which could mimic the buzzing of bees. Oliver's imagination was fuelled, motivating him to continue the interaction (Oldfield & Franke, 2005). Being able to maintain a similar game over several sessions supported him to "link previous experiences and create a line that connects past, present, and future" (Epstein et al., 2020). This linkage seemed important, given the multiple changes he was experiencing in his life.

Even though his cognitive and language skills were relatively well-developed, Oliver continued to need support to develop self-regulation (Epstein et al., 2020; Greenspan & Wieder, 2006). Despite experiencing difficult circumstances and emotions, he was not only able to engage in music therapy sessions but also appeared to bring, and to begin to process, issues that were important to him. His desire to "save the bee, and let it out" and to "look after the frog," gave Karen openings to gently nurture and care for him during sessions in a range of ways. She describes inviting him under a blanket where he felt secure, singing about ants in the rain while gently and rhythmically tapping "raindrops" on his body; and later improvising a song about a baby bird coming out of its nest, to encourage Oliver to come out from under the blanket. Even when a child is not actively participating in music making, the addition of music in role play can result in them appearing less anxious and more in control of their emotions (Epstein et al., 2020; Thompson & Elefant, 2019).

Epstein et al. (2020) found that music therapists attune to children during musical games by varying dynamics, intonation, timbre, pulse, and pitch, and using vocal interventions such as vocal sound effects, decrescendos, and whispering to create anticipation or tension and to emotionally expand and enrich the children's play. When singing a song about a train, Karen used the volume of her voice to indicate its proximity, i.e., "pretending the train was far away and quiet, then coming near and very loud, then modulating back to quiet." Similarly, she attunes to Oliver's actions and adds vitality to his play by "using a quiet, slow, mysterious voice"; "becoming increasingly animated as she varied her dynamics"; and "reducing the volume of her chant until he moved close to her." When Oliver seemed "flat and sad," she imagined the wooden "frog" instrument he was holding was also sad and sang "Little Brown Frog" in such a way that Oliver was able to experience and demonstrate empathy for the frog.

> Musical games within the context of music therapy emphasise the relational value of mutually created and shared world of meaning between the therapist and the child. The child's verbal strengths are not simply acknowledged: they become the foundation for musical-play experiences that aim to expand their repertoire of social and relational experiences. (Thompson & Elefant, 2019, p. 347).

Music therapists working with children who are verbal, often improvise songs to create a musical narrative, or introduce familiar precomposed songs with themes that match the play ideas of the child (Epstein et al., 2020; Salomon-Gimmon & Elefant, 2019; Thompson, 2018). Verbal tamariki takiwātanga introduce imaginative stories and ideas into music therapy sessions more frequently than nonverbal children, but their play-narratives are often disorganised, nonlinear, and therefore difficult to understand (Epstein et al., 2020; Thompson & Elefant, 2019). Therefore, when verbal tamariki takiwātanga are involved in dramatic play or storytelling, "the music therapist has an important role to play in addressing more foundational qualities, such as supporting emotional, arousal and attention regulation, a sense of continuity, and vitality" (Epstein et al., 2020, p. 87).

From the brief descriptions of Oliver's sessions, it seems that ideas for the play came predominantly from Karen, who was able to provide the infrastructure and "platform for interaction that both therapist and child could access and therefore co-create a [...] coherent play narrative" (Epstein et al., 2020, p. 83). Thompson and Elefant (2019) argue that "developing the quality of play in the context of relational dynamics can be a relevant focus for children on the autism spectrum, even when they have substantial verbal language skills" (p. 354). This is reinforced by Oldfield's (2018) suggestion that music making and drama "are so strongly linked that it is difficult to separate the two [...] Both music therapists and drama therapists are primarily interested in the quality of the communication and dialogue that occurs through the combination of music and drama" (p. 126).

After Oliver listened to the train song several times he was relaxed and moved enough to tell Karen he loved her. Mike was concerned with Karen's response that she loved Oliver too, arguing that tamariki takiwātanga can have an abstract understanding of emotions and that the exchange might be hard for him to process. Yet Freyer was "very moved" by the event. These diverse responses to the exchange are not surprising since the notion of love remains controversial within the psychological therapies. Many practitioners embrace the word as an important factor in the therapeutic relationship, while others are cautious or even see it as taboo (Charura & Paul, 2015).

Charura and Paul (2015) suggest love in the therapeutic relationship is a "dynamic, living energy which can be safely experienced because it is therapeutically boundaried [...] a non-possessive love, compassionate love, openness to work with the other as they are, as well as the potential of what they could be" (p. 7). Mike's concern that Oliver might not be able to process the message of love is perhaps mitigated if we accept that love in the therapeutic relationship is not just about tender and positive feelings, including empathy, warmth, and acceptance but also about the struggle to connect (Charura & Paul, 2015). More about therapeutic boundaries is included in Chapter "The Nature of Music Therapy with Tamariki Takiwātanga in New Zealand (Aotearoa)."

References

Charura, D., & Paul, S. (2015). What has love to do with it? In D. Charura & S. Paul (Eds.), *Love and therapy: In relationship* (1st ed.). Routledge. https://doi.org/10.4324/9780429476907

Epstein, S., Elefant, C., & Thompson, G. (2020). Music therapists' perceptions of the therapeutic potentials using music when working with verbal children on the autism spectrum: A qualitative analysis. *The Journal of Music Therapy, 57*(1), 66–90. https://doi.org/10.1093/jmt/thz017

Greenspan, S. I., & Wieder, S. (2006). *Engaging autism: The floortime approach to helping children relate*. Da Capo Press.

Oldfield, A. (2018). Humour, play, movement and kazoos: Drama in music therapy with children and families. In A. Oldfield & M. Carr (Eds.), *Collaborations within and between dramatherapy and music therapy* (pp. 113–128). Jessica Kingsley Publishers.

Oldfield, A., & Franke, C. (2005). Improvised songs and stories in music therapy diagnostic assessments at a unit for child and family psychiatry: A music therapist's and a psychotherapist's perspective. In F. A. Baker & T. Wigram (Eds.), *Songwriting: Methods, techniques and clinical applications for music therapy clinicians, educators and students* (pp. 24–44). Jessica Kinsley.

Reynolds, M. (1957). Morningtown ride. In *Hide & seekers* [1964 Album]. W&G Records.

Salomon-Gimmon, M., & Elefant, C. (2019). Development of vocal communication in children with autism spectrum disorder during improvisational music therapy. *Nordic Journal of Music Therapy, 28*(3), 174–192. https://doi.org/10.1080/08098131.2018.1529698

Thompson, G. A. (2018). Dramatic role play within improvisational music therapy: Joey's story. In A. Oldfield & M. Carr (Eds.), *Collaborations within and between dramatherapy and music therapy* (pp. 31–51). Jessica Kingsley Publishers.

Thompson, G. A., & Elefant, C. (2019). "But I want to talk to you!" Perspectives on music therapy practice with highly verbal children on the autism spectrum. *Nordic Journal of Music Therapy, 28*(4), 347–359. https://doi.org/10.1080/08098131.2019.1605616

10

"JAMES"—"Seeing This Made Me Smile"

Background

James was a 6-year-old New Zealand European boy, who was interested in music and dance, Lego, Star Wars, and animals. He was able to communicate verbally but would sometimes become mute when anxious. James began taking medication for hyperactivity towards the end of his programme of therapy, which appeared to significantly increase his capacity to participate.

James' music therapist, Mary, was highly experienced. Twenty-three sessions, typically weekly, took place in Mary's studio. Sessions closed when James indicated he wanted to finish, at a time which also coincided with changes in family circumstances. James gave feedback about the sessions at the beginning and at the end of each session, on formal evaluation forms (not included with the case study), and his mother attended two formal review meetings to discuss goals and evaluate the programme. The initial music therapy goal was to support James' confidence and reduce his anxiety, and in turn to develop his communication, self-expression, and play.

D. Rickson, *Music Therapy with Autistic Children in Aotearoa, New Zealand*, https://doi.org/10.1007/978-3-031-05233-0_10

The Music Therapy Process

In the first vignette James is seated at the piano, playing a few notes quietly, and glancing at Mary for cues. When she asks, "How do you want to say hello?," he begins to play a short musical phrase on the upper registers of the piano using the white keys. She responds with an answering phrase on the lower register, and they begin a playful and light-hearted duet. James looks at Mary frequently as they play. When she introduces short, detached notes, he immediately imitates this new style of playing. He then takes the lead and initiates several changes in the music by introducing the black keys and exploring the whole keyboard, sliding up and down the notes. The music becomes loud and energetic before coming to an end. Following this James says his first words of the session… "Done… Done… Done…" Mary replies, "All done on the piano" and they move on to something else.

In the second example James is energetic. He grabs a pair of drumsticks and begins to play freely on the drum kit in a loud and explosive manner. Mary joins him immediately from the piano, playing the tune of their Hello Song. He looks briefly at her and smiles. James' playing is initially self-directed. He explores the different instruments within the kit, and Mary is providing musical structure in the form of clear steady rhythmic pulse and a familiar melodic line. James is still not looking at her, but his playing eventually becomes more organised and structured. They share a musical pulse and begin taking turns to lead and follow each other, connected in the music. The music remains lively as they segue briefly to another familiar theme before returning to the Hello Song. When Mary plays two repeated dominant chords James seems to recognise a potential ending. He closes with a cymbal crash, while Mary embellishes the music with a glissando (sliding up and down the piano keys). They are synchronised in their actions, sounds, and emotional states as they end together with a flourish, smiling at each other. There is a brief pause before Mary declares "That's awesome for a Hello Song."

The third description begins with both Mary and James standing at the drum kit for the "Hello Song." James counts them in and plays rhythmically with Mary for a few bars. Mary begins to chant and sing, eventually incorporating "Let's sing hello to James…" into her song.

James spontaneously replies with "Let's sing hello to Mary," looking at her as he does so. She begins to improvise on the words "Hello to James" and he responds, "Hello to Mary." They play, mirroring each other's actions, and matching the inflections and affective quality in each other's voices. After a while, when Mary drops the volume to sing and play softly, James initiates an ending to the song. But not before he brings the volume back up and leads them to an almost perfectly timed flourished ending.

> Mary noted that James was demonstrating more confidence, through his spontaneous use of voice and increasingly complex music making.

In the final description Mary was playing the guitar. James had chosen the hand drum and was sitting on the piano stool with Mary in front of him, on the floor. When she asked him what they should sing, he started to play a rhythmic sequence, which sounded like "If you're Happy and You Know It." As she began to sing this song, he quickly shook his head. They took a moment to think about what they might sing. James suggested "about my cat." Mary provided a rhythmic and melodic structure, and James offered spontaneous ideas for the lyrics: "They are so cute," "Cats are so cute." When Mary sang, "What colour is your cat?" he replied, "Black and white and grey… and they are so cuddly." James sang comfortably with her, simultaneously and alternately, and they ended the song singing the last lyric together.

Commentators' Interpretations of James' Case

Most commentators who didn't know James was impressed with the immediate connection that was created between James and Mary. They suggested that trust was established quickly (Vivian, Freyer) and that the "attunement " and "synchronisation" that occurred as part of the musical relationship contributed significantly to the establishment of rapport (Dana, Ruella, Freyer). James' grandmother, however, felt that the primary factor in the developing relationship was time spent together. She argued that although James seemed to develop confidence and was able to speak more, this "had little to do with the music and more to do with the time spent with Mary" (James' grandmother). In contrast, others were aware of significant non-verbal *and* musical communication (Vivian, Freyer, Ruella), his smiles and other indications of fun and enjoyment (Vivian, Freyer, Dana), and his ease and willingness to experiment with the instruments (Vivian).

> The medium of music allowed him to have a safe interactive form of communication where he was able to influence the direction it took without the pressure of verbal social cues [...] I loved seeing the way he mirrored Mary's actions and words [...] it must have been very rewarding for her to feel such synchronicity between them. (Freyer)

Commentators who did not know James noticed that he initially seemed to "flit from one instrument to the next" and that he was "losing interest quite quickly if the momentum wasn't kept up" (Dana). However, from the second clip his ability to "tune in," and to keep the beat and rhythm was evident; and in the third and fourth examples, he was demonstrating "increasing levels of comfort and confidence" and had begun to use his voice (Vivian, Freyer). He was self-directed and motivated (Vivian, Hilda) and showed sustained engagement (Vivian). Ruella noticed once he attuned to Mary, he began to play together with her, listening and responding. His playing was more organised, and he seemed to settle and become more regulated through the course of playing music together.

Commentators also highlighted James' developing spontaneity, creativity, and leadership skills (Dana, Freyer, Mike), and "his increasing social engagement, which for someone on the spectrum at six years of age, was a strong social development" (Mike). Freyer noted the strong sense of accomplishment James seemed to show as he and Mary created their "genuinely interactive duet." It was therefore evident that he made progress towards the goals of developing confidence and reducing his anxiety (Hilda, Freyer, Mike, Vivian, Ruella) as well as communication, including increase in verbal language (Freyer, Mike) and play (Hilda, Ruella).

> Overall, this case study showed an anxious young man gain confidence and self-expression. Over the course of the therapy James develops from being verbally reticent to willingly engaging in interactive communication through music. He was clearly regulating his actions in response to his therapist's musical cues. (Freyer)

> Over time, he (remains) playful and seems to gain confidence, particularly in his use of voice. This culminates in the final learning story where he is comfortable enough to initiate a song improvisation about his cat [...] providing the lyrics for the song. (Ruella)

On the other hand, Hilda observed that, like many autistic children, James' use of verbal language seemed to diminish under stress (Hilda). She and James' family friend both agreed that James seemed less anxious in the music therapy environment but questioned whether this could be sustained in other settings.

> It is hard to tell from these short videos whether music therapy was beneficial in helping reduce James's anxiety. The fact that he got to the stage where he didn't want it anymore indicates that his interest in this had passed. (However) regardless of the end results, James being exposed to new experiences like this is a good thing." (James' Family Friend)

> I don't know whether this transferred to his life outside the sessions, or whether it was sustained afterwards. But it seemed that the well-focused, hard work of the music therapist, for a few months, helped a little autistic boy to be less anxious and feel safe using new skills to express himself. It is so nice to see an autistic child smiling and enjoying what they are doing." (Hilda)

Similarly, while Dana made many positive comments about the music therapy process, she seemed less impressed with James' engagement during sessions and his progress overall. She observed that when he began therapy, he already appeared to be a young man who knew what he wanted and could make his own decisions. She agreed that James appeared to be enjoying music therapy, had developed good rapport with Mary, and "for the most part was able to remain in sync with her," and suggested that an improvised approach which provided opportunities for James to explore the instruments and create simple tunes seemed somewhat helpful.

Dana also noticed that James' engagement increased over time, as more structure was introduced into the music therapy sessions. However, she argued that his short attention span and tendency to "flit from one instrument to the next" could be addressed through a variety of structured activities which had the same learning focus. Moreover, she suggested that Mary's "constant questioning regarding what shall we do next" was not helpful and that she might need to demonstrate more enthusiasm, to counter James' potential boredom. Her observations were somewhat reinforced by statements from family members who suggested that while James seemed to have establish a positive relationship with Mary, he was not always enthusiastic about attending music therapy.

> (If James) doesn't want to do something he won't do it and he tires of things quickly. So, for him to stay in the room with Mary told me a lot. He certainly had his off days where he cut the sessions short or had to be bribed or encouraged to do it but overall, he enjoyed it. (James' mother)

> Over time he got more relaxed with Mary as he normally does. James started off exploring the different instruments and he seemed to enjoy this kind of exploration. He was very happy playing and singing at first but after a while he started complaining he didn't want to go anymore as it was boring. (James' grandmother)

In contrast Freyer believed James was aware that he had "the agency to express his opinion and (the understanding) that it will be listened to."

> I felt proud that James felt safe enough with his therapist that he could reject her suggestion and see that he had a voice that would be heard. I was pleased to see his therapist was willing to make great use of pause and wait for a response from James. All too often people rush in to speak for

> people with ASD instead of waiting for them to process their thinking and express themselves. (Freyer)

Integration of Findings from Descriptions and James' Questionnaires

The results from the Likert questionnaires confirm the commentators' considerably diverse responses to this case. Five of the six expert commentators who did not know James were positive about all aspects of his music therapy, while Dana and some family members expressed considerable doubts.

Firstly, all commentators agreed that the stated goals seemed appropriate for James, and that music was important in these interactions. However, while family members generally agreed that the way Mary facilitated the sessions was important, and that James was positively engaged, and enjoying the music therapy sessions, they were less certain whether he was developing skills that would help him learn, about how important and meaningful music therapy was for him overall, and whether he was making progress towards his goals. Dana expressed doubts about the approach used, suggesting that a more highly structured programme of activities might have served James better, and while family members noted that James gained some positive benefits from the music therapy programme, they also conveyed that overall, they did not feel it went well for him.

On the other hand, there are contradictory statements in the descriptive data suggesting family members were unclear about the music therapy process and outcomes. For example, his aunt claims that music therapy has not helped James, yet notes the process was able to "break the ice … and bring him out of his shell to be able to give it a go." Similarly, James's mum suggests she didn't notice any changes in him yet goes on to say she was impressed by his ability to stay on task during sessions.

> To be honest I didn't notice any changes in James. From watching the videos, I see Mary is teaching him a lot, such as following a pattern, focusing on one thing at a time, slowing down and participating and so

> forth. Normally he is all over the place so to follow Mary's lead for half an hour was impressive to see and shows just how much he was enjoying it. (James' mother)

Perhaps those who knew James were commenting on his ability to manage in wider contexts, whereas the commentators who didn't know him could only comment on progress indicated in the case study data. It seems family members' hopes, and expectations may have been high, particularly regarding generalisability. For example, James's aunt alluded to music therapy "working well for others," and his grandmother said:

> I was hoping it would give James great enjoyment and (he would) become more relaxed and calmer in general, however it didn't calm him, and he was the same right through. He is now on Ritalin which has calmed him down so much more as well as able to concentrate more. I feel this therapy didn't work in the way I had hoped for James. I am glad he got to relax and speak more to Mary though. (James' grandmother)

Like James' grandmother, other family members, tended to attribute positive change to the introduction of medication rather than the music therapy. In contrast, those who didn't know James suggested that medication gave him more opportunity to engage with the therapy which in turn influenced his development. For example, three of the commentators included relatively detailed descriptions of how musical interaction supported the developing therapeutic relationship, reduced James's anxiety, and increased his ability to attend. Freyer argued that this occurred "irrespective of medication changes" (Freyer) while Mike wrote "I still think the music therapy intervention has been extremely helpful."

Commentators agreed that Mary had developed a good rapport with James, and this was important. Some, including his mother, described experiencing their own warm feelings while observing the work including "it is so nice to see an autistic child smiling and enjoying what they are doing" (Hilda); "I'm delighted to see James' increased sense of confidence and his use of expressive language" (Mike); "it feels like a really lovely way for him to interact and naturally support his communication, both verbally and non-verbally" (Ruella); and "to see him smiling and enjoying himself without a digital device was really good" (James' Family Friend).

> James is in general a difficult child to bring up. He not only has ASD but Developmental Dyspraxia, high anxiety and ADHD. He is now on Ritalin which has been a big help [...] But seeing my son in the videos made me smile... He enjoyed it, he loved Mary, so as his mum that to me is the main thing I wanted for him. (James' mother)

Music Therapist's Summary

> In music therapy sessions James worked with intention and was creative and joyful in his self-expression. As his anxiety reduced, he became more confident, and creative. James would benefit from involvement in group music therapy, as well as other music activities, in future.

My Reflections on James' Case

James' music therapy goals, to increase confidence and reduce anxiety, and in turn to develop communication, self-expression, and play, were not expressed specifically in musical terms. However, Mary's account of James' music therapy process focusses on their musical interactions and the quality of James' musical expressions, and there seemed to be an understanding that increased *musical* confidence, communication, and self-expression would be considered primary outcomes. And so, while Mary did not "label" her approach at all, it seems clear that it is not only child-centred but also aligns with music-centred music therapy. In music-centred music therapy, children are supported to experience and express themselves in music, and their process is described in musical terms, because musical experience and expression are the goals of therapy (Aigen, 2014). Goals are achieved *within* the music making, and the clinical significance of the work is determined by the quality of the child's musical engagement. Behavioural outcomes become secondary (Aigen, 2014).

In the first vignette James is playing tentatively but, as Mary joins him, he becomes energised and fully engaged, varying his phrasing, staccato, pitch, and dynamics, and expressing himself until he is seemingly emotionally replete, perhaps satisfied, and relieved, but certainly "done." In second and third vignettes, James is more involved from the beginning. He seems stronger, more able to musically assert himself. In the second vignette, for example, he begins loudly and energetically, releasing an "explosion" of emotion. In the beginning he needs the strength of the piano and drumkit to express himself but is eventually able to use his voice—a more personal instrument—and becomes relaxed enough to use it in a conversational way, in the music. With Mary's musical support in the form of steady rhythmic pulse and familiar melodic line, he was able to engage in musical dialogue before ending with a "flourish." Interestingly, while flourish might be defined in musical terms as an ornamental embellishment, it is also a concept employed by positive psychology (Seligman, 2011) to encapsulate happiness and well-being. The third example demonstrates that James is more readily able to engage in a steady musical dialogue, which was articulated calmly and confidently.

When making music with children, music therapists can sense how genuinely motivated and engaged they are. Mary has demonstrated that careful description of the musicking, not only of what happened but also what it felt like, can also highlight children's developing emotional and communication skills. Importantly, it seems that many of the commentators, who might not understand musical terms, were also able to get a strong sense of the quality of James' musical engagement from the descriptions, and the video examples. Apart from Dana, those who didn't know James suggested that trust was established quickly and were aware that the "attunement" and "synchronisation" that occurred as part of the musical relationship contributed significantly to the establishment of rapport. The work appeared to "resonate" with them.

On the other hand, Mary's crafting of the music and James' motivation to be involved, led Dana to suggest that he was doing ok throughout and therefore hadn't made much progress. She, and James' grandmother, judged the success of the programmes by his behaviours surrounding the musicking, which included his occasional reluctance to attend, and relatively low level of impetus. From a music-centred perspective, however, the point of the therapy would be for James to experience the benefits inherent in musical experiences. Then, as he increasingly benefitted from opportunities for musical expression, his ability to manage himself in non-musical interactions might also improve. Some commentators recognised this, valuing the immediate connection and non-verbal communication that Mary and James established, and his enjoyment of musicking.

Those who knew James also argued that positive change could be attributed at least in part to the time he spent with Mary and to the medication that was introduced during the music therapy programme. This is of course very likely. As it is with many forms of therapy, extricating factors that contribute to music therapy outcomes can be difficult. Regarding "time spent," for example, it is well-known that "common factors such as empathy, warmth and the therapeutic relationship [...] correlate more highly with client outcome than specialised treatment interventions" (Lambert & Barley, 2001, p. 357). However, rather than specifically arguing that music therapy was the catalyst for James' development, the case study demonstrates how musicking supported his ability to experience and express himself differently.

Mary reported that James gave formal feedback at the beginning and end of each session, but his input is not highlighted in the case study. This is disappointing from two perspectives. Firstly, it would have been interesting to hear his voice, to directly understand how he experienced the sessions. Secondly, while Mary's descriptions provide very clear evidence of their musical collaborations, the potential benefits of James' broader participation in their music therapy programme should not be ignored. There can be significant advantages for all parties when takiwātanga are invited to share their experiences of music therapy (Jeong & Darroch, 2021). When children are encouraged to think for themselves, share ideas, and make decisions, they develop an awareness of their abilities, an increased sense of agency, and are better understood by others.

References

Aigen, K. (2014). Music-centered dimensions of Nordoff-Robbins music therapy. Music Therapy Perspectives, 32(1), 18–29. https://doi.org/10.1093/mtp/miu006

Jeong, A. A. Y., & Darroch, B. (2021). Using letter boards in client-centred music therapy: "Autistics can teach if some are ready to listen". *New Zealand Journal of Music Therapy, 19*, 34–53.

Lambert, M. J., & Barley, D. E. (2001). Research summary on the therapeutic relationship and psychotherapy outcome. *Psychotherapy Theory Research & Practice, 38*(4), 357–361. https://doi.org/10.1037/0033-3204.38.4.357

Seligman, M. E. P. (2011). *Flourish: A visionary new understanding of happiness and well-being*. Free Press.

11

"EMMA"—"Takiwātanga Communicate in Many Ways"

Background

Emma was a 10-year-old girl of New Zealand European ethnicity. She was described as a cheerful girl who has a sense of fun. She loves music, especially from Disney movies, and dancing. Emma was enrolled in a special school but was located at a satellite class, which enabled her to get the specialist teaching she needed in a regular school environment. Her team included Occupational and Speech and Language Therapists.

Emma was non-verbal but was successfully using a Speech Generating Device (SGD) for communication, which enabled her to request preferred items from adults. She reportedly had good receptive language and could follow simple instructions. Emma experienced sensory differences which resulted in her mouthing, putting her fingers in her ears, and running and flapping to regulate herself. She also experienced challenges with body awareness and balance and had a short attention span.

Her music therapist, Lisa, was a beginning therapist in this context. She employed a child-centred approach, encouraging active music making and spontaneous play to promote autonomy and growth. Music was predominantly improvised, but structure was employed to

D. Rickson, *Music Therapy with Autistic Children in Aotearoa, New Zealand*, https://doi.org/10.1007/978-3-031-05233-0_11

help Emma to understand what was going to happen during music therapy sessions. Routine transitional activities such as greetings and farewell songs were included to provide security.

Music therapy was provided approximately weekly. Thirty-nine individual sessions took place in a small classroom away from other children, where Emma felt secure. The initial music therapy goal, drawn from the Key Competencies, was "Relating to Others." Early sessions therefore included classmates, but later Emma's team agreed that individual music therapy "to increase and develop interpersonal communication and interaction in a one-to-one relationship" would be likely to be beneficial.

The Music Therapy Process

At the beginning of the first example Emma was quiet and appeared shy. She was sitting away from Lisa; eyes averted, physically and emotionally distant, and reluctant to become involved. Lisa tried to engage her in simple rhythm and body percussion activities by improvising simple songs describing what Emma was doing. Emma seemed to be listening but continued to put things in her mouth. Eventually she stood and moved closer to Lisa, making eye contact, and smiling. She began to explore the instruments that were laid out in the music case by mouthing them. As she held a shaker egg, Lisa modelled movement for her while singing and emphasising "shake the eggs UPPPP!" and (pause) "shake the eggs DOWNNN!" Emma was happy to stand still and experience the feel, colour, and taste of the shaker egg. However, when Lisa introduced a Disney tune, she came closer, quietly, maintaining eye contact, picked up a beater, and began to tap the bongo drums. At the end of the session when Lisa asked, "How does that make you feel—can you show me on your device?" Emma used her communication device to answer, "sad."

Lisa surmised that Emma was engaged in a lot of solitary play and there did not seem to be any emotional connection between them. Moving forward, Lisa would aim to support Emma with her social interaction and spontaneous use of language.

The second description is from a session which took place three months later. The primary focus for sessions had been refined, and the aim was to sustain Emma's interaction.

Lisa looked at Emma, inviting her to come and engage with her, while playing a sequence of major chords on the keyboard. Emma walked purposefully over to the keyboard indicating interest. She struck keys in the upper register in a decisive movement, playing loudly in response to the invitation. Both Lisa and Emma were standing, and as Emma began to make exaggerated, fast-paced movements, Lisa matched with similar energy and vitality in her body movements. Emma returned to the keyboard and struck it, producing single notes and clusters of sound, and as Lisa matched her a playful dialogue emerged. At one point during the improvisation Emma briefly took Lisa's hands to direct her playing, and at another she accidentally struck the rhythm function on the keyboard activating a rock beat which provided rhythmic ground for the improvisation. Emma reintroduced her "dance," and Lisa sang, matching and extending Emma's musical ideas. Emma was watching and listening, leading the dialogue with her musical responses, movement, and gestures. Emma then took Lisa's hands and placed them around her (Emma's) head, all the while giving direct eye contact. Later she took Lisa's hands and indicated she should clap them together, before striking the keyboard to create a new musical shape. At the end of the session when Emma is asked "How did that make you feel?" she selected "Crazy."

Lisa surmised that goals to extend social skills, encourage emotional expression and increase levels of sustained active participation were well met in this session. She recognised that the keyboard was motivating for Emma and suggested it could be used more regularly to develop her independence. She would continue to focus on developing Emma's independence, but also supporting her to sustain interaction and to transition from one activity to the next.

In the next example, Emma independently selected a green shaker and pink tambourine with a strawberry picture on it, from the music case. With her finger in her ear, she acknowledged Lisa by looking at her, before beginning to move rhythmically in anticipation of their musical interaction. She seemed fully engaged, listening to, and making sustained eye contact with Lisa. When Lisa asked, "are you ready to sing hello?" Emma tapped her shaker against the guitar. She transferred the shaker into her left hand so she could play the guitar with her right and began to explore the instrument. She was smiling and laughing, while also concentrating hard, as she explored the sounds of the guitar. Lisa allowed the music to emerge naturally according to what Emma was doing, and it seemed that Emma was enjoying the interaction. When Emma turned to the pink tambourine, and Lisa sang "Emma likes the pink tambourine, the pink tambourine, the pink tambourine. Emma likes the pink tambourine …and the strawberries 1, 2, 3!" —Emma pointed to the strawberry and licked the tambourine.

Lisa surmised this session was significant as Emma was able to move to a new activity without sitting down or losing interest. She demonstrated sustained attention, and shared emotional expression. The sessions have begun to flow more seamlessly as Emma is increasingly motivated to take more responsibility in the shared relationship. Further, Emma's increasing ability to focus on another person appeared to help mitigate her sensory needs.

The fourth description comes from a follow-up session. The regular music therapy programme had finished four weeks previously, but Lisa met Emma again to determine whether learning had been consolidated and development sustained. In this session, Emma had been asked to choose a "music therapy" song using the icons on her SGD. Instead, she chose the "Secret Life of Pets" Disney icon. Lisa knew this meant she would like to hear the song "Welcome to New York." But Emma was reluctant to put her device down and was playfully teasing Lisa. When she eventually put it down and moved the guitar onto her own lap, they began tapping the back of the guitar together while Lisa sang the song.

The playful interaction continued. Emma kicked her left leg out in time with the rhythm and leaned closer to Lisa before putting her knee on the guitar and vocalising. When Lisa imitated her sound, Emma vocalised again and touched Lisa's face, near her mouth. As they continued to tap the guitar together, in time to Lisa's singing, Emma again began to sway, pressing into the guitar. She looked at Lisa, pulled the guitar closer to her body and turned it around seemingly inviting Lisa to play. As Lisa helped to stabilise the instrument, Emma began to scratch the guitar again, and Lisa imitated the movements. Emma smiled at Lisa, shook her head, and laughed. Lisa laughed too as Emma turned the guitar over again and leaned in to smile at her, resting her toes on Lisa's shoe. Emma vocalised again, and Lisa copied her. Emma began to explore the guitar strings, but then tapped and paused—again seemingly requesting Lisa's response—but drew the guitar closer to her face and laughed. Lisa and Emma shared several minutes of playful interaction before Emma moved her fingers over the strings of the guitar, intentionally exploring the sounds she could make and fully concentrating on the sensory experience.

> Lisa surmised this session involved substantial shared and meaningful interaction. Emma demonstrated sustained attention and led most of the communication. She acted with intention, and shaped and led the dialogue. She demonstrated a willingness to explore, to engage in purposeful movement, vocalisation, and emotional expression. She was relaxed about Lisa's' physical proximity and the videoing that was taking place. Lisa and Emma experienced mutual joy and understanding of each other in the moment.

Commentators' Interpretations of Emma's Case

Commentators agreed that music therapy was an effective way for Emma to develop a meaningful relationship and to interact with others. The child-centred approach, and the patience and intuitiveness of Lisa, especially during initial sessions, were considered crucial to Emma feeling comfortable and confident enough to fully engage (Vivian).

> Emma has developed a bond with the music therapist over the period that she had music therapy sessions. She has learnt to trust Lisa and that music therapy is fun. This bond naturally leads to better engagement and more communication, which is part of the goal we had decided on. (Emma's mother)

Once trust was developed, Emma was able to engage in a variety of activities in music therapy (Emma's teacher). She began to develop her listening (Ruella), to offer sustained eye contact (Emma's teacher, Dana, Emma's mother, Ruella) had clearly gained confidence (Dana) and could even remain engaged while transitioning between activities (Ruella). "From a child who ran away after striking a chord (literally), Emma started to show incredible amount of interest [...] and sustained attention" (Vivian), and concentration (Emma's teacher). She began to engage in spontaneous interaction (Dana) and the quality of her interactions became richer as she moved from fleeting moments of connection to leading sustained periods of playful communication (Ruella). Emma and Lisa were "engaging in shared play" (Ruella), "'in the moment' together, working synchronously" (Freyer). "The trusting relationship is exemplified in the final learning story, as Emma moves close to Lisa to explore the guitar together" (Ruella).

> I loved the eye contact and the moment when their foreheads were together, and I found Emma's laughter infectious [...] it was a real strength of these sessions to see the therapist reacting to child led choices and using them to further capture interest. (Freyer)

Commentators noticed Emma's increasing use of gestures, including her directing Lisa's arm to an instrument. They observed that she was able to express preferences, for example, choosing percussion instruments and the music she wanted to engage with (Dana, Ruella) and to lead the direction of the therapy (Dana). Vivian and Mike were impressed with the vocabulary she was able to draw on to express her emotions "bordering on sophistication when using a word like 'crazy'" (Vivian). The fact that Emma chose different emotions for different sessions suggests an increasing level of engagement and understanding (Mike). Her ability to follow instructions (Dana) and her "obvious watching, processing and participating" led Hilda to suggest that "autistic children such as Emma understand more than is apparent to adults" (Hilda). Moreover, the resulting increase in agency (Dana, Mike) contributed to her ongoing use of her SGD (Hilda, Dana, Vivian, Emma's mother).

> It was lovely to see Emma move from being distant and uncertain, to engaged, interactive and using communicative intent. [...] She developed her use of her SGD with Lisa to make choices (student agency and voice), and to express her thoughts. These are great gains for Emma who tends to focus on her own agenda and needs with little awareness of others. (Emma's teacher)

Commentators considered the management of Emma's use of the SGD, as well as other visual aids, to be a crucial part of the music therapy process. Emma's mother, aunt, and teacher all expressed appreciation for her use of the device in and beyond the therapy space. However, Freyer also noted "while communication is an important goal, assistive technology can sometimes limit spontaneity and is not necessarily needed in all contexts." In contrast, Vivian suggested that it might be harder for Emma to generalise "turn-taking," "initiating," and "responding to peers" to the classroom setting without the device. Her suggestion that the use of the SGD would result in more sustainable outcomes, was borne out by Emma's mother.

> Lisa was very proactive in utilising Emma's talker during sessions, and we added some relevant items [...] specifically for these sessions. However,

> we found that she also refers to these at home as a request for Mum to sing the songs of her choosing, which has increased (our) interactions with Emma at home. Emma has also worked out she can request these songs to be played on the TV, which has expanded her choices of entertainment at home. (Emma's mother)

However, it is important too that music therapy supported Emma to develop other forms of intentional communication (Freyer). Commentators observed that she was able to communicate and express her feelings through the medium of music and dance (Dana), as well as vocal sounds (Freyer) and "she surely started opening up in terms of the emotions physically" (Vivian). These opportunities were particularly valued since Emma is "not easily understood in day-to-day life outside her close family" (Emma's Aunt). Emma's teacher reported that her sensory issues were significantly impacting on her ability to engage with other people, and with cognitive tasks. During classroom music, for example, Emma would sit away from the group and engage in what was described as self-stimulatory behaviour (Emma's Teacher). Hilda noted that:

> (Emma) might be experiencing the world as an overload of sensory experiences rather than be lost in her own world or have intellectual impairment. She appears to try to control the sensory input by such activities as fingers in her ear, licking, tasting, and smelling objects, looking intently and closely, and shaking her limbs […] In these music therapy sessions these actions are accepted and even incorporated into the sessions—and in doing so indicating that the music therapy environment is safe for her. She imitates and copies Lisa at times and Lisa imitates her shaking and flapping. It is clearly dynamic communication. (Hilda)

The music therapy environment provided opportunities for Emma to have her sensory needs met, and in turn to regulate her emotions and behaviour (Dana). She was able to explore the instruments and use them in her own way, and her enjoyment was obvious (Aunt, Dana, Freyer, Emma's mother, Emma's teacher). There was no evidence of her "(feeling) fearful, or throwing or destroying objects, hitting objects or self-harming, or trying to get away as autistic children such as her frequently do when under stress" (Hilda). Further, it seems that the gains Emma made with sensory regulation and communication may have been generalised. Following her programme of music therapy, her teacher and mother both reported significant progress regarding Emma's need to put things in her mouth or fingers in her ears. Her mother wrote:

> Emma has also shown a lot more interest during this time in making various sounds from musical instruments, rather than just putting them in her mouth or banging them. She has discovered a new way to play with them. When we go to the toy library, she now readily chooses musical instruments, whereas before it was difficult to get her to make a choice. (Emma's mother)

> It was great to see the way Emma reacted and interacted during her music therapy. Clearly it brings her great joy and is a part of her happy childhood life. Music therapy is a clever and wonderful way to help Emma with communication and for enabling her to trust and enjoy her interactions with others. (Emma's aunt)

Commentators expressed "admiration" for Lisa's planning, flexibility, and patience (Dana); found the case "heart-warming," "wonderfully engaging," and "encouraging" (Freyer) and were "delighted at Emma's increased engagement and agency" (Mike). Emma's teacher wrote, "If all children with autism had the opportunity to work with a music therapist, I would be a very happy teacher."

> I feel like music therapy has been an important part of Emma's year, and excellent progress has been made towards her goals. I feel that Lisa has worked very hard to interact with Emma in a way that makes sense to her (her unique way of being) and at her pace, allowing time for Emma to respond and initiate her own ideas. I think this has led to the formation of a strong, trusting therapeutic relationship, which has been vital to the success of the music therapy sessions. (Ruella)

Integration of Findings from Descriptions and Emma's Questionnaires

Eight of the nine commentators of this case somewhat agreed, agreed, or strongly agreed, with the positive statements, while Vivian disagreed or strongly disagreed with seven of the ten statements.

Vivian suggested the sessions provided space for Emma to become comfortable which gave her the confidence to interact physically with Lisa. However, she disagreed with Lisa's thought that Emma was initially maintaining an emotional distance, arguing "I got a sense that she was emotionally present throughout." She also had a sense that Emma was using her communication device "reasonably well" from the beginning, and that she would already have had a means of expression she could use across settings. She argued therefore for fewer goals that were more focussed on choice making, turn-taking, and sustained attention, suggesting they would result in more specific outcomes. She also felt that Emma might have been more able to manage these tasks if she was offered less choice, e.g., choice of two instruments rather than a full array.

Others were much more impressed with Emma's positive responses.

> Overall, this was a really rewarding case study to review. It was lovely to see the therapeutic relationship develop, and the detailed transcripts were invaluable in helping see the progress Emma was making. The standout observation for me was the way all the people in her life understand and support Emma's 'way of being'. (Freyer)

> Emma has always had a love of music and movement, so it was a natural choice for her to participate in music therapy […] It was lovely to see Emma engaging and participating with Lisa. Not only is she having fun, but she is also increasing her interactions and communication. Initially I was hopeful that her verbal communication may increase and although I am disappointed this has not happened, I can see other developmental changes in her […] Music therapy has been beneficial. (Emma's mother).

Music Therapist's Summary

Emma demonstrated increased and improved skills with social interaction including listening, joint attention and focused attention, participation, leading and initiating, thinking, and predicting, turn taking, and communicating ideas. She appeared to develop increased tolerance for sound, and awareness of her body in space (increased proprioceptive and kinaesthetic awareness). She also seemed to develop more strength with fine motor skills. She was more able to manage her emotions, demonstrated improvements in emotional expression and growing responsibility and personal commitment to relationship.

My Reflections on Emma's Case

Lisa's descriptions of Emma's sessions situate her as a child-centred, improvisational music therapist, who considers the work from a music-centred perspective at times. However, she writes less about the detail of the music, and more about the ways she and Emma are situated in the room, the quality of their movements, and how they eventually connect through improvised dance, movement, and music. The music therapy sessions took place at school and, as a newly qualified music therapist, Lisa was carefully guided by the school team.

Context would have played an important part in the ways Lisa planned and executed the work, including the focus on a "Key Competency" from the curriculum, and the use of Speech Generating Device (SGD) in the therapy context. According to the "Key Competencies," Emma's goal, "relating to others," refers to "interacting effectively with a diverse range of people in a variety of contexts," including the ability to "listen actively, recognise different points of view, negotiate, and share ideas." While Emma reportedly had good receptive language, it seemed music therapy would afford her opportunities to express her thoughts, feelings, and emotions and to develop reciprocity.

Just as Mary did for James, Lisa was able to underline some of the ways Emma was able to demonstrate the development of these skills through musical expressions. For example, when she describes Emma at the keyboard, she highlights the reciprocity that developed by emphasising the way they call and respond to each other, Lisa calling with a sequence of chords, Emma striking keys in response, and a short burst of synchronised movement emerging before Emma returns to the keys, striking single notes and clusters which invite Lisa to join her. Descriptions of Emma's "decisive movement," loud playing, "exaggerated face-paced movements" convey the energy in the room and demonstrate her motivation and commitment to the interaction. When she initiates dance moves Lisa follows her, her accompaniment containing and supporting Emma's musical ideas.

In other places, however, Lisa's description of the interaction is less overtly music-centred. That is, she tells us that the music is "playful," that Emma is "watching and listening," "leading the dialogue," but does not give detailed description of the musicking. In the third example she describes how Emma invites her to play by moving rhythmically and tapping her shaker against the guitar. She also shares important information about Emma transferring the shaker from one hand to another, smiling and laughing, concentrating, giving eye contact, and engaging in imaginative play (pointing to an object and demonstrating understanding, i.e., licking the "strawberry"). Here Lisa is giving holistic consideration to Emma's physical, social, emotional, cognitive, musical, and adaptive functioning. It seems she was aiming to help her gain greater awareness of self, others, the environment, and the self in relation to others and the environment, and so her approach also aligns well with Developmental Music Therapy (Boxill & Chase, 2006, p. 101).

The description of the fourth session also provides a relatively detailed account of Emma and Lisa's interpersonal interaction, without conveying the expressive and emotional content of the music. For example, there is little qualitative information in the description of Emma and Lisa tapping the back of the guitar while Lisa sang, Emma vocalising and touching Lisa's face, or Emma beginning to explore the guitar strings before tapping and pausing. On the other hand, Emma's relaxed demeanor was beautifully conveyed as she "kicked her left leg out in time with the rhythm and leaned closer to Lisa," "began to sway, pressing into the guitar," "rested her toes on Lisa's shoe," and "drew the guitar closer to her face and laughed."

While commentators appeared to highly value Emma's musical interaction, they also drew attention to how she was managing in wider contexts. For example, most considered Emma's use of the SGD to be a crucial part of the music therapy process not only because it provided her with opportunities to communicate with Lisa but also because she needed to practice using the device to manage it more effectively in the classroom and at home. This is logical in a school environment where the emphasis is on supporting children's learning needs across contexts. Moreover, verbal communication in music therapy, especially when children initiate it, is important (Thompson & Elefant, 2019). However, musical interaction also provides opportunities for children to demonstrate communicative intent beyond the use of the SGD.

The premise that music therapy affords participants communication beyond words underpins many approaches (Aigen, 2014), and music therapists can sometimes feel uncomfortable when musical interaction becomes secondary to verbal interaction (Thompson & Elefant, 2019), or other developmental tasks. Freyer did suggest that Emma's SGD might sometimes limit spontaneity, hinting that more space might have been created for musical interaction. Yet she also recognised that "tailored environmental adaptions" contributed to Emma's developing interpersonal communication and emphasised "how important it is to recognise that people with ASD communicate in many ways" (Freyer).

It is important to note too that Emma and Lisa's communication was frequently grounded in mediums of gesture, movement, and dance. Perhaps this was driven by Emma's cheerful and fun-loving personality to a certain extent, but many music therapists incorporate movement and dance (Marquez-Garcia et al., 2021; Oldfield, 2006) and playfulness and drama (Thompson & Elefant, 2019) in sessions with tamariki takiwātanga. While Emma's flapping and running were presumed to support her sensory integration, in many situations her movements would prevent or limit her from engaging fully in beneficial activities, including interaction with peers (Church et al., 2000). In music therapy, however, her movements became part of her "dance" with Lisa, a purposeful and integral part of the activity with the music providing an "auditory frame of reference" for her movements (Ockelford, 2000, p. 204). Takiwātanga may have difficulty attending to the timing of sensory information, suggesting that activities which challenge interpersonal synchrony and synchronising to external cues may be helpful (Kawakami et al., 2020; Morris et al., 2021).

Simple rhythm and body percussion activities and improvised songs described and reinforced what Emma was doing, and she became intrigued, motivated by the synchronicity she was experiencing. As Kim et al. (2009) note, musical attunement happens in non-verbal and multimodal contexts, including vocal and instrument exchanges, facial expressions, eye contact, and synchronous movement and gestures (p. 390). Moreover, enabling and encouraging her movements might not only have helped Emma to manage at the moment but might also contribute to a reduction in stereotypic behaviours in the longer term (Tse et al., 2018).

References

Aigen, K. (2014). Music-centered dimensions of Nordoff-Robbins music therapy. *Music Therapy Perspectives, 32*(1), 18–29. https://doi.org/10.1093/mtp/miu006

Boxill, E. H., & Chase, K. M. (2006). *Music therapy for developmental disabilities* (2nd ed.). Pro-Ed.

Church, C., Alisanski, S., & Amanullah, S. (2000). The social, behavioral, and academic experiences of children with Asperger syndrome. *Focus on Autism and Other Developmental Disabilities, 15*(1), 12–20. https://doi.org/10.1177/108835760001500102

Kawakami, S., Uono, S., Otsuka, S., Yoshimura, S., Zhao, S., & Toichi, M. (2020). Atypical multisensory integration and the temporal binding window in autism spectrum disorder. *Journal of Autism and Developmental Disorders, 50*(11), 3944–3956. https://doi.org/10.1007/s10803-020-04452-0

Kim, J., Wigram, T., & Gold, C. (2009). Emotional, motivational and interpersonal responsiveness of children with autism in improvisational music therapy. *Autism, 13*(4), 389–409. https://doi.org/10.1177/1362361309105660

Marquez-Garcia, A. V., Magnuson, J., Morris, J., Iarocci, G., Doesburg, S., & Moreno, S. (2021). Music therapy in autism spectrum disorder: A systematic review. *Review Journal of Autism and Developmental Disorders*. https://doi.org/10.1007/s40489-021-00246-x

Morris, P. O., Hope, E., Foulsham, T., & Mills, J. P. (2021). Dance, rhythm, and autism spectrum disorder: An explorative study. *The Arts in Psychotherapy, 73*, 101755. https://doi.org/10.1016/j.aip.2020.101755

Ockelford, A. (2000). Music in the education of children with severe or profound learning difficulties: Issues in current U.K. provision, a new conceptual framework, and proposals for research. *Psychology of Music, 28*(2), 197–217. https://doi.org/10.1177/0305735600282009

Oldfield, A. (2006). *Interactive music therapy: A positive approach*. Jessica Kingsley Publishers.

Thompson, G. A., & Elefant, C. (2019). "But I want to talk to you!" Perspectives on music therapy practice with highly verbal children on the autism spectrum. *Nordic Journal of Music Therapy, 28*(4), 347–359. https://doi.org/10.1080/08098131.2019.1605616

Tse, C. Y. A., Pang, C. L., & Lee, P. H. (2018). Choosing an appropriate physical exercise to reduce stereotypic behavior in children with autism spectrum disorders: A Non-randomized crossover study. *Journal of Autism and Developmental Disorders, 48*(5), 1666–1672. https://doi.org/10.1007/s10803-017-3419-3

12

"ELIJAH"—"Speaking His Language"

Background

Elijah was a six-year-old Filipino boy, born in New Zealand, who loved Micky Mouse Clubhouse television programmes. He was non-verbal and used a core board, gestures, and sign language to communicate in the classroom. He demonstrated sensitivity to sounds, particularly low frequency, and tended to mouth or bite objects. He also experienced high levels of anxiety, avoided eye contact, and had difficulty staying in his classroom at school.

His music therapist, Anna-Maria, was a "beginning therapist" in this context. She had worked for three years, but with only one child, and that child was also takiwātanga. Anna-Maria employed a child-centred improvisational approach with Elijah. Music therapy was typically provided weekly, in the family home initially, then at his school, for a total of 28 sessions. The initial music therapy goals were to develop Elijah's play skills, vocalisation (through singing), independence, and turn-taking skills.

D. Rickson, *Music Therapy with Autistic Children in Aotearoa, New Zealand*, https://doi.org/10.1007/978-3-031-05233-0_12

The Music Therapy Process

The first vignette begins with Anna-Maria placing her percussion instruments on a piece of material on the floor. Elijah immediately went over to the music space and began to skid across the floor with the material under his feet. Anna-Maria accompanied his movement playing one of his favourite television themes, on the glockenspiel. He stopped suddenly, and looked up at the ceiling, pausing for a second, before walking over to a small plastic toy and picking it up to bite it. He then ran to the trampoline and jumped on it. Anna-Maria took her stretchy rope and began to play "Row, row, row your boat" with his mother, singing to encourage him back. Elijah returned to them and jumped into the rope as if he were skipping. As he did this he was blowing and making an "f" sound. This was the first time his mother had heard him making a sound of any kind other than "Dadda," and she appeared very excited. Suddenly again, Elijah turned his attention to the triangle and was able to play fleetingly while Anna-Maria accompanied on the glockenspiel. Then he ran away again.

In the second description Elijah is in a bedroom hugging cushions. When Anna-Maria calls from the music space, singing his name, he eventually comes into the room, stands on the couch, and hums the two pitches of "Hello Elijah" (G-C). Anna-Maria picked up the guiro and played while simultaneously singing "Hello Elijah." He stopped, looked up at the ceiling and paused. She made the "f" sound. He came up behind her, grabbed her, and put his face near her mouth, smiling briefly.

> Anna-Maria noted this was the first time he had smiled at her. While he immediately jumped away, they had made a connection.

In the next example, Anna-Maria began with a drum and beater. Working with his mother, she modelled "Your turn mummy" and then "Your turn Elijah." Elijah became agitated when his mother lifted his hand to help him hit the drum, and Anna-Maria suggested she let him do it himself. When they resumed the game Elijah picked up two beaters and played them one at a time on the drum as she accompanied him on the ukulele. Elijah's mother appeared really pleased, saying she had never seen him use beaters like that before. They gave Elijah the "thumbs up" signal and praised him, before Anna-Maria played a calming lullaby on the ukulele, to give him a break. He lay in his mother's arms and was able to calm himself. A few minutes later they successfully repeated the turn-taking exercise after which Elijah was rewarded with his favourite TV programme.

The next description involved a venue change, with the music therapy taking place at Elijah's school. When Anna-Maria handed Elijah two beaters, he immediately began to play the drum. She joined him, slapping her hands on her knees before accompanying with the guiro. After a brief pause, she tried to re-engage him verbally. Elijah smiled but did not respond when she said, "Your turn." However, when she playfully tapped his drum Elijah picked up the triangle beater and hit the drum too. He then took Anna-Maria's wooden beater and played, listening to the different sounds he was making. In time he started to hum. Next, he hit the two beaters together, paused, and looked up with a sense of recognition. Anna-Maria resumed singing "Hello Elijah" while playing the guiro. Eventually she surprised him, hitting the drum with a beater while calling his name. Elijah immediately responded by hitting the drum, while simultaneously saying his name too. When Anna-Maria repeated the game, Elijah again picked up the beater and said his name.

The classroom in which the therapy took place has a swing. In the next description, Anna-Maria is improvising a song, "Elijah likes to swing." The melodic shape matched the up and down action of the swing. As he swung to the song, Elijah smiled and laughed out loud. A short time later he began making bird-like sounds, which Anna-Maria copied. Elijah paused and looked up. He then went independently to the piano and began to play, sounding single notes from the bottom end of the piano to the top. When Anna-Maria tried to join him, he moved away to something else.

In the penultimate description, Anna-Maria is playing three different rhythms on a bell drum to distinguish the names of mother, Anna-Maria, and Elijah. Elijah was curious about this. He focussed and looked at her as she played each rhythm and chanted the names. When she showed him how to play the drum he looked up at the ceiling, paused, and then played it again with two sticks, one after the other, seemingly enjoying the sound. Elijah played the bell drum using an even action and it was easy for Anna-Maria to accompany him with another drum. They played simultaneously and alternately, taking turns.

In the final example, Elijah was sitting at the piano when Anna-Maria asked him to copy her sound. When she sang "Ooh-wah" he copied it immediately with a croaky, husky sound. For the next few minutes, she repeated the sounds, which he sometimes copied back. Towards the end of the session, he paused before making some of his own sounds, incorporating the "Ooh-wah" into his phrase.

Commentators' Interpretations of Elijah's Case

Commentators observed that Elijah had begun to feel secure, to warm to Anna-Maria, and to trust her. This was demonstrated in his ability to maintain physical closeness and to interact with her musically. Her playful approach attracted his attention and kept him engaged until he felt safe to interact. Thus, music therapy helped to reduce his anxiety (Hilda) and he was increasingly able to attend (Freyer, Hilda, Mike), to listen (Vivian), maintain eye contact (Freyer), take turns (Freyer), and vocalise for intentional communication (Freyer; Mike). He demonstrated "a keenness to explore" and the "ability to tolerate change" in this setting (Vivian). Several commentators highlighted improvements in Elijah's communication (Ruella, Vivian, Elijah's mother, and father). Specifically, "Elijah moved on from basic echolalia" and was becoming "more interactive with others" (Freyer).

> One has to see Elijah's achievements in the context of ASD being a complex and extraordinary spectrum of challenges and strengths. Elijah started this process with high anxiety, nonverbal, and offering little to no eye contact. By the end, with prompts like striking

> the drum with a beater, Elijah said his name at home, and he could high-five both his mum and the therapist. Whilst I don't know how long the programme was, this is to me extremely strong progress. (Mike)

Elijah's drumming was reportedly "impressive. [...] he had very good rhythm" (Dana). Ruella noticed Elijah's preference for independent activity and his resistance when his mother attempted to help him beat the drum. Similarly, Dana seemed to suggest that more progress might have been made if Elijah's mother had not been present in sessions. Mike, on the other hand, recognised how very exciting it must have been for Elijah's mother to hear him make new sounds and to say his name for the first time. Music therapy was a place where he began to recognise that his voice was a tool for communication (Freyer) and, at home, he continued to use his voice to have conversational, turn-taking, exchanges of sound (Elijah's mother and father). Dana and Vivian both observed that he needed time to process sounds and to formulate a response but was "then able to initiate the sound on his own" (Dana).

> The 'Ooh-wah' was a very enjoyable interaction to watch. It was not initially clear if Elijah was deliberately repeating the 'Ooh-wah' sound, but as the clip progressed, he became more intentional in his vocal sounds. His eye contact changed from moving around the space to become more directional towards his therapist and (with) the echolalia he appeared to be making a communicative connection in response to her. The high five at the end was a positive indication that Elijah was engaged in the activity. (Freyer)

Throughout the time he was attending music therapy Elijah continued to demonstrate a need for vestibular, tactile and/or proprioceptive, and oral stimulation which was, according to commentator reports, well managed. Elijah showed promise in tolerating people and noises (Vivian), and the use of the swing was helpful, as it "gave Elijah the "vestibular stimulation" he may have needed prior to the session. (Moreover) the therapist's ability to improvise made the session a little more exciting" (Dana).

> Elijah appeared to learn the 'rules' of copying sounds in tandem with banging instruments and being part of an activity involving others. He clearly needs to seek sensory input while engaged in these tasks, such as using the swing or mouthing the blocks, but is able to be distracted from those activities and be redirected to the activities being modelled. (Freyer)

Elijah's caregiver believed the music therapy helped him to gain more motivation to explore his environment, suggesting that music therapy "opened his senses and […] opened him up to more experiences (which he is) sometimes willing to share with other people." However, he also suggested that while Elijah has become more interested in his auditory environment, his active participation in music has not been readily sustained. While he used to "sing" when was attending music therapy sessions, Elijah became "more interested in hearing people singing his songs rather than singing himself" (Elijah's caregiver). In contrast, he, as well as Elijah's mother and father, noticed ongoing improvements in Elijah's communication, including his vocalisations, that they attributed to music therapy.

> I noticed that he has a lot more eye contact and his interest in music has increased. He is now vocalising and seems to be in an almost conversational exchange of sounds with us at home. [...] When I call his attention, he also has sort of conversational babbles (or baby talk) which he did not use to have. (Father)

> Elijah's interaction skills have had significant positive impacts on his social capabilities. He is more inclined to interact with people he is not familiar with and develop relationships further with those he already is connected to. […] He has become more responsive to people when we talk or play with him. (Elijah's caregiver)

> Teachers and teacher aides at school have told me that Elijah has been more sociable at school. He has joined mat time and will tolerate other children being near his personal space a bit more. And when the teacher plays music in the classroom (especially on wet days when they are all confined in the room), he will usually calm down and just be happy. (Elijah's mother)

Commentators noted that music therapy was enjoyable for Elijah and helped to reduce his anxiety. Mike who has lived experience of ASD wrote:

> It was an extraordinary privilege to watch this work. I feel that this relationship has been extremely beneficial to Elijah's progress, and I am feeling a strong sense of the joy that his family must have been feeling when he made that progress. (Mike)

> Sessions helped Elijah vocalize a bit more, say his name, and learn to take turns like in a conversation. So, (I believe) music therapy will definitely help other children struggling to communicate [...]. I feel so blessed that he was able to be part of this study. (Elijah's mother)

Integration of Findings from Descriptions and Elijah's Questionnaires

Nine people evaluated Elijah's case, including three who knew him well, and all but one (Hilda) felt that music therapy was important for him. However, while Hilda disagreed that music therapy was important for Elijah, she also provided the following contradictory statement.

> Anything that helps to de-stress autistic kids is important in helping them get through the rest of their day. I hope he continues to have access to such empathetic music therapy as it appears to work well with his sensory needs. (Hilda)

All commentators agreed that Elijah was developing skills that would help him learn, that music therapy interactions were meaningful for him, and that he seemed to enjoy music therapy overall. They felt that the stated goal seemed appropriate for him and that he made *timely* progress. Yet Dana was unsure whether he made progress towards his stated goals, presumably because she was focussing on the development of independence. The qualitative data clarifies that she queried the presence of Elijah's mother, perhaps anticipating that more progress might have been made if he had worked independently with Anna-Maria.

> From what was observed, music therapy is effective for Elijah because he appears to enjoy it. (However) I would've liked to have seen sessions where mum wasn't present to see what his engagement would look like, so to compare the outcome. Mum is amazing; she's loving, patient and is very much part of the session. Its clear mum wants to be involved and I think it's wonderful. However, I do wonder if Elijah would be able to cope without mum being present or whether it will have an impact on the therapy sessions. (Dana)

Music Therapist's Summary

> Elijah demonstrated increased interest in exploring and creating sounds on musical instruments including voice. His understanding of cause and effect improved from an auditory perspective (he was able to understand that if he hit a beater on a drum, he created a particular sound and if he hit two sticks together it was different), and he began to explore how he could make various vocal sounds (high and low sounds with his voice, and by moving his lips). He is engaging for longer periods, has begun to take turns, and generally appears more relaxed and happier.

My Reflections on Elijah's Case

The use of the voice is a key factor when attempting to engage tamariki takiwātanga in reciprocal interaction (Salomon-Gimmon & Elefant, 2019). The vocal play, accompanied by appropriate facial expressions and gestures that Anna-Maria and Elijah engaged in, contains many features common to parental and music therapy interaction and will be familiar to music therapists around the world. As Oldfield (2020) notes, the utilisation of "babbling" vocal exchanges which typically occur between carers and infants, and the incorporation of children's vocalisations and musical sounds into interactive improvised musical exchanges, is important in supporting speech development.

> Both music and baby talk have similar melodic, rhythmic, and dynamic expressive features, which include repetition, exaggeration, and elaboration as well as variation in volume, pitch, and speed. One can even find spontaneous vibrato and glissandi in some mothers' utterances to babies. (Dissanayake, 2012, p. 6)

The timing, phrasing, and intensity of the musical exchanges can help the child to become more synchronised, organised, and regulated, and the adult to feel intimately connected to the child. The mutual influence of "infant-directed singing," or non-verbal "conversation," therefore creates a sense of togetherness and promotes bonding and attachment (Edwards, 2014) and the child begins to develop a sense of self, to expand communication, social, and emotional abilities (Stern, 1985). For tamariki takiwātanga, the development of cognitive ability, gestures, and imitation, as a precursor to expressive language (Luyster et al., 2008) sensory and emotion regulation, and relational skills (Epstein et al., 2020), is crucial. They may therefore need a stronger emphasis on nonverbal input than children without the diagnosis (van Ijzendoorn et al., 2007, p. 605).

The success of techniques such as infant-directed singing requires sensitive attunement to the child's signals (Edwards, 2014). Anna-Maria repeated the musical and non-musical characteristics Elijah's vocalisations to "form a continuous chain of mutual vocal behaviours"; repeated them with variations, to change the character of the vocalisation and extend the communication; and introduced vocalisations that were attuned to his emotional state; just as parents and infants do (Salomon-Gimmon & Elefant, 2019). Like other music therapists she "expanded and developed the pitch, the melodic line, the rhythm, the outline, and the intensity" (Salomon-Gimmon & Elefant, 2019, p. 186) of his vocalisations. This is important, because even when tamariki takiwātanga's vocalisations are echolalic (repetitive of other's past words or sounds), they are likely to have a purpose to regain emotional equilibrium; maintain focus; explore sounds; to block or mask others; to express strong emotion; or to initiate or maintain communication (Dromi et al., 2018; Marom et al., 2018). It is not surprising then that Elijah's caregiver noticed Elijah preferred at times to listen passively to music that was sung to him yet continued to actively respond to carefully presented musical "motherese." These are contrasting activities, and simply presenting music in the environment is unlikely to promote the engagement of tamariki takiwātanga (Preis et al., 2016).

When music therapy takes place in the child's home environment the music therapy is often family-focussed, both in orientation and goals (Edwards, 2014). The music therapist is not only concerned about outcomes for the child, but also for the families (Allgood, 2005; Thompson & McFerran, 2015b). Musical Interaction Therapy (MIT), for example, focusses specifically on the interaction between tamariki takiwātanga and their caregivers, with the music therapist supporting their timing with live improvised music to create an experience resembling the preverbal interaction described above (Wimpory & Gwilym, 2019). Thompson (2012) adds that when family-centred practice occurs in natural settings such as the home environment, families can be supported to embed therapeutic activities into the child's daily routines.

In contrast, during Elijah's at-home sessions his mother appears to be predominantly positioned as an observer and a role model, providing a secure base for Elijah to go back to when he needed additional emotional support, rather than a recipient of the therapy focus. Anna-Maria used the principles of infant-directed singing to communicate directly with Elijah, helping him to feel secure, while perhaps considering his need as a six-year-old to function independently from his mother, at home and at school. While not specifically stated, this possibility is reinforced by the decision to move music therapy sessions from home to school, and Dana's suggestion that it might have been better if mum had not been present at all. While Dana suggests "it was clear she wanted to be involved," we don't know from Anna-Marie's account of the music therapy whether or how this was negotiated.

Parents need to be ready to take on the role of partner in the therapy process. Whole family systems are impacted when a child is takiwātanga, with stress, anxiety and social isolation commonly reported (Blauth, 2017). Primary caregivers of tamariki takiwātanga have higher stress levels than both the general population, and parents of children with other developmental disabilities (Blauth, 2017) and this can counteract potential positive outcomes of intervention programmes, particularly those that are time intensive (Osborne et al., 2008). Some parents become dependent on therapists (Forsingdal et al., 2014; Oldfield, 2006) and they and others might not always be ready to take on highly collaborative roles. Sometimes too, parents feel insecure; the skills of the music therapist can feel threatening (Blauth, 2017; Oldfield, 2006); and being actively involved in music therapy sessions can feel risky, either in terms of learning how to support their child musically, or letting a child make their own choices (Allgood, 2005).

van Ijzendoorn et al. (2007) found that while parents of tamariki Takiwātanga are as sensitive to their children's needs as other parents, their children tend to be less secure and disorganised, and less involved in play, so that even sensitive parental behaviours may at times be too low-keyed to reach them. It can therefore take more time and effort for tamariki takiwātanga and their parent/s to develop predictable and well-matched interaction patterns. The parents tend to initiate, suggest, or give instructions for games more frequently and to lead the play more than parents of other children (Freeman et al., 2006; Patterson et al., 2014), and might appear more physically intrusive (van Ijzendoorn et al., 2007). When the child initiates an interaction, however, joint attention tends to be more "responsive" giving the child further opportunities to initiate (Patterson et al., 2014).

Music therapists can work in gentle, non-intrusive ways to support parents to attend positively to their children's appropriate social and play behaviours (Edwards, 2014; Ginn et al., 2017; Hernandez-Ruiz, 2018). When Anna-Maria felt the need remind Elijah's mother to let him play the drum by himself, his mother accepted this readily, and her ongoing comments demonstrate that she continued to appreciate his involvement in music therapy. Difficult or painful moments in music therapy can be managed in a constructive way, and positive moments can be highlighted (Oldfield, 2006). Parents appreciate a more positive assessment of their child (Warwick, 2019) and in music therapy they often see them in a more positive light (Oldfield, 2006; Rickson et al., 2015b; Thompson, 2012; Thompson & McFerran, 2015a). Elijah's mother seemed excited to hear him progressing his vocal sounds in music therapy and beyond.

Music therapists undoubtedly have a role to support families of takiwātanga directly (Blauth, 2017; Thompson, 2012). Nevertheless, Elijah's case study shows that even when the focus is on the individual child, gains in interpersonal communication can be made and generalised to other contexts, in turn improving family life. The playful use of techniques such as infant-directed singing is made meaningful in the music therapy context and, as Elijah's father's comments suggest, observers can understand, appreciate, and continue to use them in other settings. He had clearly embraced opportunities to capture "teachable moments" and embed learning opportunities into everyday activities (Zwaigenbaum et al., 2015).

References

Allgood, N. (2005). Parents' perceptions of family-based group music therapy for children with autism spectrum disorders. *Music Therapy Perspectives, 23*(2), 92–99. https://doi.org/10.1093/mtp/23.2.92

Blauth, L. (2017). Improving mental health in families with autistic children: Benefits of using video feedback in parent counselling sessions offered alongside music therapy. *Health Psychology Report, 2*(2), 138–150. https://doi.org/10.5114/hpr.2017.63558

Dissanayake, E. (2012). The earliest narratives were musical. *Research Studies in Music Education, 34*(1), 3–14. https://doi.org/10.1177/1321103X12448148

Dromi, E., Rum, Y., & Florian, J. G. (2018). Communication, language, and speech in young children with autism spectrum disorder (ASD). In A. Bar-On, D. Ravid, & E. Dattner (Eds.), *Handbook of communication disorders* (pp. 811–828). De Gruyter Mouton. https://doi.org/10.1515/9781614514909

Edwards, J. (2014). The role of the music therapist in promoting parent-infant attachment/Favoriser l'attachement parent-enfant: rôle du musicothérapeute. *Canadian Journal of Music Therapy, 20*(1), 38–48. https://doi.org/10.1037/0003-066x.46.4.333

Epstein, S., Elefant, C., & Thompson, G. (2020). Music therapists' perceptions of the therapeutic potentials using music when working with verbal children on the autism spectrum: A qualitative analysis. *The Journal of Music Therapy, 57*(1), 66–90. https://doi.org/10.1093/jmt/thz017

Forsingdal, S., St John, W., Miller, V., Harvey, A., & Wearne, P. (2014). Goal setting with mothers in child development services. *Child Care Health and Development, 40*(4), 587–596. https://doi.org/10.1111/cch.12075

Freeman, L., Caserta, M., Lund, D., Rossa, S., Dowdy, A., & Partenheimer, A. (2006, March 1). Music thanatology: Prescriptive harp music as palliative care for the dying patient. *American Journal of Hospice and Palliative Medicine, 23*(2), 100–104. https://doi.org/10.1177/104990910602300206

Ginn, N. C., Clionsky, L. N., Eyberg, S. M., Warner-Metzger, C., & Abner, J.-P. (2017). Child-directed interaction training for young children with autism spectrum disorders: Parent and child outcomes. *Journal of Clinical Child & Adolescent Psychology, 46*(1), 101–109. https://doi.org/10.1080/15374416.2015.1015135

Hernandez-Ruiz, E. (2018). Music therapy and Early Start Denver Model to teach social communication strategies to parents of preschoolers with ASD: A feasibility study. *Music Therapy Perspectives, 36*(1), 26–39. https://doi.org/10.1093/mtp/mix018

Luyster, R., Kadlec, M., Carter, A., & Tager-Flusberg, H. (2008, September). Language assessment and development in toddlers with autism spectrum disorders. *Journal of Autism & Developmental Disorders, 38*(8), 1426–1438. https://doi.org/10.1007/s10803-007-0510-1

Marom, M. K., Gilboa, A., & Bodner, E. (2018). Musical features and interactional functions of echolalia in children with autism within the music therapy dyad. *Nordic Journal of Music Therapy, 27*(3), 175–196. https://doi.org/10.1080/08098131.2017.1403948

Osborne, L. A., McHugh, L., Saunders, J., & Reed, P. (2008, July). Parenting stress reduces the effectiveness of early teaching interventions for autistic spectrum disorders. *Journal of Autism & Developmental Disorders, 38*(6), 1092–1103. https://doi.org/10.1007/s10803-007-0497-7

Oldfield, A. (2006). *Interactive music therapy: A positive approach.* Jessica Kingsley Publishers.

Oldfield, A. (2020). Book Review. In P. Kern & M. Humpal (Eds.), Early childhood music therapy and autism spectrum disorder. *British Journal of Music Therapy, 34*(2), 108–120.

Patterson, S. Y., Elder, L., Gulsrud, A., & Kasari, C. (2014, July). The association between parental interaction style and children's joint engagement in families with toddlers with autism. *Autism, 18*(5), 511–518. https://doi.org/10.1177/1362361313483595

Preis, J., Amon, R., Silbert Robinette, D., & Rozegar, A. (2016). Does music matter? The effects of background music on verbal expression and engagement in children with autism spectrum disorders. *Music Therapy Perspectives, 34*(1), 106–115. https://doi.org/10.1093/mtp/miu044

Rickson, D. J., Molyneux, C., Ridley, H., Castelino, A., & Upjohn Beatson, E. B. (2015b). Music therapy with people who have autism spectrum disorder—Current practice in New Zealand. *New Zealand Journal of Music Therapy, 13,* 8–32. https://www-proquest-com.helicon.vuw.ac.nz/docview/1897698669?accountid=14782

Salomon-Gimmon, M., & Elefant, C. (2019). Development of vocal communication in children with autism spectrum disorder during improvisational music therapy. *Nordic Journal of Music Therapy, 28*(3), 174–192. https://doi.org/10.1080/08098131.2018.1529698

Stern, D. N. (1985). *The interpersonal world of the infant*. Basic Books Inc.

Thompson, G. A. (2012). Family-centered music therapy in the home environment: Promoting interpersonal engagement between children with autism spectrum disorder and their parents. *Music Therapy Perspectives, 30*(2), 109–116. http://ezproxy.massey.ac.nz/login?url=http://search.ebscohost.com/login.aspx?direct=true&db=ccm&AN=2012088717&site=eds-live&scope=site

Thompson, G. A., & McFerran, K. S. (2015a). Music therapy with young people who have profound intellectual and developmental disability: Four case studies exploring communication and engagement within musical interactions. *Journal of Intellectual & Developmental Disability, 40*(1), 1–11. https://doi.org/10.3109/13668250.2014.965668

Thompson, G. A., & McFerran, K. S. (2015b). "We've got a special connection": Qualitative analysis of descriptions of change in the parent–child relationship by mothers of young children with autism spectrum disorder. *Nordic Journal of Music Therapy, 24*(1), 3–26. https://doi.org/10.1080/08098131.2013.858762

van Ijzendoorn, M. H., Rutgers, A. H., Bakermans-Kranenburg, M. J., Swinkels, S. H. N., van Daalen, E., Dietz, C., Naber, F. B. A., Buitelaar, J. K., & van Engeland, H. (2007, March–April). Parental sensitivity and attachment in children with autism spectrum disorder: Comparison with children with mental retardation, with language delays, and with typical development. *Child Development, 78*(2), 597–608.

Warwick, A. (2019). Prelude: The unanswered question. In H. Dunn, E. Coombes, E. Maclean, H. Mottram, & J. Nugent (Eds.), *Music therapy and autism across the lifespan: A spectrum of approaches* (pp. 15–34). Jessica Kingsley Publishers.

Wimpory, D., & Gwilym, E. (2019). Musical interaction therapy (MIT) for children with autistic spectrum conditions (ASCs): Underlying rationale, clinical practice and research evidence. In H. Dunn, E. Coombes, E. Maclean, H. Mottram, & J. Nugent (Eds.), *Music therapy and autism across the lifespan: A spectrum of approaches* (pp. 97–136). Jessica Kingsley Publishers.

Zwaigenbaum, L., Bauman, M. L., Choueiri, R., Kasari, C., Carter, A., Granpeesheh, D., Mailloux, Z., Smith Roley, S., Wagner, S., Fein, D., Pierce, K., Buie, T., Davis, P. A., Newschaffer, C., Robins, D., Wetherby, A., Stone, W. L., Yirmiya, N., Estes, A., ... Natowicz, M. R. (2015, October 1). Early intervention for children with autism spectrum disorder under 3 years of age: Recommendations for practice and research. *Pediatrics, 136*(Supplement 1), S60–S81. https://doi.org/10.1542/peds.2014-3667E

13

"SOPHIA"—The Development of Verbal Language Through Musical Play

Background

Sophia was a 6-year-old girl, who attended a regular school with teacher's aide support. She responded positively to music making and was noted to have abilities with rhythm, melodic phrasing, and pitch matching. She was verbal but had difficulty articulating words, used short sentences, and was not confident talking outside of her home or family environment.

Her music therapist, Lianne, was an experienced therapist in this context. The music therapy was provided approximately weekly, for a total of 29 sessions, in a music therapy room in the community. Sophia's mother attended the first 11 sessions. The referral was for support with speech development and social skills. Initial music therapy goals were to develop Sophia's ability to engage in shared interaction including:

- Imitating, reciprocating, expressing, sharing, taking turns, negotiating
- Using voice and singing lyrics

D. Rickson, *Music Therapy with Autistic Children in Aotearoa, New Zealand*, https://doi.org/10.1007/978-3-031-05233-0_13

The Music Therapy Process

In the first description Sophia is using the harmonica to blow the rhythm of syllables and phrases. She began by using it to communicate "mum" during greeting song, then throughout the session she continued to play in dynamic ways, attempting to communicate ideas. At first, she seemed to be testing Lianne and her mother's tolerance for noise, but the interaction morphed into a playful and interactive exchange between Lianne and Sophia. For example, she was blowing loudly and quietly to create anticipation and playing long sustained notes to make or emphasise a point.

> Lianne noted Sophia was able to demonstrate sustained attention when leading, and to represent specific sounds (such as animal noises) on her instrument.

In the second description from session ten, Lianne and Sophia both had a kazoo. The kazoo had been introduced because this instrument gave her greater capacity to vary her pitch and be expressive, to mimic speech and conversational exchange. Sophia used the kazoo fluently, imitating speech patterns through the modulation of pitch, phrasing, and accent. She also began to talk through the kazoo, confidently repeating her sounds until they could be understood and engaged in call and response games using the kazoo. Later in the session when "building" a structure with instruments, she verbalised "house," and sang a packing up song with Lianne.

In the third description Sophia had removed the xylophone keys which were inscribed with letter names. Lianne introduced an alphabet song while Sophia verbalised a word for every letter of the alphabet. She did this with ease and was able to remember almost all the words when they repeated the song. When she was not able to be understood, she was able to laugh and continue with the activity.

Lianne noted that Sophia was demonstrating creativity, humour, persistence, resilience, and an ability to remain self-regulated.

In the fourth description Sophia is "conducting." She had learnt that she could influence Lianne's music in this way and was enjoying opportunities to lead. When conducting, Sophia shared sustained eye contact with Lianne. However, when Lianne tried to lead the game Sophia became resistant. Towards the end of this session when Lianne spontaneously and humorously waved the beater, Sophia responded—slowly at first, but eventually with dynamic movements, repeating certain gestures, and conveying emotion in her "dance."

The therapist surmised that Sophia was demonstrating trust and was beginning to take risks and to relinquish control. She was less inhibited and showed potential to interact creatively.

Commentators' Interpretations of Sophia's Case

Commentators noted clear evidence of progress over time particularly with interpersonal skills (Mike, Ruella, Vivian) such as making eye contact, taking turns, listening, responding, and leading and following (Ruella). Sophia learnt to "navigate the space around her, respond to her environment and to compromise" (Sophia's mother). Sophia enjoyed conducting and leading, but over time she became more tolerant of allowing the therapist to lead and was more willing to be the "follower" (Sophia's mother; Ruella; Vivian).

> I can see that Sophia has demonstrated growth in regulating herself and responding to things around her. She had been given space to respond

> naturally and to see where that response took her. She could see when her response produced reciprocation, further interaction, or nothing. She learned [...] that she could play and interact meaningfully with the therapist or have some time to herself, while still keeping up some kind of interaction to let the therapist know she was still aware of her and wanted to continue some communication. (Sophia's mother)

Sophia's mother noted that she was attending for longer periods and was more able to participate in sustained play. As Sophia explored the instruments with Lianne, rapport was established (Dana, Mike) and trust grew (Freyer). Sophia was increasingly engaged with Lianne (Dana, Sophia's mother, Ruella) and gained the confidence to communicate verbally as well as musically (Dana, Freyer, Ruella, Vivian, Sophia's grandmother). Her social skills developed as she moved from parallel, to imitative and interactional play (Hilda). Vivian also suggested that skills such as "transitioning ease from one instrument to the other," and "exploring emotions through the various instruments" were very positive outcomes of therapy for Sophia. Music therapy provided a safe space where she could develop necessary confidence and begin to understand her capability (Vivian).

> I can see how her confidence and independence has developed throughout the year. At home, she has always demonstrated confidence, but I recognise that during this year of music therapy, she has developed independence. Being at home with us, we tend to wrap her around cotton wool, and when she is at my home and surrounded by her uncle and aunties, we tend to do everything for Sophia (out of our love for her). (Sophia's grandmother)

Commentators agreed that music therapy had a positive impact on Sophia's developing speech and communication skills (Hilda, Mike, Ruella, Sophia's grandmother). "She became less reliant on her mother as her interpreter and more willing to take risks and overcome frustration if she was not always immediately understood" (Freyer). "Sophia was able to use the instruments to communicate with Lianne, when she didn't want to communicate directly," (Sophia's mother). "Over time, she seemed to become more confident in using her words and less frustrated when she was not understood by Lianne. She filled in gaps in songs and sang along with familiar songs" (Ruella).

> Sophia thrived in this space. Music therapy provided opportunities for her to make sounds, to communicate a sound, to interact with another person, while she was still trying to find the ability/confidence to do the same with her own voice. Sophia was given access to a variety of instruments in each session and was able to use them freely in her own way to express and aid her in her communication. (Sophia's mother)

> Sophia enjoyed the ease with which she was able to mimic speech sounds (with the Kazoo). This was a great example of a safe and playful barrier that Sophia (could use) to allow her to feel safe to interact with the therapist. But at the same time, it allowed Sophia to explore the sounds and movement of her mouth in the pronunciation of words as she tried to communicate words clearly through the kazoo to the therapist. Music therapy for Sophia provided a safe and playful environment where she was able to explore sounds (no pressure for the sound to be coming from her!) and experiment with sounds. (Sophia's mother)

That said, Dana felt that Sophia's progress was relatively slow given the number of music therapy sessions she attended. She suggested Lianne needed to challenge Sophia more, arguing that "it was unclear why Sophia chose not to speak during most of her music sessions." She thought that Sophia "had a lot more to offer in terms of her musical aptitude, but she appeared reluctant to reveal her true musical potential." Similarly, Mike felt that Lianne "missed an opportunity to really use Sophia's interests and be truly child-centred" arguing that even more might have been done with the Kazoo to encourage her speech.

> It seems to me that Sophia, when feeling comfortable, was happy to use speech. I was a little sorry that the therapist didn't continue the work with the kazoo, because [...] Sophia demonstrated how much speech she had using the kazoo; and given what we know about ASD and the

> specialised interests that even young children on the spectrum demonstrate, I wasn't surprised that when the kazoo wasn't being used there was less verbal engagement. (Mike)

> Music therapy should continue for Sophia but at an advanced level. She needs to be coached by someone who will nurture her musical talents. She should be in a gifted and talented programme as I think her mind needs to be stimulated and she needs to be challenged. [...] The tasks set out for Sophia were simple and I think she would've advanced significantly if she was challenged [...] I would suggest Sophia has the potential to be an accomplished musician and using music as a vehicle will certainly lift her confidence and encourage her to socialize with people other than her immediate circle (parents/family). (Dana)

Nevertheless,

> This case study had clear measurable goals that helped to demonstrate the progress Sophia made over the course of the music therapy [...] Towards the end of the therapy Sophia was showing increased eye contact and reciprocal play and there was evidence to suggest that she was beginning to generalise some of those skills into other contexts in her life. (Freyer)

Integration of Findings from Descriptions and Sophia's Questionnaires

While video was not able to be included with this case study, the description was rich enough for Sophia's grandmother to spontaneously write "I can picture most of the things described in the report." All commentators noted that the narrative demonstrated that Sophia made important and positive progress in her interpersonal communication with the therapist. They agreed that she was clearly developing skills that would help her learn, that music and the way the therapist facilitated the sessions were both important factors, and that music therapy was important for Sophia overall.

However, while most commentators felt there was evidence of progress towards the initial referral goal "to support speech development," Mike and Dana both thought more could have been achieved. As Mike argued, Sophia was already verbal, so perhaps the goal may have been to increase speech output and was not well expressed. Interestingly, Lianne had noted that "fostering social interaction and fundamental communication skills might provide Sophia with confidence to explore her verbal language." In contrast, it seems that Sophia's enjoyment of the non-verbal musical interaction might have delayed motivation to use verbal communication, in the music therapy setting at least.

Nevertheless, Dana argued that progress was slow and that the music therapy programme might have included some more direct challenges for Sophia. She went as far as suggesting that Sophia might benefit from a "gifted and talented" programme, but this seems like a bold statement to make given that no video material accompanied the study. Similarly, with no video material to view, and her perception that Sophia's engagement and confidence was increasing, it was surprising that Dana suggested Sophia was not necessarily enjoying the music therapy interaction.

Mike also suggested that lack of information regarding Sophia's cultural background may have influenced commentators' perceptions of the case. This and his perception that she could have been more overtly challenged, might also explain why he disagreed with the statement that music therapy interaction would have been meaningful for Sophia.

Music Therapist's Summary

Lianne summarised that Sophia demonstrated steady progress in her ability to engage in shared play (to share, take turns, and negotiate). In music making she learnt to lead and to follow; to imitate, reciprocate, and express herself. Her vocal confidence increased, and she began to say single words, eventually adding words to familiar songs, and singing simultaneously with the therapist. Over the period of the therapy Sophia demonstrated reduced need for control both within and outside of sessions. She appeared to experience herself as an able communicator.

My Reflections on Sophia's Case

The case of Elijah, presented in chapter twelve, demonstrates how music therapy can support takiwātanga to develop conversational vocalisations. In contrast, while she was reluctant to talk, Sophia began her therapy with a sophisticated ability to communicate through sound and to confidently engage in non-verbal conversations, particularly when using a musical instrument other than voice.

The playful ways Lianne facilitated the sessions, including returning to activities that promoted non-verbal communication, such as kazoo conversations and the conducting game, drew on Sophia's creativity and humour, ensured that she remained confidently involved, and, as Vivian noted, more aware and trusting of her own abilities. Eventually she gained the confidence to talk to Lianne in music therapy sessions. Sophia's mother was convinced that the creation of a safe and playful environment where Sophia felt able to explore and experiment with sound, without pressure to perform in a particular way, was a "natural approach" that underpinned the progress she made in using verbal language. And she was surprised and delighted by this outcome. On the other hand, Dana and Mike seemed to have less patience with this approach, suggesting that it might have been helpful to challenge Sophia more directly with speech goals, even if, as Mike suggested, the focus continued to include playful interaction using the kazoo.

Takiwātanga frequently experience difficulties with verbal language, especially with the use of pitch (prosody), using language in plausible ways (pragmatics) and understanding the meaning of words, signs, or sentences (semantics) (Lim, 2009). However, they appear to be able to receive linguistic information more readily when it is embedded in music, and in turn to use this information to develop speech (Lim, 2009, 2010). The "cognition of music is far less neurologically demanding than the processing of language, and is a developmental precursor" (Ockelford, 2019, p. 670). Sophia was able to communicate musically, playfully, and expressively varying her use of dynamics, rhythm, pitch, and duration, until she was confident enough to "talk" into the kazoo. Eventually she was verbalising within sessions, introducing a word for every letter of the alphabet, prompted by letter names of xylophone.

These outcomes strongly support Amelia Oldfield's (2018) argument that the kazoo is effective with tamariki takiwātanga because they are easy to play and provide opportunities for the therapist and child to interact on equal terms; the exchanges are often humorous, leading to shared laughter; therapist and child use their voice in expressive ways without relying on language; and they promote interactive spontaneity (p. 126).

Great variability exists in terms of tamariki takiwātanga's communication, language, and speech abilities, with each child presenting a unique clinical profile, and it is crucial to know the child well before specific goals are decided (Dromi et al., 2018). In Sophia's case, it seemed her paucity of speech may have been related to anxiety or lack of confidence. By focussing on supporting her interpersonal or socio-communication, i.e., her engagement in shared and reciprocal play, Lianne was not only taking time to come to know Sophia but helping her to develop skills that underpinned maintenance of social relationships and verbal language development (Paul et al., 2015). "When we learn language, the music of speech comes first. [...] Language acquisition thus lies at the crossroads of music and language" (Brandt et al., 2019, p. 583). It can be argued that Lianne was using Sophia's natural affinity for music and rhythm-based tasks to motivate her to use her voice in music therapy, and in turn to develop skills with sung and spoken language. Providing an environment where Sophia could draw on her creativity and humour, to develop self-regulation which can in turn lead to persistence and resilience, was viewed as an entirely credible endeavour.

Dana made the positive suggestion that Sophia's musical talents might be nurtured, with a view to her becoming an "accomplished musician." Many takiwātanga have described ways in which music has not only mediated their challenges but enriched their lives (Bakan, 2018; Farmer, no date). Music making can provide an alternative channel for expressing ideas and emotions that cannot be otherwise expressed, enable connections with people with whom one would otherwise never have connected, and lead to lifelong friendships (Farmer, no date). It can help takiwātanga to "be in the world more" (Grace, in Bakan, 2018, p. 81), "a hobby and a powerful stress relief when needed" (Gibson, in Bakan, 2018, p. 131) or "a welcome refuge from the interpersonal engagements that (have to be) endure(d) in the outside world" (Rindale, in Bakan, 2018, p. 45). Rindale explains, "the music did not laugh, or judge, or make nasty comments, or quizzical facial expressions and gestures at the sight of some unexpected behavioural tendencies, among other things" (p. 45). Farmer (no date) is convinced that his gradually increasing comfort and confidence in connecting with other people in social situations can be attributed to his continual involvement in performing and composing music, and that other takiwātanga are experiencing the same benefits. Being a musician can be just as much a part of one's identity as being takiwātanga and, as, performers and collaborators, autistic musicians can give significant pleasure, support, and knowledge to others.

References

Bakan, M. B. (2018). *Speaking for ourselves.* Oxford University Press. https://doi.org/10.1093/oso/9780190855833.003.0005

Brandt, A., Slevc, L. R., & Gebrian, M. (2019). The role of musical development in early language acquisition. In D. A. Hodges & M. Thaut (Eds.), *The Oxford handbook of music and the brain* (pp. 567–597). Oxford University Press. https://doi.org/10.1093/oxfordhb/9780198804123.013.23

Dromi, E., Rum, Y., & Florian, J. G. (2018). Communication, language, and speech in young children with autism spectrum disorder (ASD). In A. Bar-On, D. Ravid, & E. Dattner (Eds.), *Handbook of communication disorders* (pp. 811–828). De Gruyter Mouton. https://doi.org/10.1515/9781614514909

Lim, H. A. (2009, Sep). Use of music to improve speech production in children with autism spectrum disorders: Theoretical orientation. *Music Therapy Perspectives, 27*(2), 103–114. https://doi.org/10.1093/mtp/27.2.103

Lim, H. A. (2010). Effect of "Developmental Speech and Language Training Through Music" on speech production in children with autism spectrum disorders. *Journal of Music Therapy, 47*(1), 2–26. https://doi.org/10.1093/jmt/47.1.2

Ockelford, A. (2019). The neuroscience of children on the autism spectrum with exceptional musical abilities. In D. A. Hodges & M. Thaut (Eds.), *The Oxford handbook of music and the brain* (pp. 671–695). Oxford University Press. https://doi.org/10.1093/oxfordhb/9780198804123.013.31

Oldfield, A. (2018). Humour, play, movement and kazoos: Drama in music therapy with children and families. In A. Oldfield & M. Carr (Eds.), *Collaborations within and between Dramatherapy and Music Therapy* (pp. 113–128). Jessica Kingsley Publishers.

Paul, A., Sharda, M., Menon, S., Arora, I., Kansal, N., Arora, K., & Singh, N. C. (2015). The effect of sung speech on socio-communicative responsiveness in children with autism spectrum disorders. *Frontiers in Human Neuroscience, 9*, 555–555. https://doi.org/10.3389/fnhum.2015.00555

14

BEN—Play, Pretense, and Performance

Background

Ben was a 5-and-a-half-year-old Pacifika (Cook Island / Māori / Samoan) boy who was very interactive, communicative, and curious. He reportedly had speech and language difficulties, but initiated conversations and shared thoughts and feelings during music therapy assessment sessions. Ben preferred to engage in games that were familiar to him, was inclined to follow others rather than lead, and experienced what was described as "afternoon burnout" after trying to "fit in" with peers at school. He has a diagnosis of Global Developmental Delay as well as ASD.

His music therapist, Annabelle, was an established therapist in this context. She employed a child-centred and improvised approach in her work. Music therapy was provided weekly, for 12 months. Sessions were held in a community centre, and the initial goal was to increase Ben's confidence in leading and responding and to help him to become more self-expressive.

D. Rickson, *Music Therapy with Autistic Children in Aotearoa, New Zealand*, https://doi.org/10.1007/978-3-031-05233-0_14

The Music Therapy Process

The first example opens with Ben asking Annabelle if she knew the song "Remember Me" (Anderson-Lopez & Lopez, 2017) from the movie Coco (Unkrich, 2017). He said he wanted to play the song "right now!" like Miguel who is the guitarist in the movie. Annabelle found the score and began to sing, accompanying herself at the piano while Ben strummed the guitar. After just a few seconds, Ben stopped playing. Annabelle continued singing, conveying her interest and enjoyment of the song, and Ben rejoined, playing what sounded like a well-formed musical chord. Annabelle introduced melody in lieu of playing chords, to give Ben the sense that he was accompanying her on the guitar.

> Annabelle noted that this was the first time Ben had initiated a musical idea.

In the next example Ben asked Annabelle whether she knew of the movie "Rampage" (Peyton, 2018). Ben had seen it recently and talked excitedly and passionately about the "gorilla, alligator and the wolf." As he described it, he drew a picture of a big animal on the board he had brought with him. He also depicted the appearance of the gorilla in the movie by drawing it in the air with his finger as Annabelle reflected the image with heavy and loud chords on the piano. When she asked Ben to tell her the story, he beat his chest saying, "The gorilla was mad." Annabelle sang his words, accompanying with music which conveyed madness and anger. Ben continued to beat his chest before introducing a throwing action. After confirming that the Gorilla "threw everything" he shared that the alligator was "mad" too. When Annabelle reflected "poor alligator" Ben corrected her, reinforcing that he was "mad." Throughout, Annabelle actively listened and watched his actions, creating music that was congruent with his story and movements.

Annabelle noted that it was significant that the activity was based on his idea, and that he was able to both lead and respond the dynamic interaction.

In the third description Ben introduces "New Rampage" to tell a different story. In it "the gorilla, the alligator and the wolf" are still present, but they are "destroying the city" and "destroying the people and the soldiers." As Annabelle began to set the mood for the new story Ben joined her, playing in time on his drum. He suddenly decreased the volume and looked at her as if he was asking her to follow him. As their music subsided, she asked him what happens next. Ben described the characters "climbing up the giant tower" on their "claws." As he talked, he enriched his story with actions. When he heard Annabelle begin to sing his lyrics, he looked at her with glaring eyes, and depicted the action of climbing by playing the drum gradually louder and faster. Annabelle followed the extreme changes in his speed and dynamics with her music.

The next example begins with Annabelle playing the Jurassic Park theme (Williams, 1993) on the piano. As she played Ben began tapping the rhythm on the castanets. Then he chose to play the melody on the kazoo. Annabelle continued to accompany him, and the music became gradually more adventurous. Variations on the theme led to increasingly colourful improvisations as they adjusted their playing to each other to create a shared piece of music. At one moment Ben picked up the horn and, deliberately holding it the wrong way, blew it. The pair looked at each other and giggled, appreciating his humour, before Ben reintroduced the theme on the kazoo.

In the fifth example Ben seemed interested in the songbook—Animal Boogie (Penner, 2011). He began to speak the lyrics of the song into a microphone, saying "it's a bear" or "monkey." When he heard his voice, he smiled excitedly. After singing three words of the chorus ("shake, shake, Boogie") he suddenly stopped. He seemed to lose confidence but continued to hold the microphone while making long "ah" sounds and saying short words. Annabelle continued to support him by playing the song, giving him as much as time he needed to tentatively express himself using the microphone. Eventually he began to sing the chorus again, repeating the word "shake" continuously and for a long time. He then blew the horn into the microphone and became very excited to hear the sound. Annabelle improvised lyrics to invite him to continue. He blew again, enjoying sharing the funny sounds he discovered. He laughed a lot as he contributed to their interactive music making.

Commentators' Interpretations of Ben's Case

Commentators suggested Ben showed development in his abilities to engage with others (Freyer), to actively listen (Freyer) and to use initiative (Ruella). They were impressed with the way in which the music therapy process could be used to bring Ben's imagination to life through the medium of music, song, and dance (Dana, Ruella) and to safely explore using humour in his interactions (Freyer). "There is strong evidence of him actively listening and determining the course of his interactions with Annabelle" (Freyer). He became "freer in his expression, increasingly leading the musical interactions" (Ruella).

> (In the latter sessions) Ben interacted in ways like any other child would do and (this) was a vast improvement to the interactions he demonstrated in the first story. It was clear that he was making rapid progress towards the goals and the intuitiveness and wide-ranging repertoire of Annabelle was very evident in this case study. It was not only the interpersonal interactions, but Ben's musical interests also seemed to be taking big strides. (Vivian)

> As the sessions progressed there was definite evidence of Ben's increased listening and involvement in activities. The altered volume of the drumming in story three in response to his narrative appeared to help him gain confidence [...] his actions appeared to be interactive and responsive as well as deliberate. (Freyer)

> Ben has developed essential leadership skills, developed another way to engage with people and another way to communicate where he

> doesn't have to communicate verbally. He has also gained confidence to communicate with other people other than his own family. (Ben's aunt)

"Over the course of the therapy a tremendous amount of learning and development was demonstrated (in terms of) increased confidence in leading and responding, trust and security" (Mike). Ben's mother argued that the non-judgemental and child-centred nature of the music therapy space, where he could focus on his interests, was crucial to this developing confidence. Ruella agreed:

> The musical excerpts showed Ben attuned with Annabelle, where they played together, listening, and responding to one another and matching pitch and tempo. In the final learning story, Ben showed clear enjoyment in using the microphone to play a horn and to speak and sing a little [...] this demonstrated an increase in his confidence to express himself. (Ruella)

Initial videos showed a rather tentative child who is interested in but wary of the instruments on offer, but Ben gradually develops confidence as Annabelle works hard to find what motivates him (Hilda). By story five he had become quite comfortable with the physical proximity of Annabelle (Freyer, Vivian), was making good eye contact and vocalising more (Freyer), and demonstrated a very trusting relationship with Annabelle (Ben's aunt, Freyer, Mike, Vivian). "Increased musical mutuality was very much in evidence and again demonstrated his improving active listening skills. [...] He was willing to take more risks because he felt he was in a safe space and relationship" (Freyer).

> Music therapy became a safe space for Ben to 'be himself', engage in interactive play in a way where he felt comfortable to lead the activity, initiate his own ideas, and express himself. This links with the identified goals for therapy, which were to increase Ben's confidence in leading and responding and build trust and security so that he could become more self-expressive. (Ruella)

> Once Ben has that trust or has created a relationship with someone, he tends to share what is important to him with the person. For example, the

> 'Remember Me' song is a very important song to Ben as we first watched this with his nana. [...] With him being able to share this with someone other than his family indicates that he has developed trust with his music therapist. (Ben's aunt)

Ben's mother argued that music therapy was "definitely helping him to explore his feelings and be expressive" and "to think calmly—not in an overloaded way." He would have had significant auditory and tactile feedback as he expressed himself on the drums and this likely helped him to deal with stress (Hilda). Hilda concluded "from my perspective as an outsider with a glimpse into his music therapy journey, he certainly appears to become more self-expressive" (Hilda). In the music therapy setting:

> (Ben) is temporarily removed from the stress caused by his peers and has the full focus of a skilled and attentive adult [...] Music therapy is very valuable for tamariki takiwātanga like Ben as it provides a little oasis of positive one-on-one therapy that is enjoyable and sensory in a positive way without any problematic peers or puzzling school routines. (Hilda)

Ben gained a new perception of himself as someone who could express himself through music (Ben's mother). He has an interest in music, and he is very good at singing so music therapy helped increase his confidence (Ben's aunt). Ben's aunt went on to say, "music is a portal where he can channel his inner thoughts and emotions and express them freely" so it is "vital in his development as an individual." His auditory and musical abilities are resources that can be used to develop turn-taking and cooperation with peers (Freyer).

> Ben's family understand that it is very difficult for him to communicate with others, to connect with others and to trust others. [...] After watching the videos, I felt emotional, happy and a sense of relief. The reason for this is that kids and people on the autism spectrum are treated differently in society and for a stranger to take interest in Ben's development is heart-warming. (Ben's aunt)

As can be seen in the above quote, Ben's aunt found aspects of the case "heart-warming" while others found it "enjoyable" (Dana, Mike), "pleasurable" (Freyer), and "lovely" (Hilda) to watch. Annabelle "created a fun environment, was energetic and creative" (Dana); and "flexible, responsive and attuned to Ben" (Ruella); to "enable Ben's unique personality to emerge as he gained confidence" (Freyer). His mother was proud and full of aroha (love) as she watched her son lead the conversation at music therapy—"the world through his lens." Freyer argued that Ben's story "really showcased how effective music can be as a conduit for helping takiwātanga to build a social connection and begin to have confidence to work collaboratively with a trusted partner" (Freyer).

Integration of Findings from Descriptions and Ben's Questionnaires

This was an uncomplicated case with all commentators agreeing that Ben made timely progress towards appropriately determined goals. They agreed that he seemed positively engaged in meaningful interaction and was enjoying himself while developing skills that would help him learn. There was unanimous agreement that the way Annabelle facilitated this interaction was important. There was also unanimous agreement that music therapy was important for Ben, overall. This is reinforced by the qualitative data which describes significant progress in terms of developing relationships, confidence, and self-expression.

> Ben really stood out for me as a student for whom music therapy was indeed a very useful form of intervention. (Vivian)

Music Therapist's Summary

Annabelle suggested Ben's music making moved from 'restricted' to become more dynamic, expressive, responsive, and joyful. As he developed confidence he began to share thoughts and ideas, as well as emotions and feelings. He demonstrated determination and increasing independence; and over the period of therapy his interactions became more genuine and real.

My Reflections on Ben's Case

Music therapists often use movement, music, playfulness, and drama in sessions with tamariki takiwātanga, allowing them to take control in constructive ways (Epstein et al., 2020; Oldfield, 2006). The therapists create music that incorporates and conveys the emotion in the children's words, adding vitality to their verbal initiatives and play, and increasing dramatic effect (Epstein et al., 2020). The music fosters the child's sociodramatic or imaginative play, creates meaning, enhances connections, and understandings between the therapists and children, and nurtures verbal expression (Epstein et al., 2020).

Ben's music therapy sessions were strongly imaginative and dramatic, focussing on his interest in enacting scenes from his favourite movies. In the first vignette he was able to play the guitar and imagine himself as the guitarist in the movie. In the second he began by talking excitedly and passionately about a movie plot, drew pictures on a board and with his finger in the air, before engaging in dramatisation, embodying the protagonist gorilla. Annabelle encouraged and supported by accompanying with strong and loud chords, signifying the heaviness of the gorilla and his powerful chest pumps. She continued providing musical and emotional attunement as he enacted madness and anger, and when Annabelle tried to contribute an idea, Ben was able to assert himself, correcting her to ensure that *his* story was sustained.

Annabelle's scaffolding of the musical interaction (Geretsegger et al., 2015) was giving him agency to engage in highly expressive dramatic play. Her musical responses helped Ben to "create a continuous narrative [...] (of) creative, verbal, or dramatic play-plots" (Epstein et al., 2020, p. 83). As Annabelle created musical motifs to support Ben's expressions the pair were beginning to develop a repertoire of collaborative experiences, or a "shared musical history" (Geretsegger et al., 2015, p. 271). In the subsequent session Ben was not only motivated to continue this work but also began to illustrate the story with his own drumming. During this process, loud and energetic music that accompanied stories of dangerous and disruptive animals eventually gave way, albeit fleetingly, to steadier more organised "climbing." Later, still drawing on the themes that Ben has introduced, Annabelle is able to take more of a lead. Ben is able to join her using range of musical instruments and, without escalating the theme to dramatic, potentially uncontained, heights, was able to create "adventurous" music to complement their colourful collaborative improvisation.

The synchrony and timing of attuned interaction, supports the child's ability to regulate and enables them to maintain optimal levels of affective involvement (Nind & Powell, 2000; Stern, 1985). For example, Mossler et al. (2013) describe work with tamariki takiwātanga which begins with the child demonstrating physical aggression towards his therapist. While needing to physically protect herself initially, his therapist was eventually able to take over and attune to the high level and quality of his affect by screaming dramatically and singing his name, with glissandos. The child was intrigued and began to laugh while looking at the movements of her mouth, and they were eventually able to engage in playful musical, including vocal, interaction (Mossler et al., 2013).

Channelling emotions into songs can help takiwātanga to "get feelings under control," "come to terms with reality," and "find peace of mind and inner strength through alternative emotional release" (Farmer, no date). His mother noticed that Ben was beginning "to think calmly—not in an overloaded way." He began to use his voice to "sing," contributing lyrics and sounds of pre-existing works. While he was still somewhat self-conscious, it seems significant that Ben is now able to be himself, communicating directly rather than through a fictional persona. As his mother noticed, he not only "gained a new perception of himself as someone who could express himself through music" but gave others a glimpse into "the world through his lens." This adds support to Thompson's assumption that within "attuned, musical-play space, there are opportunities for developmentally rich learning experiences" (Thompson, 2018, p. 34).

Thompson (2018) also describes work with a 6-year-old child who had excellent verbal skills, which had a very similar trajectory to Annabelle's work with Ben. "Joey" only fleetingly used musical instruments, preferring to express himself through movement, action, drama, and storytelling. Like Annabelle and Ben, Grace and Joey were engaged in dramatic role play, "as if (they) were collaborators in a musical theatre production" (Thompson, 2018, p. 33). In each improvised session, themes and motifs from previous sessions would reappear. However, in Joey's case he began to bring real-life events into their storytelling, while Ben began to ease out of the dramatic play and into the real world.

Play, pretence, and "performance" are particularly important for tamariki takiwātanga. Physical gesturing and gesticulating alone are important in the development of thinking and talking, while dramatic play can develop self-awareness, empathy, understanding, and togetherness (Neelands, 2009; Trowsdale & Hayhow, 2013).

> Playing is what we all do as children, pretending is in essence at the heart of empathy—imagining what it is like to be in someone else's shoes—and performing is being conscious of being witnessed doing something in front of another. [...] The person, like the actor in rehearsal, is sensing what it is like to be in another's shoes; they are exploring other versions of themselves using instinct and body, never truly losing themselves. The significance for the person, especially one with a learning disability, is that the sense of 'me in another state of being/feeling' awakens awareness of what more he or she is capable of. (Trowsdale & Hayhow, 2013, pp. 74–75).

References

Anderson-Lopez, K., & Lopez, R. (2017). Remember me. In *Coco (Original Motion Picture Soundtrack)*. Walt Disney.

Epstein, S., Elefant, C., & Thompson, G. (2020). Music therapists' perceptions of the therapeutic potentials using music when working with verbal children on the autism spectrum: A qualitative analysis. *The Journal of Music Therapy, 57*(1), 66–90. https://doi.org/10.1093/jmt/thz017

Geretsegger, M., Holck, U., Carpente, J. A., Elefant, C., Kim, J., & Gold, C. (2015). Common characteristics of improvisational approaches in music therapy for children with Autism Spectrum Disorder: Developing treatment guidelines. *Journal of Music Therapy, 52*(2), 258–281. https://doi.org/10.1093/jmt/thv005

Mossler, K., Gilbertson, S., Kruger, V., & Schmid, W. (2013). Converging reflections on music therapy with children and adolescents: A collaborative seminar on diverse areas of music therapy practice and research. *Voices: A world forum for music therapy, 13*(2). https://doi.org/10.15845/voices.v13i2.721

Neelands, J. (2009). Acting together: Ensemble as a democratic process in art and life. *Research in Drama Education, 14*(2), 173–189. https://doi.org/10.1080/13569780902868713

Nind, M., & Powell, S. (2000). Intensive interaction and autism: Some theoretical concerns [Article]. *Children & Society, 14*(2), 98–109. http://helicon.vuw.ac.nz/login?url=http://search.ebscohost.com/login.aspx?direct=true&db=a2h&AN=12063702&site=ehost-live

Oldfield, A. (2006). *Interactive music therapy: A positive approach*. Jessica Kingsley Publishers.

Penner, F. (2011). *Animal Boogie*. Barefoot Books.

Peyton, B. (2018). *Rampage* Warner Brothers.

Stern, D. N. (1985). *The interpersonal world of the infant*. Basic Books Inc.

Thompson, G. A. (2018). Dramatic role play within improvisational music therapy: Joey's story. In A. Oldfield & M. Carr (Eds.), *Collaborations within and between Dramatherapy and Music Therapy* (pp. 31–51). Jessica Kingsley Publishers.

Trowsdale, J., & Hayhow, R. (2013). Can mimetics, a theatre-based practice, open possibilities for young people with learning disabilities? A capability approach. *British Journal of Special Education, 40*(2), 72–79. https://doi.org/10.1111/1467-8578.12019

Unkrich, L. (2017). *Coco* Walt Disney Pictures.

Williams, J. (1993). Jurassic park theme. On *Jurassic Park*. MCA Records.

15

"LUCAS"—Feelings Are Very Confusing

Background

Lucas was a 6-year-old boy who had good cognitive skills and was competent with speech and language, reading, and maths. However, his fine motor skills were underdeveloped and as a result he had difficulty handwriting. He experienced proprioceptive dysregulation as evidenced by his seeking of deep pressure. Lucas struggled to pay attention, was anxious, needed to maintain control, had difficulty managing change, liked rules, and wanted to be "perfect." He experienced complex family dynamics and had limited interaction with peers. As a result, perhaps particularly of his sensory experiences, he would sometimes express himself loudly and forcefully and was seen to be oppositional.

His music therapist, Rachael, was an "established therapist" in this context. She had worked for seven years in school and centre settings and with five tamariki takiwātanga. She employed a playful, semi-structured, child-centred approach which involved the use of precomposed songs and music, as well as verbal interaction. Music therapy sessions were held mostly weekly, in the school library during term time, and at home during holidays. The agreed goals were for Lucas to improve

D. Rickson, *Music Therapy with Autistic Children in Aotearoa, New Zealand*,
https://doi.org/10.1007/978-3-031-05233-0_15

his fine motor skills using musical instruments; to play alongside peers and learn to take turns, to recognise his feelings, and to manage them appropriately.

Lucas had two teachers, both of whom commented on his case. In the following paragraphs they are identified as Teacher Chris and Teacher Diane.

The Music Therapy Process

The first example begins with Lucas picking up a shell horn and blowing it, before saying “it sounds like the Titanic!” He then found a book of boats from the library shelves. Rachael began to sing “Under the Sea,” inviting Lucas to identify and name the sounds of sea creatures pictured in the book. While previously he would ask her to stop, he allowed her to sing and joined with a whale sound. However, when she asked him what sound the Dolphin might make, he suddenly became very quiet. With further prompting he suggested the request made him “nervous.” When Rachael attempted to reassure him with “we can’t know everything,” he became less anxious, even smiling and laughing. However further talk highlighted the difficulties Lucas had with understanding feelings when at one point he declared “onions make you sad because they make you cry.”

In the second example Rachael and Lucas are improvising. Lucas’ music, like his speaking voice, was often loud. As Rachael played loud and soft sounds on the chimes Lucas began to imitate the volume saying the words “LOUUUUD and soft.” When Rachael talked to him about it afterwards, she discovered he thought it was necessary to be loud to gain and maintain people’s attention. Later Rachael was wrapping Lucas in a very soft blanket, so he could “snuggle in” for their goodbye song. In this session he wanted *her* to be wrapped in the blanket, while she played live music. They began to explore sounds that might be “relaxing” or might “wake (her) up!” Lucas enjoyed this activity and giggled when Rachael “woke up!” to louder sounds. When they were packing up, he suggested there were a lot of emotions in the world and began to name some before saying “sometimes you can feel lots at once, it’s very confusing.”

Rachael surmised Lucas had begun to think about how people could 'feel' based on what they 'heard'. He also recognised that he could feel multiple emotions simultaneously, which could be confusing.

In the third example, Lucas was playing the keyboard, loudly at first. Gradually he began to introduce a variety of dynamics, first fast, and then slow, loud, soft, high, and low, while Rachael gave him the language for what he was doing. He discovered how the recording function on the keyboard worked and enjoyed listening to recordings of his creations. This enabled him to reflect on the sounds he was making, and he was taking ideas from one improvisation into the next. Lucas then asked Rachael to play him a song (something he didn't often let her do), adding that it should be something "without words." He was still and quiet as she played Fur Elise for him. He then asked to record it, and as they played it back, he climbed into her lap and told her to "snuggle up." He took several audible deep breathes and she felt his body relax.

Rachael surmised, being able to play and to understand the impact of varying dynamics and being able to ask for a song without words to help him relax, seemed important outcomes for Lucas. In addition, the use of the keyboard would support the development of his fine motor skills.

In the fourth example Lucas was keen to show Rachael that he had learnt "Jingle bells" by ear. He stayed focussed on this one task for some time. When he got a note wrong, he kept going, testing out other notes to find the right one, without getting frustrated and returning to the beginning. However, as the session was due to finish, he became quiet. When Rachael questioned him, he said "I don't want you to go." She continued "was it because you didn't want the music to finish because we were having fun?" When he answered "yes" she was able to explain that it was helpful to hear him say that. He was then able to help her to tidy up and finish the session successfully.

Rachael felt this was important because he had answered her rather than walking away. She surmised that Lucas was demonstrating the ability to regulate his behaviour, to verbalise the reason for his mood change.

Prior to the final example Lucas had continued to play by ear but still found it hard to let others play. He began the session by telling Rachael that his dad had played the piano since he was 11. He then started to play Fur Elise, something he had continued to enjoy since it had become his "snuggle in song." He played in a focussed way for 13 min, occasionally asking for support from Rachael. Suddenly he turned to her saying "How about you play? When they had finished playing, Lucas helped Rachael to pack up the room and was able to finish the session without needing his tight hug, before walking calmly to class.

Rachael noted that Lucas' invitation for her to join in, without any prompting, was important. He wanted to share, which was very different from the beginning of the year when he would ask her to "please stop" (singing/playing instruments). He was able to remain calm, without the need for additional proprioceptive feedback.

Commentator's Interpretations of Lucas' Case

The rapport between Lucas and Rachael was clear in the video clips (Vivian, Ruella). Lucas responded positively and it was clear their relationship grew at each session (Dana). Commentators were impressed by Rachael's spontaneity and her ability to think on her feet (Dana); to accommodate Lucas' sensory preferences by introducing the blanket (Ruella); to remain calm and ignore his oppositional behaviour (Freyer); and to maintain the expectation that he would help her pack up (Freyer). "I loved the very special moment between Lucas and Rachael when he eventually allowed them to play music together on the keyboard" (Freyer). Mike, who is takiwātanga, was very moved by Lucas' case.

> What a remarkable relationship! The reactions I am having to this story are incredibly strong because Lucas reminds me of me. The introduction (to the case study) reads almost word for word as a description of me when I was six. Lucas is clearly articulate and bright and the skilful use of an intervention like music therapy has potential to mean a tremendous amount, positively, as he grows into adolescence and adulthood. (Mike)

> Lucas is typical of autistic children today, who go to mainstream schools but usually with little one-on-one support. Like many other autistic children, he's bright and articulate but anxiety generated from lack of predictability and inability to control situations makes him fearful and anxious and causes him issues at school and with others. (Hilda)

Lucas was perceived to have made significant progress in his ability to regulate his emotions (Hilda, Freyer, Mike, Ruella, Lucas' mother, Lucas' teacher Chris). Music therapy gave him the opportunity to explore how different qualities of music can evoke different feelings (Ruella). He developed the ability to engage and focus for longer periods of time (Ruella) to tolerate imperfection (Freyer) to take greater risks (Freyer) and to understand and cope with negative emotions (Ruella, Lucas' teacher Chris) as well as growing confidence in talking about emotions and how he was feeling in the moment (Freyer, Ruella). Freyer was intrigued by Lucas' response to music being played to him, and the effect it had on his breathing and ability to self-calm. She suggested music therapy helped Lucas to begin to understand more about his emotional responses to auditory stimulation and recommended that music be used to help him remain calm in other contexts.

> I loved the way sound and tactile sensory information were used in conjunction with each other and was interested in Lucas' responses to the concepts of 'soft' and 'loud' sounds and the provision of the soft and secure tactile sensory input of the blanket. It was a lovely moment when he made the connection between what we hear and how we feel. His

> comment "sometimes you can feel lots at once—it's very confusing" is a perceptive observation from any 6-year-old. (Freyer)

> The use of a tactile tool like the blanket in conjunction with familiar music cues had a noticeable effect on Lucas's ability to regulate his emotions. [...] He appeared to show a greater willingness to place himself in situations where he did not need to be 'perfect' and was prepared to take greater risks. [...] As the therapy progressed Lucas showed a reduction in oppositional and challenging behaviour, particularly around transitions. He retained his preference to have control in a session, but gradually became more accepting of working with Rachael and allowing her to be more interactive. (Freyer)

Dana sensed that Lucas was a little agitated in the fourth example and noted that Rachael calmly de-escalated a potentially stressful situation by engaging in "the natural act" of listening and talking to connect with tamariki takiwātanga (Dana). Lucas' mother reported that before he started music therapy, it was very difficult to manage him when he became upset and that his abilities to be reasoned with when he was told "no" or when instructed to do something he does not want to do have "vastly increased."

> Lucas would have continued with his uncooperative behaviour to the point where he would then become destructive—he would have started to rage and probably would have thrown chairs about and knocked books off the shelf, because he could not or did not know how to identify and verbalise his feelings. (Lucas' mother)

> Early in therapy Lucas could say he felt 'nervous' when prompted, because he didn't know the answer to a question and did not want to get it wrong. [...] Later, when he was trying to learn Für Elise on the keyboard, he persisted when he made mistakes and didn't get upset. This shows development in accepting that making mistakes is okay and that things do not have to be perfect. [...] There were (also) several instances where he was able to articulate how he was feeling and discuss and reflect on feelings. Over time he became better at managing his feelings and consequent behaviour about finishing music therapy sessions. (Ruella)

"Through the course of music therapy, Lucas has gradually been able to let go of the 'total control' he had to have over everything in order for him to stay safe" (Teacher Dianne). He made important progress in managing transitions (Hilda, Teacher Chris). He became noticeably less anxious (Vivian) and generally prepared to be more social and interactive in sessions (Freyer, Hilda, Ruella, Teacher Chris) developing important social skills like turn-taking and responding to direction (Mike, Teacher Chris, Teacher Dianne). His teacher, Dianne, reported he is no longer leaving the classroom without any explanation and is returning to class after breaks with less supervision.

> (Lucas) has repeatedly said he wants friends but did not know how to begin being part of their world and allowing them to be part of his. In class and at times in the playground he is now able to play with other children with a lot less adult support. Turn-taking has been an area where I have particularly noticed an improvement. (Teacher Dianne)

Lucas' mother also noticed that in the initial stages of therapy he tended to regress following his music therapy sessions, but he became increasingly settled and cooperative as the year progressed.

> Initially, his ability to process much after sessions would rapidly decline [...] and remain unstable for a couple of days thereafter; until about Friday (His sessions were on Tuesdays). His irritability, sensory tolerance and communication would decrease – then a few days later, a happy and more resilient Lucas would reappear. It was as if he went into regression mode to progress but would come back with massive improvements. Now, a year after the first sessions, I do not notice any regressive or stressed behaviours on "Rachael Day", only happy reports from Lucas. He looks forward to his time with Rachael and now it is almost like a recharge for him rather than emotionally taxing. (Lucas' mother)

Lucas' teacher, Chris, expressed pride in Lucas' accomplishments explaining "Lucas' social and emotion growth in 2018 was huge. It is great to look back and remember how far he has come and how these sessions have helped him" (Teacher, Chris). His mother was "filled with confidence" because Lucas was beginning to "(take) on board the necessary social and personal life skills needed… delivered and facilitated in a mode that he particularly responds to—music."

> If Lucas had not received music therapy last year, I do not think he would be in the same place emotionally and able to self-regulate as well as he can now. (He has) begun to understand that his actions can also affect other people's emotions and reactions. It has made such a massive improvement in his life and our family life in general, that we have continued with Rachael, funding the sessions privately. (Lucas' mother)

Integration of Findings from Descriptions and Lucas' Questionnaires

Commentators agreed that the music therapy process was important and meaningful for Lucas, that he seemed to enjoy the music therapy sessions overall, and that he was, considering his background, positively engaged. They agreed that the goals for him seemed appropriate and that he made timely progress towards his goals.

They also agree that Lucas was clearly developing skills that would help him learn. Vivian argued that "this was by far the most interlinked case study in relation to music therapy interventions and classroom behaviours. The learning stories clearly show the progress made in relation to the three goals (as outlined)" (Vivian). Despite this, Vivian disagreed that music therapy was important for Lucas. It seems that while she recognised the progress he made; she was unable to link it specifically to the music therapy. Rather, she felt the improvements might be attributed to the verbal exchanges Rachael had with Lucas.

> Lucas did appear to be less anxious in these sessions, and anxiety was one of the concerns in the profile provided. […] There was finger dexterity in the way he played the piano and Rachael related the transference of these improved skills to the classroom. […] However, it was hard to ascertain if there were improvements to his short attention span, being loud and needing to be in control. There were some profound learning moments described, but I was not able to make the causal link to the therapy

> per se. More seemed to come from the dialogues between Rachael and Lucas, and partly because Lucas is extremely articulate. [...] This case study demonstrates that music therapy is equally a powerful intervention even for those in the high end of the spectrum, but these students can have better outcomes, when combined with more cognitive therapeutic interventions, as the music therapist has tried to do in places. (Vivian)

Interestingly Mike recorded that he "disagreed" that the way Rachael facilitated this interaction was important. Yet in his qualitative description Mike notes that "the therapist has been skilful in thinking about the key learning areas for Lucas"; that she was "highly skilled in using music as a 'lever' to discuss and explore complex emotions"; and that "the skilful use of an intervention like music therapy has potential to mean a tremendous amount positively as (Lucas) grows into adolescence and adulthood." The considerable incongruence between data sources suggests he may have ticked a box in error.

Music Therapist's Summary

> Rachael noted that Lucas learnt verbalize his feelings and to understand emotions, and in turn to manage his emotions. From needing to be in control, he developed an ability to play alongside and to allow her to contribute; and was eventually able to work with a peer. His writing and fine motor skills also improved.

My Reflections on Lucas' Case

Music therapy is a holistic approach which invites tamariki takiwātanga to participate in activities which involve physical movement, cognition, affect, and interpersonal communication. A constant theme in music therapy literature is the importance musical attunement, which involves music therapists providing empathic and supportive musical structures to help motivate children's interaction (Geretsegger et al., 2015; Wigram & Elefant, 2009), development of sensorimotor skills (Mössler et al., 2017), and emotional responses (Kim et al., 2009).

> Although there are different approaches within the field of music therapy, therapists practicing in each methodology and approach are focused on using or working in music to help children with ASD reach their full developmental potential. These music therapy interventions allow children with ASD to experience the world in a different way, with the intention of improving their functional skills and everyday lives. (Carpente & LaGasse, 2015, p. 300)

Lucas' case emphasises the importance of the holistic approach. For example, one of his goals was to develop fine motor skills. Motor skills are important, and, in the vignettes, we read of Lucas playing the keyboard, engaging with precomposed music that would demand specific fingering, rehearsing fine motor skills as he accessed individual and clusters of notes, and varying finger pressure to create expressive dynamics. This in turn led Hilda to suggest that playing musical instruments seems to have contributed to his making significant progress with his fine motor skills. On the other hand, fine motor skills build on gross motor skills which are dependent on reliable sensory input. And it seems that the difficulties that Lucas was having with integrating sensory input on a broad scale, would be having a more significant impact on his well-being than his immediate difficulty with fine motor skills.

Some researchers emphasise the role that movement differences play in autism, and the potential for rhythm to support motor coordination, motor planning, and functional motor skill development (Hardy & Lagasse, 2013; Janzen & Thaut, 2018; Morris et al., 2021). Sharda et al. (2018) for example, argue that social communication impairments may result from disconnections in sensorimotor and cognitive functions, which are building blocks of later social skills (p. 9). So, instead of making the development of fine motor skills a specific behavioural target within sessions, support for Lucas' fine motor challenges was built into the broader therapeutic context. That is, Rachael chose to engage Lucas in child-centred music therapy, which can make use of a range of musical materials and activities while targeting not only sensorimotor integration (Mössler et al., 2017; Nordoff et al., 2007; Sharda et al., 2018) but also emotion regulation (Mössler et al., 2017). In work with takiwātanga it can be helpful to come from a position of trying to understand sensory and cognitive functions, including multisensory integration (Berger, 2002; Ronconi et al., 2016).

The ability to self-regulate, i.e., the ability to manage behaviour according to social rules, is dependent on being able to process external and internal sensory information in typical ways. It is well-known that takiwātanga often experience and process sensory input differently and are prone to under- or overreact to basic sensations such as light, sound, smell, taste, or texture (Brondino et al., 2015; Ministries of Health & Education, 2016). Many, like Lucas, have difficulty making sense of the kinesthetic, or proprioceptive, information which comes from muscles, joints, and tendons (Ministries of Health & Education, 2016).

> Motor planning relies directly on the interaction and integration of vestibular with proprioception input. When it is lacking or deficient, the autistic child has difficulty remaining stable, complying with directives, learning to write, manipulating items, and achieving other tasks involving motor planning. (Berger, 2002, p. 67)

Sensory and/or cognitive differences also contribute to and shape emotional experiences and expressions, and can limit tamariki takiwātanga's emotional insight, access to expressive verbal and nonverbal communication strategies, and their ability to gain emotional support from others (Mazefsky & White, 2014; Neuhaus, 2020). Difficulties with processing and interpreting sensory information would have wide-ranging implications for the way Lucas was viewed and for his everyday functioning. His propensity to outbursts, forceful expressions, and reported oppositional behaviour is, as his team suggests, likely to be strongly underpinned by his difficulties with understanding and naming how he is feeling.

The combination of atypical sensory processing, alexithymia (inability to identify and describe one's own emotions), and intolerance of uncertainty can lead to emotion dysregulation (South & Rodgers, 2017).

Lucas clearly had difficulty understanding what he was feeling, as evidenced in his statements "onions make you sad because they make you cry." Yet, as Freyer noted, his comment "sometimes you can feel lots at once—it's very confusing" was a perceptive observation for a 6-year-old" and according to Ruella, "over time he became better at managing his feelings and consequent behaviour." He began to "make the connection between what we hear and how we feel" (Freyer).

Over 80% of tamariki takiwātanga experience high levels of anxiety, which can be expressed through tantrums, irritability, and aggressive behaviour (Neuhaus, 2020). Their emotional responses can vary from day to day (Mazefsky et al., 2013), and, because regulatory processes are reliant on individual goals and contextual demands, their responses can also fluctuate as goals and demands change (Gillespie, 2015; Lunkenheimer et al., 2017). Lucas' mother explained that he experienced patterns of decline and improvement over time which may have mirrored the varying levels of environmental demand that he was trying to manage. However, while listening, exploring, and listening again to a range of music, Lucas was afforded opportunities to explore how the qualities of music can evoke different feelings (Ruella), and while this was likely to have been challenging for him at times, commentators observed that he was positively engaged and calmed by the music overall. The child-centred music therapy approach that valued his personality, interests, and the ways he was adapting to the world, encouraged him to try new things.

But was it all about the music? Vivian argued that "more seemed to come from the dialogues between Rachael and Lucas […] partly because Lucas is extremely articulate." Lucas' first vignette mirrors others in this series, where the music therapists have engaged children, particularly those who are verbal, in imaginative musical play according to their interests. When Lucas' horn "sounded like the Titanic" and he chose a book of boats from the shelf, Rachael was "thinking on her feet" (Dana) as she introduced the song "Under the Sea." Taking a holistic approach which included attending to his cognitive and sensory needs Rachael was able to "use music as a 'lever' to discuss and explore complex emotions" which may have, in turn, contributed to his ability to manage himself in his classroom (Teacher, Dianne, Vivian) and to make friends (Teacher, Dianne).

> The child's personality and presenting behaviours, in the moment, provide a therapist with the opportunity to view and assess specific physiologic and holistic needs leading to successful treatment. Choice, task initiation, decision-making, and individuality are prime elements in activating the child's motivation to reorganize and undertake unfamiliar things. Music elements play a role in influencing responses and behaviours. They can relax the system from physiologic or psycho-emotional stresses, opening the gates to cognitive centres. (Berger, 2002, p. 150)

References

Berger, D. S. (2002). *Music therapy, sensory integration and the autistic child*. Jessica Kingsley.

Brondino, N., Fusar-Poli, L., Rocchetti, M., Provenzani, U., Barale, F., & Politi, P. (2015). Complementary and alternative therapies for Autism Spectrum Disorder. *Evidence-Based Complementary and Alternative Medicine, 2015*, 258589–258531. https://doi.org/10.1155/2015/258589

Carpente, J. A., & LaGasse, A. B. (2015). Music therapy for children with autism spectrum disorder. In B. L. Wheeler (Ed.), *Music therapy handbook* (pp. 290–301). The Guilford Press.

Geretsegger, M., Holck, U., Carpente, J. A., Elefant, C., Kim, J., & Gold, C. (2015). Common characteristics of improvisational approaches in music therapy for children with Autism Spectrum Disorder: Developing treatment guidelines. *Journal of Music Therapy, 52*(2), 258–281. https://doi.org/10.1093/jmt/thv005

Gillespie, L. (2015, July). It takes two: The role of co-regulation in building self-regulation skills. *Young Children, 70*(3), 94–96.

Hardy, M. W., & Lagasse, A. B. (2013). Rhythm, movement, and autism: Using rhythmic rehabilitation research as a model for autism. *Frontiers in integrative neuroscience, 7*, 19–19. https://doi.org/10.3389/fnint.2013.00019

Janzen, T. B., & Thaut, M. H. (2018). Rethinking the role of music in the neurodevelopment of autism spectrum disorder. *Music and Science, 1*, 1–18. https://doi.org/10.1177/2059204318769639

Kim, J., Wigram, T., & Gold, C. (2009). Emotional, motivational and interpersonal responsiveness of children with autism in improvisational music therapy. *Autism, 13*(4), 389–409. https://doi.org/10.1177/1362361309105660

Lunkenheimer, E., Kemp, C. J., Lucas-Thompson, R. G., Cole, P. M., & Albrecht, E. C. (2017). Assessing biobehavioural self-regulation and coregulation in early childhood: The parent-child challenge task. *Infant and Child Development, 26*(1), e1965. https://doi.org/10.1002/icd.1965

Mazefsky, C. A. P. D., Herrington, J. P. D., Siegel, M. M. D., Scarpa, A. P. D., Maddox, B. B. M. S., Scahill, L. M. S. N. P. D., & White, S. W. P. D. (2013). The Role of emotion regulation in Autism Spectrum Disorder. *Journal of the American Academy of Child and Adolescent Psychiatry, 52*(7), 679–688. https://doi.org/10.1016/j.jaac.2013.05.006

Mazefsky, C. A., & White, S. W. (2014). Emotion regulation: Concepts & practice in autism spectrum disorder. *Child and Adolescent Psychiatric Clinics of North America, 23*(1), 15–24. https://doi.org/10.1016/j.chc.2013.07.002

Ministries of Health and Education. (2016). *New Zealand Autism Spectrum Disorder Guideline* (2nd ed.). Ministry of Health. https://www.health.govt.nz/publication/new-zealand-autism-spectrum-disorder-guideline

Morris, P. O., Hope, E., Foulsham, T., & Mills, J. P. (2021). Dance, rhythm, and autism spectrum disorder: An explorative study. *The Arts in Psychotherapy, 73*, 101755. https://doi.org/10.1016/j.aip.2020.101755

Mössler, K., Gold, C., Aßmus, J., Schumacher, K., Calvet, C., Reimer, S., Iversen, G., & Schmid, W. (2017). The therapeutic relationship as predictor of change in music therapy with young children with Autism Spectrum Disorder. *Journal of Autism and Developmental Disorders, 49*(7), 2795–2809. https://doi.org/10.1007/s10803-017-3306-y

Neuhaus, E. (2020). *Emotion dysregulation in Autism Spectrum Disorder* (1 ed.). Oxford University Press. https://doi.org/10.1093/oxfordhb/9780190689285.013.20

Nordoff, P., Robbins, C., & Marcus, D. (2007). *Creative music therapy: A guide to Fostering Clinical Musicianship with CD (Audio)*. Barcelona Publications.

Ronconi, L., Molteni, M., & Casartelli, L. (2016). Building blocks of others' understanding: A perspective shift in investigating social-communicative deficit in Autism. *Frontiers in Human Neuroscience, 10*, 144–144. https://doi.org/10.3389/fnhum.2016.00144

Sharda, M., Tuerk, C., Chowdhury, R., Jamey, K., Foster, N., Custo-Blanch, M., Tan, M., Nadig, A., & Hyde, K. (2018). Music improves social communication and auditory-motor connectivity in children with autism. *Translational Psychiatry, 8*(1), 231–213. https://doi.org/10.1038/s41398-018-0287-3

South, M., & Rodgers, J. (2017). Sensory, emotional and cognitive contributions to anxiety in Autism Spectrum Disorders. *Frontiers in Human Neuroscience, 11*. https://doi.org/10.3389/fnhum.2017.00020

Wigram, T., & Elefant, C. (2009). Therapeutic dialogues in music: Nurturing musicality of communication in children with autistic spectrum disorder and Rett syndrome. In S. Malloch & C. Trevarthen (Eds.), *Communicative musicality: Exploring the basis of human companionship* (pp. 423–445). Oxford University Press.

16

Findings from Questionnaires

Process

As I analysed the descriptive data provided by the commentators, I consistently referred to the findings from the questionnaires to consider whether they corroborated or contradicted my interpretations of the narratives. Each of the case studies contains a brief explanation of the relationship between the narrative and the findings from the questionnaires. However, the findings from the questionnaires were also able to answer broader questions of whether music therapy was perceived similarly or differently according to the position/lens of the observer (i.e., people who knew the child, and people who didn't know the child) and the combination of the data sets, to a certain extent, enables speculation as to why.

Each commentator was asked to note whether they "Strongly Agreed" (6), "Agreed" (5), "Somewhat Agreed" (4), "Somewhat Disagreed" (3), "Disagreed" (2), or "Strongly Disagreed" (1) to the following statements.

D. Rickson, *Music Therapy with Autistic Children in Aotearoa, New Zealand*, https://doi.org/10.1007/978-3-031-05233-0_16

1. The child made progress towards their stated individual goal
2. The child is clearly developing skills that will help them learn (Key Competencies)
3. In the light of the background provided, music therapy is important for this child
4. In the light of the background provided, the interaction would be meaningful for the child
5. The child seemed to enjoy music therapy sessions overall
6. In the light of the background provided, the child appeared positively engaged
7. The music was important in these interactions
8. The way the therapist facilitated this interaction was important
9. In the light of the background provided, the child made timely progress towards their individualised goal
10. The stated goal seemed appropriate for this child

For writing ease, in this chapter I have called the commentators who knew a child "familiar" expert, and those who didn't know a child, "other" experts. "Familiar" and "other" experts can have different opinions. For example, while mean scores suggest music therapy was rated highly in all areas by *both* groups, familiar experts rated music therapy more highly (see 16.1). In particular there was significant difference in agreement between groups with regard to questions seven (Q7) "the music was important in these interactions" [$t(9) = -2.830$, $p = 0.0197$]; and ten (Q10) "the stated goal seemed appropriate for this child" [$t(9) = -2.627$, $p = 0.0275$].

When the data was reduced to binary "agree" or "disagree," it was possible to see that all twenty-six people who knew a child (100%) agreed to a certain extent that the music was important in these interactions. Of the six other experts, four also agreed that the music was important in the interactions in all cases; while one agreed it was important in 9/10 cases and the other agreed it was important in 8/10 cases. Commentators who knew the children (familiar experts) are likely to have already been aware of the children's positive responses to music, and the affordances that brings (see Chapter 19, p. 164). However, the case studies also contain

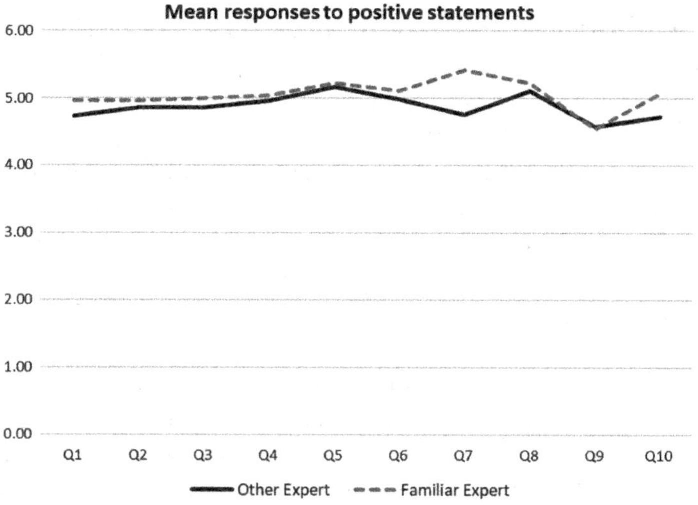

Fig. 16.1 Mean responses from questionnaires (n = 85) (1 = strongly disagree; 2 = disagree; 3 = somewhat disagree; 4 = somewhat agree; 5 = agree; 6 = strongly agree)

many examples of music therapists engaging tamariki in verbal interaction, drama, and play, as well as musical interaction. While most of the other experts were also able to see how important the music was to the interactions, at times they would have been more aware of the multiple skills the music therapists brought to the facilitation of music therapy sessions (see Chapter 18, p. 165).

Similarly, when the data was reduced to binary "agree" or "disagree," it was possible to see that all twenty-six people who knew a child agreed to a certain extent that the stated goal seemed appropriate for that child (100%). Of the six other experts, three agreed that the stated goal seemed appropriate for the child in all cases; two agreed it seemed appropriate in 9/10 cases; and the other agreed it seemed appropriate in 8/9 cases. In the few instances where the commentators could not agree the goal was appropriate for the child, it seems likely it was not stated clearly enough for them (see chapter 19, p. 144).

Viewing the Work Through Different Lens'

The patterns in the numbers highlighted three other interesting issues. Firstly, Dana, one of the "other" experts, disagreed with many of the positive statements, across cases, particularly regarding whether children were making progress towards their stated goals, in a timely way. Secondly, Vivian, also one of the "other" experts, was unsure about Emma's music therapy process, arguing that fewer and more focussed goals, within a more structured programme, might result in more specific outcomes. Both Dana and Vivian seemed to find the child-centred, flexible approaches to be somewhat chaotic at times, and indicated a preference for more organised and precise facilitation of sessions, and perceptible outcomes. This may have been because they were viewing the work through medical or educational lens', which anticipates more "measurable" developmental or academic outcomes (see Chapter 19, p. 148).

The third thing that the numbers highlighted, was the complexity and outlying nature of James' case. As noted on "Commentators' Interpretations of James' Case," commentators had considerably diverse responses to this case with five of the six expert commentators who did not know James being positive about all aspects of his music therapy, while Dana and some family members expressed considerable doubts. When examined in the context of the narrative, the findings from the questionnaires appear somewhat contradictory.

All commentators agreed that the stated goals seemed appropriate for James, and that music was important in these interactions, and family members generally agreed that sessions were well facilitated, James was positively engaged, and enjoying the music therapy sessions. His aunt agreed the music therapy process brought him "out of his shell to be able to give it a go" and his mum was impressed by his ability to stay on task during sessions which "shows just how much he was enjoying it" (James' mother).

Yet they were less certain whether he was making progress towards his goals and developing skills that would help him learn and, crucially, about how important, and meaningful, music therapy was for him overall. Three of the four people who knew James did not agree that he

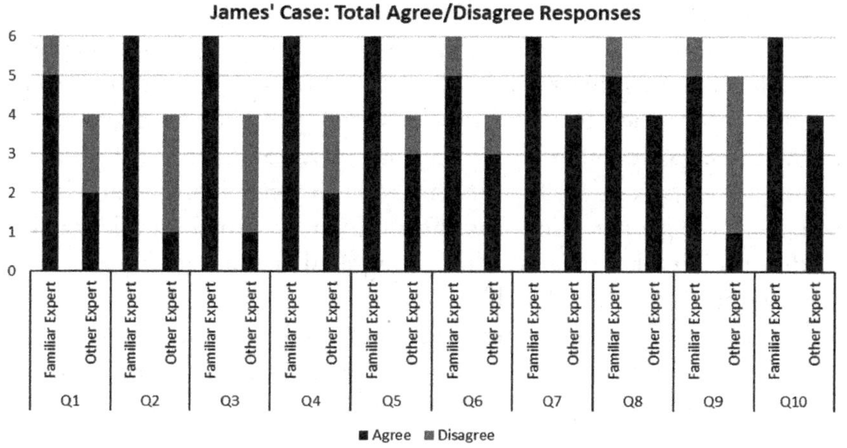

Fig. 16.2 James' case: A potential outlier with mixed agreement across eight of ten questions

was developing skills that would help him learn; that music therapy was important for him; or that he made timely progress towards his individualised goals (see Fig. 16.2). However, when the "Agree/Disagree" binary is discarded in favour of more detail, it is evident that people who knew James only *somewhat* disagreed with statements two, three, and nine.

Moreover, a major factor in how James' case was interpreted was the introduction of the medication, Ritalin. Family members tended to attribute positive change in James to the fact he was taking the medication and therefore, understandably, found it difficult to argue the positive benefits of music therapy. Further, as suggested in James' case study, family members may have had high expectations that music therapy would have a bigger impact on James' life outside of music therapy.

Summary of Questionnaire Findings

There were high levels of agreement among commentators that:

1. Music therapy was meaningful and important for the children (see Fig. 16.3).

2. In general, commentators agreed that the children made timely progress towards their individual goals, and they could see they were developing skills that would help them learn; skills that related to the key competencies described by the Ministry of Education.
3. They also agreed that the goals that were set by the music therapists were appropriate for the children. However, compared with the experts, the people who knew the children, i.e., their families or their educators, tended to more strongly agree that the stated goal was the most appropriate for the child.[1]
4. Similarly, while all commentators suggested that the music, as well as the way the therapists facilitated the interaction, was an important part of the therapy process; those who knew the children tended to put more emphasis on the importance of the music.
5. Importantly, both the expert and the familiar commentators agreed that the children were not only positively engaged but were also enjoying themselves (see Fig. 16.4).

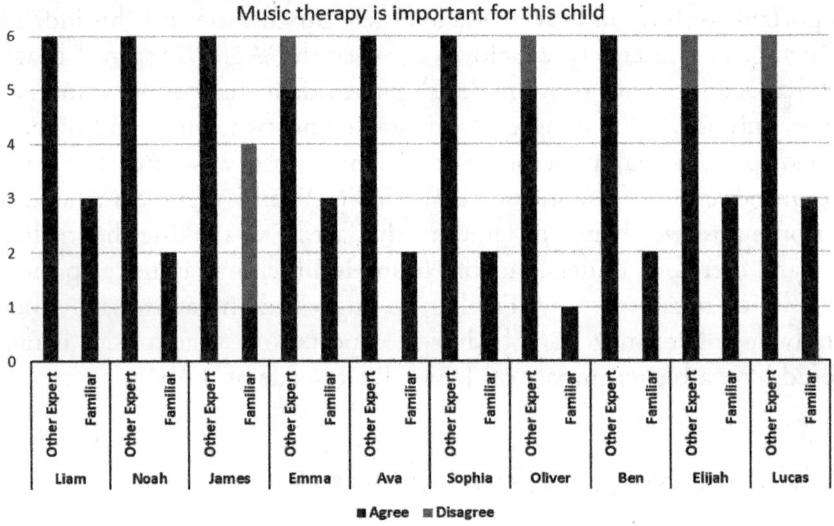

Fig. 16.3 Music therapy is important for this child

[1] "The stated goal seemed appropriate for this child". There was a significant difference in agreement between experts and those with a relationship to the child ($t(9) = -2.627$, $p = .0275$).

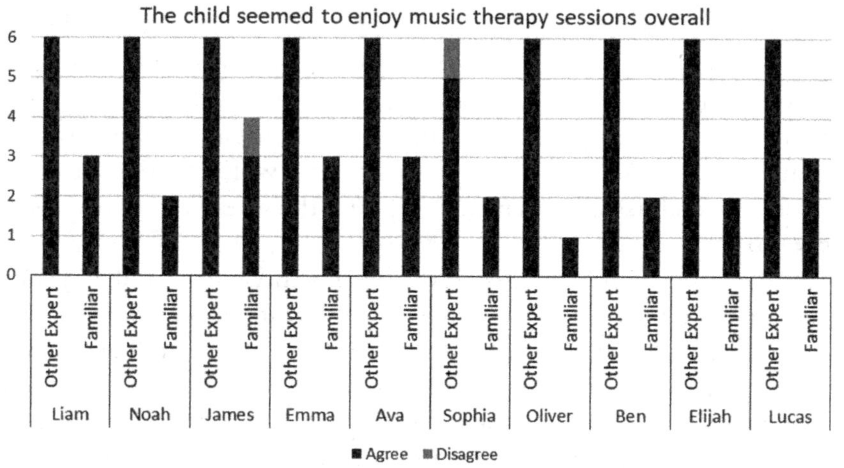

Fig. 16.4 The child seemed to enjoy music therapy sessions overall

Figure 16.4 (p. 233) shows in 83 of 85 instances, commentators suggested that the children seemed to be enjoying music therapy sessions overall. Regarding the exceptions, James' grandmother explained that there were times when he started complaining he didn't want to go to music therapy sessions anymore as it was boring. Yet all the other commentators suggested he appeared to be enjoying the sessions overall. Similarly, while Dana felt that Sophia was not being challenged enough at music therapy and "appeared reluctant to reveal her true musical potential" it was surprising that she felt she was not enjoying music therapy overall, especially when Sophia's mother claimed she "thrived in this space."

Potential Bias

Critics of case study research argue that they are a means for publicising the pre-existing assumptions of the authors (McLeod, 2010). In the current project the cases have been interrogated by thirty-two people whose pre-existing assumptions of music therapy are likely to have been extremely varied. Some, such as family members who chose music therapy for their child (e.g., parents), and others who knew a child and might support the decisions of the parents (e.g., grandparents), are likely to have begun with a positive bias. Further, with such strong positive results across nine of the case studies, it is important to also consider the impact of "acquiescence" bias, a situation in which participants tend to positively endorse all statements to please the researcher (Krosnick & Pasek, 2010).

On the other hand, in this study the potential for familiar people to feel pressure to report positively was reduced because reporting took place after the therapy had closed. Other experts were unlikely to feel pressure to report positively because they had no existing formal relationships with the researcher, families, therapists, or music therapy more widely. Some claimed to be unfamiliar with music therapy until they engaged with the project, and two were purposively chosen because they were known to be critics, unconvinced of the "scientific" value of music therapy. The high levels of agreement that music therapy was meaningful and important for the children are therefore convincing.

References

Krosnick, J. A., & Pasek, J. (2010). *Optimizing survey questionnaire design in political science: Insights from psychology*. Oxford University Press. https://doi.org/10.1093/oxfordhb/9780199235476.003.0003

McLeod, J. (2010). *Case study research in counselling and psychotherapy*. SAGE Publications Ltd.

17

Music Therapy Is Perceived to Support Regulation

From Co-regulation to Self-regulation

Self-regulation refers to our ability to evaluate and modify our behaviour, i.e., to adjust and control our energy, attention, and emotional levels, in order to participate successfully in everyday life (Loveland, 2004). Adults can help children to develop self-regulation by engaging and containing them in consistent, warm, and responsive "co-regulating" interactions (Gillespie, 2015; Lunkenheimer et al., 2017). Parents help infants to calm for example by swaddling, cooing, and rocking them, or to become aroused by bouncing, tickling, or singing to them, and drawing their attention to objects and sounds. As they grow, children typically begin to develop self-regulation, more self-control, and are gradually more able to calm or arouse themselves and to follow basic rules without direct adult support. They begin to "think for themselves," and to behave in ways that they believe they "should" behave in a particular context.

The ability to self-regulate is essential for children's learning, development, and well-being, and is especially needed if they are to successfully negotiate challenges and develop resilience in the face of adversity (Rosanbalm & Murray, 2018). The development of higher order

D. Rickson, *Music Therapy with Autistic Children in Aotearoa, New Zealand*,
https://doi.org/10.1007/978-3-031-05233-0_17

thinking, also known as executive functioning, is dependent on sensory and emotion regulation. So too is the ability to engage in reciprocal interaction, to share and take turns, to collaborate, and ultimately to socialise and develop friendships. Yet tamariki takiwātanga often have difficulty encoding, decoding, integrating and co-ordinating what they see, hear, and feel, and are therefore likely to respond in atypical ways (Berger, 2002; Loveland, 2004). They are susceptible to emotional dysregulation, which is evidenced in patterns of emotional experience and/or expression that differ in intensity and duration to the responses of same-age peers and interfere with adaptive function (Neuhaus, 2020). Many behavioural expressions of tamariki takiwātanga, including sensory seeking behaviour (such as tactile exploration) may be indications of dysregulation and/or efforts to self-sooth (Mazefsky et al., 2013).

While children are developing their abilities to manage their own thoughts, feelings, and actions with increasing independence, adults continue to provide support by recognising and responding to their cues; modelling self-calming strategies; providing physical and emotional comfort to ease distress; and decreasing demands as necessary to reduce stress and anxiety (Loveland, 2004; Rosanbalm & Murray, 2018). Supportive strategies also involve the creation of physically and emotionally safe environments which include consistent and predictable routines to promote a sense of security; and ensuring that children are aware of and supported to follow rules, using redirection, modelling, and coaching as necessary (Rosanbalm & Murray, 2018).

The reciprocal nature of music making in music therapy sessions suggests that tamariki takiwātanga and their therapists are often engaged in co-regulatory activity—that is, they mutually influence each other in their musical expressions. The therapist has a role to adjust the music in ways that will support the children to adjust their energy, attention, and levels of emotion; and give them new experiences of themselves. This in turn improves their potential to express themselves thoroughly and safely, eventually without therapist support. Commentators in this study observed that "music therapy can help children with ASD who have difficulty regulating their behaviour and emotions" (Freyer). They noticed that the structure of the music and the possibilities for repetition supported the tamariki takiwātanga, while giving them opportunities to explore, be creative, and communicate in new ways.

> Oliver's anxiety and destructive behaviours have been identified as areas of concern and music therapy appears to provide him with tools that help promote his ability to regulate. The music provided familiar patterns and repetitions that can be comforting to children with ASD. The repetition of songs and activities from earlier sessions appeared to help Oliver feel safe, especially under his blanket where he could shut out other sensory information and focus on the music and his responses to it. (Freyer)

Holistic therapeutic approaches which focus on sensory processing, movement and motor control, and synchronisation and attunement in motion and emotion, create connections that can lead to further development of social interaction and communication (Trevarthen & Delafield-Butt, 2013).

Emotion Regulation

In the cases of Noah, Oliver, James, Ava, Ben, and Lucas, emotion regulation was a primary focus, yet positive progress in the management of emotions was noted in all cases. Commentators suggested that throughout the music therapy processes, children seemed to become less stressed, anxious, annoyed, and frustrated, and increasingly able to express a range of emotions in ways that were easier for others to engage with. They learnt to compromise, to take risks, and to try new things

> I certainly see the value in music therapy in helping children [...] in reducing anxiety to reach calmness so they can connect with others by responding to and making music. From this, a possibility that the children may recognise the difference they feel from other experiences so they can reflect and develop self-awareness. (Teacher)

For example, commentators agreed Noah not only demonstrated clear improvement in his ability to calm when things did not go as he expected but also to consider the perspectives of others, to negotiate with them, and ultimately to engage in meaningful social interaction. Lucas, similarly, reportedly became less anxious and controlling and developed the ability to engage and focus for longer periods of time; to tolerate imperfection; to become more cooperative and sociable; and even developing the confidence to talk about emotions and how he was feeling in the moment. This prompted Ruella to argue that "music therapy can be an excellent way for children to build their self-confidence and practice play skills which could potentially be transferred to playing with peers in other environments"

> (The outcomes in Lucas' case) suggest music therapy may help other children with their ability to recognise and articulate their emotions and regulate their behaviour accordingly. Additionally, they may learn how music can evoke different emotions and find adaptive ways to use music to support their emotional regulation (such as listening to slow, quiet music to help calm). (Ruella)

While James' family suggested he was not always enthusiastic about attending music therapy, other commentators noticed that he appeared more comfortable and confident as sessions progressed and as his anxiety reduced. Freyer wrote, "over the course of the therapy James develops from being verbally reticent to willingly engaging in interactive communication through music. He was clearly regulating his actions in response to his therapist's musical cues."

> The use of instruments can help with emotional regulation, both as a means of communicating emotion and also in the case of wind instruments as a way to regulate breathing which can facilitate calming strategies. (Freyer)

Music therapy helped Elijah to express himself musically while inhibiting his desire to run away. He developed an ability to tolerate physical closeness, a situation that would previously have provoked stress, anxiety, or annoyance. This has had an important impact on his ability to develop relationships. Similarly, Sophia seemed more able to overcome frustration if she was not always immediately understood (Freyer), and Ben was more able "to think calmly—not in an overloaded way" (Ben's mother).

Commentators also suggested that music therapy might have helped Ava to feel less anxious, noting her decreased use of rigid speech, improved eye contact, and increased confidence in expressive use of voice. Oliver had struggled to stay on task for prolonged periods and music therapy gave him the opportunity to release anxiety through musical expression.

> The way music and tone of voice was used to help Oliver calm down and engage in structured activities shows how it is often important to use alternatives to verbal instructions to encourage cooperation from a child with ASD. (Freyer)

Sensory Integration

Sensory integration was not recorded as a goal for any of the children involved in this study, possibly because team members, and presumably music therapists, are more focussed on "emotion regulation." This might be because fearful, anxious, and aggressive behaviour—which could be the result of sensory dysregulation—is more overtly present. For example, Dana suggested "music therapy certainly has the potential to help children overcome behaviour concerns, anxiety and other underlying issues that may cause distress." Many of the "behaviour concerns" that are identified for tamariki takiwātanga can be related to the difficulties they experience with sensory integration. Takiwātanga will seek or avoid sensory stimulation to control their own sensory environment, and their responses can vary over context (Dunn, 2007). Emma's mother wrote, for example, "Emma is a very sensory child, her sensory needs tend to drive her, this means engagement for her can be very challenging as these sensory needs come above all else." And James' friend observed that in music therapy James seemed to particularly like loud sounds (and) he enjoyed the drums more than other instruments (James's Friend), whereas he may become distressed when exposed to other, especially unexpected, loud sounds.

The positive response to sound that tamariki takiwātanga demonstrate in the music therapy environment is likely, at least in part, to be because "the musical environment is a place where children can manage their own comfort levels" (Ruella). For example, as a small child Liam was always disturbed by loud noises (Aunt Amanda, Liam's grandmother) and, while his auditory sensitivity continued to be evident in music therapy (Aunt Amanda, Liam's grandmother, Mike), he seemed to "have conditioned himself to noise in the music room" and to have become "less sensitive to loud noises" (Aunt Rachelle). Family members were surprised, for example, that he seemed to be "enjoying" and "at ease" playing the cymbal (Aunt Amanda, Aunt Rachelle, Liam's grandmother). Aunt Amanda noticed that he initially seemed "quite serious while doing this activity" yet made "definite progress [...] in his ability to play the instruments (hit the cymbal/piano keys) without flinching" (Aunt Amanda).

Emma's mother and teacher also observed that individual music therapy sessions were important to enable Emma to explore the instruments and use them in her own way.

> In a large music session Emma tends to sit back and let others take over, she then tends to engage in self-stimulatory behaviour which is inappropriate. In this one-to-one situation she was able to explore the instruments and use them in her own way, her enjoyment was obvious. (Emma's teacher)

> Emma has shown a lot more interest during this time in making various sounds from musical instruments, rather than just putting them in her mouth or banging them. She has discovered a new way to play with them. When we go to the toy library, she now readily chooses musical instruments, whereas before it was difficult to get her to make a choice. (Emma's mother)

In Noah's case, while his mother argued that he still struggles when he is trying to concentrate and there is too much talking around him, or when there are sounds that can't be controlled, the sessions helped him to build up a little tolerance especially to "discordant sound." Her statements suggest Noah may also have been able to transfer his development in sensory and emotional regulation, and social skills, to wider contexts.

> I do feel that the music therapy contributed to his overall wellbeing and being able to tolerate some sensory inputs. Since these sessions he has gone to both of the boys who participated birthday parties and had a great time at both, and at each he did have a moment where he got overwhelmed (once upset at not being able to do something well, and once because the noise level in the room of very loud kids was too much for him), but was able to take himself away from the others, give himself some time, have his emotions and then return to participate when he felt ready. (Noah's mother)

Several other commentators (Freyer, Ruella, Vivian) agreed that Noah learned to use more appropriate strategies to regulate his sensory input and, like Elijah and Liam, developed an improved tolerance for noise over the period of their music therapy programmes. Similarly, Emma's teacher and Ava's family reported that sensory issues would typically have a significant impact on their abilities to engage with other people, and with cognitive tasks, yet following their music therapy programmes they were able to interact relatively freely in music sessions. Likewise, in Elijah's case:

> Music therapy, I believe, has helped him want to understand more, about what is around him. [...] I feel as though the music therapy has opened his senses which has further opened him up to more experiences (which he is) sometimes willing to share with other people. (Elijah's Caregiver)

An important contributing factor to the children's ability to manage their sensory environment was the ways in which the therapists naturally incorporated the additional sensory input the children needed, into the sessions. For example, Emma, Oliver, Lucas, and Elijah's music therapists addressed the children's tactile and vestibular sensory needs by including body movement, blankets, and a swing, in music therapy sessions. Commentators observed that throughout the time he was attending music therapy Elijah continued to demonstrate a need for vestibular, tactile and/or proprioceptive, and oral stimulation and that the use of the swing for vestibular stimulation was helpful—Elijah subsequently showed promise in tolerating people and noises. Similarly, Lucas was able to roll in a blanket when he needed to, and this enabled him to respond more easily to his environment.

> I loved the way sound and tactile sensory information were used in conjunction with each other and was interested in Lucas's responses to the concepts of 'soft' and 'loud' sounds and the provision of the soft and secure tactile sensory input of the blanket. It was a lovely moment when Lucas made the connection between what we hear and how we feel. His comment "sometimes you can feel lots at once; it's very confusing" is a perceptive observation from any 6-year-old. Lucas potentially often feels overwhelmed by a variety of sensory and emotional sensations and the recognition that these can all happen at once is a significant one that the medium of the chimes has helped him to explore. (Freyer)

In a contrasting example, when Emma was appearing to experience sensory overload and attempting to calm herself through "self-stimulation," the music therapist incorporated her physical actions into the music therapy, and the environment became "safe" for Emma (Hilda). In turn, she appeared to rely less on self-stimulation.

> Emma might be experiencing the world as an overload of sensory experiences rather than be lost in her own world or have intellectual impairment. She appears to try to control the sensory input by such activities as fingers in her ear, licking, tasting, and smelling objects, looking intently and closely, and shaking her limbs. In these music therapy sessions these actions are accepted and even incorporated into the sessions [...] indicating that the music therapy environment is safe for her. (Hilda)

Differences in organising, synchronising, and regulating sensory information not only hinder or prevent tamariki takiwātanga's development but can also feature in their unique ways of communicating and engaging with the world (Donnellan et al., 2012; Mössler et al., 2020). It seems important therefore to use the ways they interact with their environment as resources for expression, communication, and participatory sense-making (De Jaegher, 2013; Mössler et al., 2020).

Cognitive Regulation

> Children can "move from being distant and uncertain, to engaged, interactive and using communicative intent." (Emma's teacher)

Commentators suggested music therapy supported children with cognitive regulation. That is, it seemed to help them to attend, listen, concentrate, wait, turn-take, share, express preferences and make choices, take initiatives, to look for communicative clues from others, negotiate, and follow instructions. As their cognitive regulation increased some were able to engage in problem solving and other related cognitive tasks, and to demonstrate increases in expressive language. When children develop listening skills and the motivation to work collaboratively with others, they are sometimes able to demonstrate that they have more understanding than team members initially expected (Freyer). In the cases of Liam, Ava, Sophia, Ben, and Elijah, aspects of cognitive regulation were a primary focus. However, commentators also noticed important changes in James', Lucas' Noah's, and Emma's, cognitive regulation particularly as their anxiety reduced, and confidence grew.

For example, James was observed to become "quite self-directed and motivated" (Vivian). Interactions between James and Mary, his music therapist, became "more synchronised over time" as he was "listening and responding" (Ruella). There was "sustained attention" (Vivian) and his playing became more organised. Dana suggested that the narrative demonstrated James' development from being verbally reticent to willingly engaging in interactive communication through music (Dana). In Lucas' case, Dana noted that he was able to concentrate when making musical decisions, i.e., to recognise whether a pitch needed to be altered, and to make changes accordingly. While playing the piano Lucas "often corrected himself and looked to the therapist for reassurance, seemingly to see if he was on the right track." She suggested he was relying on memory, "which is common for people on the autism spectrum" (Dana).

Noah worked with peers during his music therapy sessions. In this context he was also considered to be developing skills in listening, turn-taking, and observation; with his teacher suggesting that the music therapy activities encouraged him to look for communicative (body language) cues from his partners. Similarly, Emma was noted to develop her listening (Ruella), as well as her ability to sustain attention, make choices and follow instructions (Freyer, Dana, Ruella). Freyer and Dana noticed that her confidence had "clearly" increased, which resulted in her moving from fleeting moments of connection to sustained periods of rich playful interaction (Ruella, Vivian, Dana). She was observed to be more comfortable making requests and expressing preferences, taking spontaneous "risks," and leading the direction of the therapy (Freyer, Hilda, Emma's mother). Commentators also noticed Emma's increasing expressive communication using physical gesture and her Speech Generating Device (SGD).

Commentators suggested Liam demonstrated improved cognition in the musical context, paying "keen attention to the notes" (Vivian), concentrating hard to keep in time (Liam's aunt, Liam's grandmother) and "as he progressed and gained more confidence, his music sounded more tuneful and expressive" (Liam's grandmother). As he relaxed, his confidence grew (Liam's aunt) and he was able to demonstrate his ability to listen (Hilda) take turns and wait patiently in an interactive activity (Freyer, Hilda, Ruella, Aunt); to make choices, share and negotiate (Ruella), to plan (Hilda), and to sustain concentration (Freyer, Hilda, Freyer, Ruella). His concentration was particularly evident when he was working on the CD project (Freyer) which involved him participating in a variety of tasks which engaged his logic (Hilda, Ruella). Mike also observed that it was also important that Liam could say, "I don't know" when faced with abstract choices.

Commentators noted clear evidence of Sophia (Mike, Ruella, Vivian) and Ava (Freyer, Ruella) making progress over time with their interpersonal skills. In Ava's case, as she became increasingly relaxed (Hilda, Teacher) and confident (Freyer, Dana), she was observed to offer more eye contact and her use of rigid speech decreased. She too demonstrated increased focus and engagement (Dana, Hilda, Ruella, Sophia's grandmother), improved listening, attention, and concentration, developed skills with turn-taking, and engaged in more interaction and musical collaboration (Ruella, Teacher).

Elijah appeared to enjoy his music therapy (Freyer, Hilda), which helped to reduce his anxiety (Hilda) and increase his attention (Freyer, Hilda, Mike). Specifically, he was noted to improve listening (Vivian), eye contact (Freyer), turn-taking (Freyer), and vocalisation for intentional communication (Freyer, Mike). He demonstrated "a keenness to explore" and the ability "to tolerate change" (Vivian). Moreover, "Elijah has moved on from basic echolalia to actively participating in activities like drumming and working towards the goal to become more interactive with others" (Freyer). His drumming was reportedly "impressive […] he had very good rhythm and his drumming was consistent" (Dana).

Ben too was seen to show development in his abilities to engage with others (Freyer), to actively listen (Freyer) and to use initiative (Ruella). Commentators were impressed with the way in which the music therapy process could be used to bring Ben's imagination to life (Dana, Ruella) and how he used humour in his interactions (Freyer). He became freer in his expression, increasingly leading the musical interactions (Ruella).

In Sophia's case, Ruella highlighted moments when she was making eye contact; taking turns; listening and responding; and leading and following. Hilda emphasised her development from parallel to imitative and interactional play including leading and conducting the therapist (Hilda), and Vivian her developing ease in transitioning from one instrument to the other, and her sustained attention (Vivian). Commentators also noted that music therapy had a positive impact on Sophia's developing speech and communication skills (see Communication section) and her mother highlighted Sophia's increasing willingness contribute to the music therapy play. She wrote that

> Sophia learnt to navigate the space around her, respond to her environment and to compromise with and reciprocate the therapist's attempts to interact. Sophia's ability to participate in sustained play, with a longer attention span seemed to develop over this time. (Sophia's mother)

References

Berger, D. S. (2002). *Music therapy, sensory integration and the autistic child*. Jessica Kingsley.

De Jaegher, H. (2013). Embodiment and sense-making in autism. *Frontiers in Integrative Neuroscience, 7*, 15. https://doi.org/10.3389/fnint.2013.00015

Donnellan, A. M., Hill, D. A., & Leary, M. R. (2012). Rethinking autism: Implications of sensory and movement differences for understanding and support. *Frontiers in Integrative Neuroscience, 6*, 124–124. https://doi.org/10.3389/fnint.2012.00124

Dunn, W. (2007). Supporting children to participate successfully in everyday life by using sensory processing knowledge. *Infants and Young Children, 20*(2), 84–101. https://doi.org/10.1097/01.IYC.0000264477.05076.5d

Gillespie, L. (2015, July). It takes two: The role of co-regulation in building self-regulation skills. *Young Children, 70*(3), 94–96.

Loveland, K. A. (2004). *Social-emotional impairment and self-regulation in autism spectrum disorders*. Oxford University Press. https://doi.org/10.1093/acprof:oso/9780198528845.003.0014

Lunkenheimer, E., Kemp, C. J., Lucas-Thompson, R. G., Cole, P. M., & Albrecht, E. C. (2017). Assessing biobehavioural self-regulation and coregulation in early childhood: The parent-child challenge task. *Infant and Child Development, 26*(1), e1965. https://doi.org/10.1002/icd.1965

Mazefsky, C. A. P. D., Herrington, J. P. D., Siegel, M. M. D., Scarpa, A. P. D., Maddox, B. B. M. S., Scahill, L. M. S. N. P. D., & White, S. W. P. D. (2013). The role of emotion regulation in autism spectrum disorder. *Journal of the American Academy of Child and Adolescent Psychiatry, 52*(7), 679–688. https://doi.org/10.1016/j.jaac.2013.05.006

Mössler, K., Schmid, W., Aßmus, J., Fusar-Poli, L., & Gold, C. (2020). Attunement in music therapy for young children with autism: Revisiting qualities of relationship as mechanisms of change. *Journal of Autism and Developmental Disorders, 50*(11), 3921–3934. https://doi.org/10.1007/s10803-020-04448-w

Neuhaus, E. (2020). *Emotion dysregulation in autism spectrum disorder* (1st ed.). Oxford University Press. https://doi.org/10.1093/oxfordhb/9780190689285.013.20

Rosanbalm, K. D., & Murray, D. W. (2018). *Promoting self-regulation in the first five years: A practice brief* (OPRE Brief #2017-79). https://fpg.unc.edu/publications/promoting-self-regulation-first-five-years-practice-brief

Trevarthen, C., & Delafield-Butt, J. T. (2013). Autism as a developmental disorder in intentional movement and affective engagement. *Frontiers and Integrative Neuroscience, 7*, 1–16. https://doi.org/10.3389/fnint.2013.00049

18

Music Therapy is Perceived to Improve Social Communication and Relationships

Music therapy improvisation can support communication.

Communication

Interpersonal communication occurs when people mutually influence each other during social interaction (Cappella, 1987) in their efforts to generate shared meanings and reach social goals (Burleson, 2009). However, tamariki takiwātanga often lack awareness of the emotional and/or interpersonal cues of others and are therefore unable to respond appropriately to social cues in typical ways. They may have no interest or lack the ability to influence others to develop shared meanings or achieve social goals. Markworth (2014) argues that when music therapists work with autistic people, they use "the language of music" to create unique opportunities for equal communication, shared experiences, and the development of meaningful mutual relationships. Some tamariki takiwātanga who use few or no words "have the capacity to co-opt music as a proxy language—as a fully-fledged medium of social

D. Rickson, *Music Therapy with Autistic Children in Aotearoa, New Zealand*, https://doi.org/10.1007/978-3-031-05233-0_18

interaction—and will do so given an empathetic and musically competent partner with whom to engage" (Ockelford, 2012, p. 322). In music, they can express identities, emotions, and creative freedom.

Commentators noticed that music therapists emphasise all behaviour as a form of communication (Freya) and the musical communication that occurred in sessions was sometimes described as a "language" and/or means of communication in and of itself (Freyer, Vivian). Hilda noted, "the use of words seems to be less important for many children than touching, moving or musical sounds." In Emma's case both music and dance offered important alternative means of communication and expression. "Emma is non-verbal (but this) does not impact on her ability to communicate with the music therapist" (Dana). "While she may only have made a few vocal responses during sessions, she was clearly demonstrating social-emotional reciprocity, and communicating intentionally and with purpose through eye contact, body symmetry and touch" (Freyer). Hilda argued when Lisa imitates Emma's shaking and flapping it is clearly dynamic communication. "Sometimes Emma takes the therapist's hand and uses it as a tool—an action common to autistic children who do not readily use words" (Hilda). "Emma is learning new ways to play with musical instruments, [...] interacting with the music therapist via joint attention, intentional body movements and eye contact" (Emma's mother).

> Emma's laughter was infectious. It was great to see her excitement and her anticipation when there were pauses in the music or rhythm [...]. It emphasised to me how important it is to recognise that people with ASD communicate in many ways. (Freyer)

Similarly, Sophia began by "communicating musically, playing the kazoo fluently, imitating the pitch produced by the therapist" [...] and "her expressiveness in musical (non-verbal) communication appeared to increase over time" (Ruella). Communication was a primary goal for Sophia's music therapy programme yet she "chose not to speak during most of her music sessions." Instead, she "spoke creatively, through the instruments" (Freyer), "using wind instruments as a playful way to approximate speech" (Ruella).

> Music therapy gave her opportunities to make sounds, to communicate a sound, to interact with another person, while she was still trying to find the ability/confidence to do the same with her own voice. (Sophia's mother)

Ava's teacher too reported she was "picking up skills such as pitch, singing a sequence of notes, imitating and creating rhythm; and learning to communicate with another person in a different medium" (Ava's teacher). Freyer summed up similarly explaining "music with its rhythms and patterns can be its own language, this is something that can be very effective for non-verbal takiwātanga who can communicate emotion as well as make social connections through the instruments" (Freyer). Ben's aunt argued that "music therapy has been vital in Ben's development."

> He learned to trust through music and learnt to channel his inner thoughts and emotions and express how he feels freely through music […] Through this, he has developed essential leadership skills, and developed another way to engage with people […] where he doesn't have to communicate verbally. (He) has also gained confidence to communicate with other people other than his own family. (Ben's aunt)

However, while commentators observed that the interpersonal interaction, usually musical, that occurred in music therapy was valuable for its own sake, it could also support the development of other forms of communication (Freyer, Ruella). "The playful exchanges involved in music making may support children to explore their use of voice; in singing, humming, vocalising and speaking" (Ruella) and can "potentially be used conjunction with speech therapy goals to help sound production and to help learners move from echolalia to intentional sound production" (Freyer). This is exemplified in Sophia and James cases as they both became more confident to communicate verbally as their relationship with their therapists grew (Freyer, Ruella).

> Sophia enjoyed the ease with which she was able to mimic speech sounds (with the Kazoo). […] She could explore the sounds and movement of her mouth in the pronunciation of words as she tried to communicate words clearly through the kazoo to Lianne. (Sophia's mother)

> The non-verbal quality of the music enabled James to communicate with the therapist without needing to use spoken language—interacting together in playful musical improvisations where he listened and responded. However, his use of verbal language increased over the course of therapy. Perhaps he felt more relaxed and comfortable in the music therapy setting as there was less pressure to rely on spoken language to communicate. (Ruella)

Sophia began to fill in gaps and sing along with familiar songs, used the therapist's name and asked her a question using a full sentence (Ruella). "By the end of the music therapy programme she was using much more language" (Hilda), and it seemed clear that music therapy had had a positive impact on her developing speech and communication skills (Freyer Hilda, Mike, Ruella, Sophia's grandmother). Similarly, referring specifically to Elijah's case, Freyer, Ruella, and both his parents argued powerfully that music therapy was particularly helpful for developing his vocal communication. His mother and father were extremely grateful that they were able to build on his gains, having "conversational exchanges of sounds" with him in the home setting.

> Over the course of the therapy Elijah expanded his vocal sounds and used them in a responsive way in therapy sessions. While this case study shows early emergent verbal interactions there was clearly a progression from his initial sessions to the final one where he was able to mimic sounds and turn take. (Freyer)

> He is still using a lot of babble or baby talk words when he 'talks' to me, but he has improved a lot in terms of turn taking when we do our own 'conversations'. I feel so blessed that he was able to be part of this study. (Elijah's mother)

Moreover, as noted earlier, the reduction of anxiety and the resulting increase in confidence that many children experience in music therapy can motivate them to utilise existing skills. The playfulness that occurs in musical exchanges can encourage "reluctant communicators" (Freyer).

> Ava's case shows how music therapy can be used to support children who have verbal language, but who are inhibited in its use due to anxiety or perseverating on a required response. [...] The music has its own 'language' and by responding to its rhythms and tempo through turn taking and working together to co-create songs and sounds children may feel able to take more vocal risks. (Freyer)

> I believe that other children (especially those on the autism spectrum) would benefit from music therapy because in music (especially singing), the child can expect what will happen next (sort of a routine) and will reduce the child's anxiety in communicating. I hope that other children will have the opportunity to take part in this amazing therapy to help them communicate with others. (Elijah's Father)

Assistive technology was also incorporated into music therapy sessions and was considered important in supporting communication goals (Freyer). In Emma's case, for example, Lisa set up a visual schedule, used other visual aids, and promoted her use of her Speech Generating Device (SGD). The use of the SGD enabled Emma to ask and answer questions during sessions, to demonstrate understanding, and to develop confidence in using the device, which might lead to increased use in other environments. However, Freyer also noted that the use of technology "can sometimes limit spontaneity and is not necessarily needed in all contexts" (Freyer).

In summary, some commentators valued music therapy as a "language" and/or means of communication in and of itself. Others observed the potential for it to support the development of speech and language beginning with expressive, spontaneous use of voice (Ruella) and other "early functional communication skills" (Freya); to increase communicative confidence and/or to talk with people in other contexts (Freya: Liam's Aunt, Dana, Ruella); to foster creativity, encourage social engagement, and assist language development through song (Dana). They also noted that music therapy promoted receptive communication with children developing awareness of others, improving active listening skills, and developing an interest in working collaboratively others. As Freyer suggested, their responses in music therapy can reveal that they have greater understanding than may be initially suspected.

Relationships

The Therapeutic Relationship

Commentators noticed that music therapists create trusting, secure therapeutic relationships, by providing safe spaces where children can feel comfortable to engage in play, try out new ideas, take leadership and express themselves, verbally, musically, and physically. "A trusting therapeutic relationship seemed to be a key element to the success of the therapy, and in each case, it seemed that the therapist was able to establish rapport and develop a warm and caring relationship with the child" (Ruella).

The therapists employed child-centred and/or music-centred approaches, which motivated the children's interest and ongoing engagement and enabled positive and meaningful relationships to develop. Music and dance offered important alternative means of communication and expression for the children; and the attunement and synchronisation that occurred as part of the musical relationship contributed significantly to the establishment of rapport. For example, Sophia was observed to be increasingly engaged with her music therapist as she explored the instruments and became involved in improvisation. As rapport was established and trust grew, she demonstrated improved confidence to communicate musically, as well as verbally.

Similarly, although his case was complex and involved some contradictory observations, most commentators were impressed with the immediate connection that was created between James and his therapist. Freyer argued that it was obvious, in time, that he had developed a trusting relationship with Mary that in turn gave him the agency to express his opinion, knowing that it would be listened to. "While he may not have been very verbal in the beginning, the music established early trust and his great smile was there from the start" (Freyer). His mother and grandmother, as well as other commentators (Dana, Freyer, Vivian), agreed that James enjoyed his sessions, even though he didn't always want to go. Freyer, Hilda, and Ruella were impressed by the way the developing relationship between James and Mary played out in the music making, which led to more "generalised synchronicity between them" (Freyer) and a "growing mutuality" (Ruella).

Emma's ability to engage in a variety of activities in music therapy also led commentators to suggest that music therapy was an effective way for her to begin to develop a meaningful relationship. However, the patience and intuitiveness of the music therapist, especially during initial sessions, were considered crucial to enable Emma to feel comfortable and confident enough to fully engage (Vivian). Likewise, in Lucas' case commentators suggested the therapeutic relationship was supported by Rachael's ability to think on her feet (Dana), to accommodate his sensory preferences by introducing the blanket (Ruella), and to remain calm and ignore his oppositional behaviour (Freyer). It was clear that Lucas and Rachael's relationship grew at each session (Dana) and that Emma made "demonstrable progress towards the therapeutic goals relating to building trust, developing her interpersonal communication, and working one on one" (Freyer). Lisa and Emma had a bond that "naturally leads to better engagement and more communication" (Emma's mother). Emma's mother observed that she had learnt to trust that music therapy would be fun.

Having fun was a key feature in the development of therapeutic relationships. Oliver "loved participating in music therapy and could hardly contain his excitement when Karen arrived" and Ava was seen to value her time with her therapist "because of the enthusiasm she displayed and her willingness to participate in all sessions" (Dana). Freyer witnessed the emergence of "a sense of fun and obvious trust" between Ben and Annabelle too. In Ben, the commentators saw an initially tentative and wary child who became increasingly comfortable, much more willing to take risks "because he felt he was in a safe space and relationship" (Freyer). Ben and Elijah were both observed to increase physical closeness with their music therapists. Hilda argued that Anna-Maria's playful approach was important in keeping Elijah engaged until he felt safe to interact. "Once they get to know and trust them, autistic children often enjoy the one-to-one attention of an empathetic adult" (Hilda). In Oliver and Ben's cases, their trust in their therapists was exemplified as they began to share special stories. Oliver was able to discuss things with Karen that were important to him yet not directly related to music therapy, and Ben was willing to share a song, Remember Me, that had very special meaning to him, with Anabelle.

Liam's initial responses in music therapy appeared "mechanical," and as his engagement increased the quality of relationship was "noticeably different" (Freyer). He became "at ease with Jodie" (Liam's grandmother) and the "strong connection" they had "helped capture and maintain his interest" (Freyer).

> The establishment of a successful client/therapist relationship allowed Liam to build both trust and confidence and show increasing engagement with the activities [...] He showed evidence of wanting to engage with his therapist and work collaboratively with her to try 'something new'. (Freyer)

Relationships with Peers

Even though the development of "interpersonal skills," "interaction," "social skills," "communication," "friendships," or "relationships" was important in eight of the ten cases, only Noah's sessions regularly involved peers. Peers can be helpful allies in music therapy sessions not only because their presence enables music therapists to create typical interactive music making environments but also because they can model anticipated responses (Freyer). In Liam's case, for example, the presence of his cousin in one session provided an opportunity for him to watch and learn from someone his own age.

> Peers and family members such as siblings and cousins are well placed to model preferred behaviours for children with autism. Autistic children often observe their peers very carefully, although that is often not obvious to adults. (Hilda)

Noah initially attended individual sessions, where he gained motivation and skills in relating to others, i.e., his music therapist, and the confidence to share the sessions with peers. "He enjoyed involving peers [...] and interacted positively with several partners in this setting" (Ruella). Commentators noted that he was more able to interact with others in non-verbal play, which enabled him to socialise more comfortably. He seemed to feel accepted, safe, and reassured, and more self-regulated in this context (Freyer). Commentators noticed the developing musical relationships between the young musicians (Ruella), culminating in "great interactive play. I loved how they finished together with a flourish and a great smile from Noah at the end" (Freyer).

> I feel that there would be opportunities to use music therapy to further develop social interaction skills with peers—we began to see Noah moving from playing alongside to playing together with a partner, which is an important skill for developing friendships. (Ruella)

Commentators suggested that peers might also have been involved in other cases too, if not in the sessions described, at least in future sessions. Vivian argued that "the long-term goal for any student with autism is social communication" and wondered whether another child could have joined Ben's sessions halfway through the year "to enable him to practice and generalise his learning" (Vivian). Elijah's parents were both keen for future music therapy sessions to include other children, to "teach him how to interact with children of his own age" (Elijah's mother); and Vivian felt that Lucas "may well be paired with another student to improve his turn-taking ability, but also to be able to then play alongside children in the school, which was one of the initial goals" (Vivian).

> An argument can be made for music therapy sessions [...] to be a combination of individual as well as paired or small group sessions, where children can learn in natural contexts from their peers. (Vivian)

However, while Vivian argued that it was not possible to evaluate Liam's programme of individual music therapy in the context of developing friendships, other commentators claimed the development of interpersonal skills in the music therapy room would have increased children's capacity to relate to others in wider environments. Hilda suggested, for example, that the experience of music therapy appeared to provide Liam with "a positive basis" to address his goal of developing friendships at school; while Freyer argued that Ava's growing confidence and trust in her therapeutic relationship over the course of the sessions "has potential to help Ava improve her interpersonal skills with others and become less rigid in her verbal interactions" (Freyer). Moreover, Elijah's family members were able to provide evidence that he was able to generalise his developing communication to other contexts.

> Elijah's interactions (in music therapy) have had significant positive impacts on his social capabilities. He has become more responsive to people when we talk or play with him. [...] (I can) see Elijah's progress in his gradual inclination to interact with people he is not familiar with and develop relationships further with those he already is connected to. (Elijah's Caregiver)

Further, the relationships that Noah developed with peers in music therapy were able to be fostered in other environments and, as his mother noted, he appeared to be developing genuine friendships in other contexts. "He is now socially connecting at a better level - his friends think of him and want to have him around" (Noah's mother). Noah's mother felt he would have made even more progress if peers had joined his sessions earlier.

Further discussion on the involvement of peers is provided, in the "Individual or Group Sessions."

Relationships with Family Members

"Family-centred practice" typically takes place in the home environment and focusses on supporting family members to embed therapeutic approaches into the child's daily routines (Thompson, 2012). In contrast, parents and other people who are well-known to a child can be involved in music therapy sessions to provide comfort and security, as well as enabling and modelling appropriate interactive responses.

For example, while Oliver's music therapy took place in the home setting, his music therapist, Karen, was clearly taking an "individual" approach to music therapy, directly supporting Oliver rather than supporting the family to facilitate the musical interaction. That is, while Oliver's mother was present at sessions she seemed rarely directly involved. Instead, she was a supportive presence, available to reassure and redirect him as needed, and sometimes filming the interaction between Oliver and Karen. It seemed important for his psychological well-being that she was not only physically accessible to Oliver but also that she was able to respond when he indicated he needed help. Ruella wondered whether it might have been helpful for Ava's mother also to be directly alongside, rather than engaged in other activities within the home.

> In the first learning story, it appears that Ava needed a lot of reassurance and she called out to her mother for affirmation. I wonder whether it might have been a good idea to include her mum or dad in the initial sessions as she gained familiarity with the therapist and with the music therapy sessions. (Ruella)

However, the music therapist needs to judge whether it might be more advantageous for a child to be working independently, without the support of another familiar adult. Tamariki takiwātanga are typically readily engaged in music activity, thus music therapy sessions can provide good opportunities for them to begin to work more independently. For example, Dana felt that Elijah was enjoying his sessions so much that it would have been good to see whether he could retain the same level of engagement *without* his mother's presence.

> Mum is amazing; she is loving and patient and is very much part of the session. It is clear she wants to be involved and I think it's wonderful. However, I do wonder if Elijah would be able to cope without mum being present. (Dana)

Similarly, Freyer and Hilda also questioned whether the presence of Oliver's and Sophia's mothers may have been detrimental at times. Freyer suggested "it seemed as if some of Oliver's more excitable moments also involved him seeking her reaction" and that for some tamariki takiwātanga "behaviour can escalate with their main caregiver present." Regarding Sophia, she "thought it was significant that Sophia's language 'exploded' when her mother was not present."

> This emphasises that it can often be important to have sessions without a caregiver once a child feels safe in their therapeutic relationship. Parents often unwittingly act as an interpreter for children with communication difficulties which prevents them from learning to overcome frustration when they are not easily understood by others. (Freyer)

Hilda also argued that Sophia seemed to make more progress when she was alone with Lianne.

> This is not to criticise parents, of course, but in my experience, they can have expectations or preconceptions of their children and their abilities that can be a distraction to developing a fully therapeutic relationship between a music therapist, or other professional, and an autistic child. (Hilda)

Sophia's family were Samoan, and when reflecting on Sophia's case Mike wondered whether there might be an undisclosed cultural element to the narrative "because of the continued interaction of the parents."

> I think it is really important for cultural elements to be made explicit in therapy because we know that there are cultural nuances and differences to how people understand and accept autism. It is important for therapists to be clear about those cultural nuances and for the child's interests to truly lead therapy. (Mike)

References

Burleson, B. R. (2009). The nature of interpersonal communication. In C. R. Berger, M. E. Roloff, & D. R. Ewoldsen (Eds.), *The handbook of communication science* (2nd ed., pp. 145–164). Sage. https://doi.org/10.4135/9781412982818

Cappella, J. N. (1987). Interpersonal communication: Definition and fundamental questions. In C. R. Berger & S. H. Chaffee (Eds.), *Handbook of communication science* (pp. 184–238). Sage.

LaGasse, A. B. (2017). Social outcomes in children with autism spectrum disorder: A review of music therapy outcomes. *Patient Related Outcome Measures, 8*, 23–32. https://doi.org/10.2147/PROM.S106267

Markworth, L. (2014). Without words: Music as communication for children with autism. *Qualitative Inquiries in Music Therapy, 9*, 1–42.

Ockelford, A. (2012). *Songs without words: Exploring how music can serve as a proxy language in social interaction with autistic children.* Oxford University Press. https://doi.org/10.1093/acprof:oso/9780199586974.003.0021

Thompson, G. A. (2012). Family-centered music therapy in the home environment: Promoting interpersonal engagement between children with autism spectrum disorder and their parents. *Music Therapy Perspectives, 30*(2), 109–116. http://ezproxy.massey.ac.nz/login?url=http://search.ebscohost.com/login.aspx?direct=true&db=ccm&AN=2012088717&site=eds-live&scope=site

[illegible]

19

Goal Setting and Planning in Music Therapy with Tamariki Takiwātanga

Introduction

The following paragraphs capture some of the observations commentators made about the music therapists' goal setting, planning, and timelines. Assessments which can support the development of goals, programme planning, and evaluation, are necessary as a basis for therapeutic practice (Bergmann, 2016). The music therapists who submitted data for this study were not directly asked to include information about how they assessed the children and made decisions about the goals they might work towards. However, given that none were referenced, it seems unlikely that they used specialised assessment tools such as the Assessment of the Quality of Relationship (AQR) (Schumacher & Calvet, 2007) or the Individual Music-Centered Assessment Profile for Neurodevelopmental Disorders (IMCAP-ND) (Carpente, 2014). Instead, like the music therapists in our exploratory study (Rickson et al., 2015) it seems that on receiving a referral, they engaged in a process of listening to what people think is important, aligning their wishes with what has already been documented e.g., in the learners' Individual Education

D. Rickson, *Music Therapy with Autistic Children in Aotearoa, New Zealand*, https://doi.org/10.1007/978-3-031-05233-0_19

Plan (IEP), and with broader guidelines such as the Key Competencies (Ministry of Education, 2014), and began programmes with broad goals that were refined or modified during the music therapy process. That is, they typically employed a relationship-based approach to assessment grounded in the child's ability to attend, adapt, and engage in musical play (Carpente, 2014). The goals that were eventually specified for the children were expressed in non-musical terms, which according to some theorists (Aigen, 2014b) has the potential not only to pathologise children, emphasise their (dis)abilities, and the need for remediation, but also to marginalise their perspectives and interests. However, in these cases the goals were broad, and music therapists' descriptions include examples of music-centred (Aigen, 2014a) and resource-oriented (Rolvsjord, 2010) practices which emphasise a continuous link between clinical and nonclinical musical experiences (Aigen, 2014a, p. 19).

Broad Goals

As might be anticipated, many of the goals music therapists were working on related to the diagnostic criteria for autism spectrum disorder according to DSM-V. However, Ruella suggested there was "more emphasis on fostering development in social communication (the first set of criteria) than on encouraging flexibility in terms of restricted, repetitive patterns of behaviour, interests or activities (the second set of criteria)."

> Some areas that stand out (for me) as focus areas in music therapy include encouraging social-emotional reciprocity by supporting development in initiating and responding to social interactions, promoting nonverbal communication behaviours such as appropriate use of eye contact, and fostering the development of relationships. In the diagnostic criteria for restricted, repetitive patterns of behaviour, music therapy focusses on areas related to managing transitions and supporting self-regulation regarding sensory differences. (Ruella)

Ruella went on to note:

> Broad goal areas (in these cases) tended to focus on maintaining attention and engagement, developing self-expression, using non-verbal and verbal communication skills, encouraging emotional self-regulation, and fostering social interaction skills such as sharing, taking turns, leading and following, and making choices. (Ruella)

In some cases, goals were explicitly linked to the New Zealand Curriculum Key Competencies.

> Overall, these case studies demonstrated that music therapy was relevant in terms of the Key Competencies, with goals relating particularly to the competencies of managing self, relating to others, participating and contributing, and some also focusing on promoting the use of language, symbols and text (mainly the use of spoken language in these instances). (Ruella)

Music therapy goals can also be drawn from or formulated to support specific education goals according to the children's Individual Education Plan (IEP). In Noah's case commentators drew attention to the clearly outlined goals, intended outcomes, and next steps (Freyer; Hilda) which not only aligned well with the key competency curriculum (Hilda), but were also clearly linked to his Individual Education Plan (IEP) (Freyer). This is important because:

> IEPS are so often static documents instead of the collaborative plan they are intended to represent. By including those goals into the music therapy plan the music therapist is helping them to be part of a genuine living document. (Freyer)

Assessment—Developing Specificity

On the other hand, while the broad goals established for the children aligned well with the needs of tamariki takiwātanga according to diagnostic and learning criteria (including DSM-V; Key Competencies;

and IEPs), the formulation of more specific aims or objectives was also important.

> For some children, goals were set at the beginning of music therapy, perhaps following discussions with family and/or school team, and perhaps after one or two initial music therapy sessions to gather additional assessment information. In other cases, it appeared that therapy commenced without predetermined goals, and that these were established much later during therapy, or maybe even left to see what naturally unfolded throughout music therapy. (Ruella)

In more than half of the cases, commentators who did not know the children believed it would have been helpful to assess children more formally, and/or to develop—or be more explicit—about specific goals (aims or objectives) for them. Freyer for example, argued "the overall goals for the therapy (in James' case) were quite general" and in Ben and Ava's cases the goals could be "more specific which would make them easier to measure." Dana argued that "it might have been better to have clear goals for (Lucas) each session," and even suggested "a more robust plan might have included a behaviour management plan" for Oliver. In a somewhat similar vein, in Emma's case Vivian suggested there may have been too many "lofty" goals for such a short period of time, and Mike and Vivian both agreed clearer assessment and more concise goals may have been helpful for her.

> It seems as if the therapist was less comfortable with Emma's "way of being" at the start of the relationship [...] the extent to which the therapist knew about the ways in which Emma managed self and related to others, needs to be clearer. (Mike)

> Having more focused goals over a longer period of time could have resulted in more specific outcomes for Emma in terms of her turn-taking and sustained attention, which I think were more suitable to music therapy given that she already had a communication device that she used reasonably well to express herself. (Vivian)

That said, commentators had conflicting views on how specific the goals might be. In Ava's case for example, the goals were reportedly focused, pragmatic, and well scaffolded (Vivian), "straightforward and typical for what adults would like for a child with autism" (Hilda). The music therapist co-constructed sessions with Ava and "demonstrated a very in-depth understanding of the purposes of the sessions" (Vivian). Yet Freyer, as noted above, argued that the goals for Ava could have been more specific and measurable.

When goals are more precise, outcomes can also be concisely reported. But concise reporting on a specific aspect of functional ability does not provide a full picture of the challenges a child is trying to manage. Understanding can be enhanced with the inclusion of rich description. In Noah's case the music therapist had even demonstrated how the literature had informed her choice of goals and strategies, and this contextualisation helped at least one commentator, Vivian, to develop a better understanding of his progress.

Further, Mike wondered whether it might be helpful in some cases to separate education and therapy processes because he felt the IEP might put too much emphasis on "success" (Mike). Singing, for example, can help tamariki takiwātanga to develop measurable speech and language skills, but in James's case therapeutic goals of being able to demonstrate agency and to have an outlet for self-expression were deemed to be more important. For example, his family friend noted that being able to choose and to sing about his cat "obviously made him feel good. [...] Communication does not come easily for James particularly if he is upset [...] singing about something that makes him feel happy would benefit him when he is upset" (James's Friend).

As noted in Chapter 16, there were high levels of agreement overall that stated goals were appropriate for children. All twenty-six commentators who knew a child agreed to a certain extent that the stated goal seemed appropriate for that child. Similarly, all other experts agreed to a certain extent that the stated goal was appropriate for children in eight of the cases. However, in Emma's case one disagreed, and in Sophia's case two disagreed.

Interpreting the Behaviour of Tamariki Takiwātanga

The development of specific goals requires clear understanding of children's needs. Yet in several instances, from the information made available to them, Mike and Hilda queried music therapists' interpretations and/or decisions relating to children's behaviour. For example, referring to James's case, Mike, who has lived experience of autism, cautioned music therapists to consider that when a child engages in or enjoys repetition, this might not always indicate positive progress. "We know that echolalia is something that is part of the autistic experience, so I would be careful not to over-emphasize repetition as progress because this may have been an echolalic response" (Mike).

Similarly, referring to Liam's case, Mike cautioned music therapists not to assume too much regarding children's engagement levels and potential for change, especially in early sessions. Liam's aunt agreed that it takes time to understand Liam's communication, suggesting "(He) can appear standoffish at times and as if he isn't listening, but I don't believe this to always be true" (Aunt). In Oliver's case too, Mike questioned the music therapist's interpretation of the child's reluctance to engage. Speaking to the goal "to reduce distress," he suggested:

> I would ask "whose distress" and how do we frame this. I didn't get a sense of "great distress" from Oliver, but rather non-engagement and some anger which is not uncommon for young children on the spectrum – but that is a different thing to distress. I think differentiating this would be helpful. (Mike)

Mike also argued that Ben's music therapist may have underestimated Ben's initial competence, noting that he appeared motivated and confident in the context of the difficulties outlined, especially when therapy focused on his interests. Mike suggested the music therapist's perception of Ben's "improvement" may have been related to her becoming more attuned to him over time.

> I was fascinating by the original goals set at the start of the therapy because I think even early in the therapy Ben appeared to be a confident 8-year-old given the impairments that were listed (including global developmental delay). I do really appreciate and like the fact that the therapist showed clear understanding of strategies for working with children on the spectrum e.g., regular use of visual schedules; but I would have added another focus on pragmatic language use and use of eye contact. (Mike)

Mike's reference to eye contact as a potential goal is interesting given his lived experience of autism. Ben's mother also suggested that "the therapist would have got more engagement from him if she was able to make eye contact with him during the play" (Ben's mother). Yet in three other cases Hilda questioned whether aiming for improved eye contact would be a useful or appropriate goal for children with ASD.

> Many autistic adults have indicated that eye contact is hard and stressful. It is perhaps even culturally inappropriate for some autistic people. Another goal (for Emma) such as more use of her Augmented Communication device might have been more useful. Such technology is developing rapidly and there may be a time when Emma can fully communicate using AAC, while she may still not be readily utilising eye contact […] Neurotypical culture puts a lot of emphasis on eye contact for communication […] I don't think it is a useful measure for autistic children […] (For example) it seems that Elijah is observing and taking in much of what is happening. He has those 'peripheral glances' that I have often noticed in autistic children as if they don't want to look directly at something or someone but somehow can get a better look with a sideways glance […] making and maintaining eye contact is stressful and can distract from other means of communication or learning. (Hilda)

In an environment which values neurodiversity, it might be increasingly unusual for music therapists to cite improved eye contact as a specific goal, but it is possible to assume that as sensory integration improves, so might the child's ability to offer spontaneous eye contact. As Freyer notes:

> Music therapy has potential to help increase eye contact and verbal interaction and engagement, particularly where the child is being asked to lead the direction of the session. (Freyer)

Context has a significant influence on the responses of tamariki takiwātanga and therefore on what the goals of or strategies for therapy might be. James's family friend highlighted the importance of teamwork when they suggested:

> It would be good to determine if he enjoyed the music as much if he was just playing on his own, or if he needed the assistance of someone else there to guide him. If he enjoyed playing on his own, then it would be worth pursuing this interest. If he only enjoyed playing with the teacher, then maybe the enjoyment was more about having her attention and not so much about the music itself. (Friend)

Complexities of Goal Setting

Hilda suggested that common goals for tamariki takiwātanga, such as increasing confidence to promote learning and responding, and forming trust and security to become self-expressive, can be difficult to achieve. "The world can be a puzzling and hostile place for young people with autism so developing things like confidence and trust can be a 'hard ask' for a music therapist" (Hilda). Being able to describe the music therapy process, rather than to measure outcomes, therefore seems important. In Lucas' case, for example, while goals were identified (to improve his fine motor skills; to play alongside peers; to take turns; and to recognise and manage his feelings) one of the most important outcomes seemed to be that his music therapist was able to help others understand him a little more. That is, by using a descriptive approach, Rachael was able to include an analysis of the reasons why Lucas might be oppositional and examples of his challenging behaviours.

> She identified his anxieties well and examined what he was communicating due to his uncertainty. I found it helpful to have that as a lens to read and watch the different sessions and I appreciated the fact that she

> included examples of challenging behaviour as well as capturing success. (Freyer)

Moreover, the various and conflicting views of expert commentators' views regarding the potential to make different decisions when working with children provide good examples of the dilemmas that music therapists can face, and reinforce the value of descriptive reports in which music therapists explain the choices and decisions they made. For example, Mike was curious about the goal of speech development for Sophia. He wrote, "It seems to me that Sophia, when feeling comfortable, was happy to use speech. So, I wonder if more differentiation around (targeting of) expressive speech would (have been) helpful" (Mike). Dana, too, seemed to feel that Sophia might have been challenged a little more through her music therapy programme. Yet Freyer suggested Sophia's therapist "had clear measurable goals that helped to demonstrate the progress Sophia made over the course of the music therapy." Sophia's mother also agreed that the sessions were focused and highlighted the way the music therapy *process* enabled change to occur.

> Sophia had undertaken music therapy with some goals in mind, and the sessions were tailored to work to achieving those, through natural learning methods for children – play, music, and exploring. The gradual trust-building, relationship-building and interaction are very clear to see as the sessions went on. Sophia was very much a part of the process and I think that her involvement and active guidance of Lianne's sessions would have definitely helped her develop confidence in her growth and learning. (Sophia's mother)

Commentators' thoughts on the use of communication technology within and around music therapy sessions were also diverse. For example, while Freyer suggested the technology "can sometimes limit spontaneity and is not necessarily needed in all contexts" others felt that the music therapy might have focused even more on supporting the use of assistive technology, especially before and after sessions, to enable child voice to be heard.

> Using visual aids or their communication tool before, during and after the music sessions could enable more participation by the children. From the therapists' point of view, it would be more useful to help them plan the next steps when informed by the child's voice, alongside their professional judgement of what works and why. (Vivian)

> Given that initial concerns were around communication, self-expression and play I was wondering why the iPad was not used for communication before during and after the music sessions for more understanding of James's learning from his perspective? Could it have been used as a pre and post dialogic tool to evaluate and set new goals? Apart from music therapy, could games on iPad have also boosted his communication and play skills with peers? (Vivian)

Despite the "alternative suggestions" mentioned above, music therapists were noted to be reflective and adaptive; willing to try different approaches throughout the therapy to be responsive to children's needs (Freyer). In Noah's case, Vivian highly appreciated seeing how the therapy process moved from individual to group sessions (Vivian). The therapist "developed an interesting and safe […] therapeutic space for Noah where his verbal, physical coordination, negotiation, self-regulation, musical and social skills could be developed within an inclusive school setting" (Hilda) and, at the same time, education goals were being addressed (Freyer; Noah's teacher).

> Noah's reticence around anything relating to literacy meant that other pathways could be explored that still provided the interactive skills needed to meet the therapeutic goals, but they could be achieved with a focus on music making and working collaboratively with others rather than a focus on songs. (Freyer)

The multiple opportunities that music therapy provides for supporting learning and development mean that prioritising goals, specifying aims, and choosing activities to support those aims, while maintaining a holistic child-centred approach, can be difficult. For example, by keeping their focus broad Liam and Ben's music therapists were observed to offer them "a range of learning opportunities" (Dana). Most importantly, the child-centred therapeutic approach enabled music therapists to modify activities when children become stressed or anxious. Referring to Elijah's case, Hilda wrote, "anything that helps to de-stress autistic kids is important in helping them get through the rest of their day." Similarly, Ben's aunt argued that "If Ben grew to like/trust a therapist and to have the confidence to express himself freely through doing music therapy, then is that not something in itself?"

Music therapy is influenced by multiple theoretical frameworks; music therapists apply a wide range of methods and techniques according to the context in which therapy services are provided (Geretsegger et al., 2014; Thompson, 2020); and the principles informing processes for goals and objectives are therefore broadly expressed (Thompson, 2020). In these case studies, the music therapists appeared to employ "experience-oriented strategies" which enabled them to begin with an initial understanding of the children's needs or reasons for coming to therapy, and to clarify goals as the process unfolded (Bruscia, 2014; Thompson, 2020). They employed collaborative child-centred approaches, in which the tamariki takiwātanga were encouraged to lead the direction of the therapy. Such approaches resist formally defined and measurable goals.

On the other hand, each of the therapists had identified a therapeutic focus for the work and clearly considered this to be, as Thompson (2020) suggested, a key part of their professional responsibility. Ensuring that the child, family, and team are aware of the focus of the work is also part of the therapist's advocacy for their profession since goals "work to communicate what happens in music therapy" (Thompson, 2020, p. 8). Interestingly while Dana and Vivian argued that the therapists who contributed data for this study might have articulated more concise "measurable" goals, having read the narrative case studies they seemed very aware, and generally very appreciative, of "what happens in music therapy" with tamariki takiwātanga in New Zealand. Had the music therapists been working directly with Dana or Vivian in multidisciplinary teams, they would have had to negotiate the ways in which goals were to be articulated in each context. As Thompson (2020, p. 9) notes there is considerable "complexity, nuance and depth to the way goal processes develop in music therapy practice" and "it is the therapist who attempts to balance the tensions between the actors."

The Cruciality of Process

The descriptions of practice indicate that New Zealand music therapists are, overall, more concerned with "being with" children, offering them motivating opportunities which are likely to promote their learning and development across several domains, than identifying specific targets that might lead to measurable change. Their "goals" are broad, suggestive, and open to change, according to how the children engage with the process. It seems that their primary focus is on creating autism-friendly environments, in which children are respected and trusted to thrive on their own terms. This is in line with current understanding of neurodiversity, which resists focusing on and changing "deficit" behaviours in favour of ensuring that "all children are equally valued and are equitably provided for" (Bevan-Brown, 2021).

Liam's case particularly, highlighted the debate around describing takiwātanga tamariki as "being in their own world." Yet one might ask "and why shouldn't they live in their own world, at *least* some of the time"? Jodie was working hard to help Liam develop skills that would enable him to cope with the demands of living in a world that is designed to accommodate the needs of neurotypical children. But, as Grace Thompson suggested in the foreword of this book, we have, for too long, expected autistic people to change their way of being to fit in with others. On a personal level, of the most powerful encounters I experienced with tamariki takiwātanga during my career occurred when a young boy spontaneously introduced the song "Welcome to my World" (Winkler & Hathcock, 1963) into his session. While he could speak *some* words his verbal communication was limited; yet he sang this song to me clearly, boldly and with expression that moved me profoundly. It was very easy to accompany him as he sang. I received his song as a gift—the lyrics (see Sect. "Welcome to my World") seemed to serve as an allegory, an acknowledgement of the relationship we had developed through our mutual efforts to understand each other.

Hilda offered a relatively long critique of the "problems" associated with other interventions commonly used with tamariki takiwātanga. Citing Applied Behaviour Analysis (ABA) as an example, she suggested clinicians often hold deficit views of autism, where characteristics such as "stimming" or "hands over ears" are viewed as negative behaviours that need to be fixed. Goals and outcomes are often decided without collaboration with child or family and are sometimes inappropriate. Hilda noted that children have been asked to sit for "long periods of time doing boring repetitive tasks which do not align with their interests or skills," and their compliance is motivated by "rewards and even punishments for incorrect responses. Autistic adults who have experienced such therapy as children often describe it as abusive." Hilda went on to say:

> Music therapy could not be more different. Although all these children are very different to each other there are common themes. For a start the therapists all seem to like the child and want to build a relationship with each child, to find and work with each child's interests and skills. The therapist tries to make the physical and musical environment as interesting and engaging as possible for the child. Choices are provided but often limited to avoid choice confusion. For some children all senses are involved. This child/therapist relationship is essential for developing and achieving child-specific goals. These goals will usually involve developing skills which are helpful for the child and useful in the neurotypical world such as making choices, taking turns, and making friends. These goals can also be translated into the requirements of the NZ Curriculum. (Hilda)

It might be argued that Hilda is describing historical interventions that have been superseded by more child-centred ways of doing things, and/or that it comes from just one commentator who has had difficult experiences. However, another spontaneous comment from Sophia's mother suggests, sadly, that she concurs with Hilda.

> The potential for music therapy for other children is massive. Music therapy has been a very different therapy experience for us. We are used to visibly controlled environments, repetition, forceful interaction, trying to turn all the exercises into a game so that our child stops fussing and wants to cooperate [...] Music therapy is more a natural process. Here, there was no set schedule, and sessions were only marked by the hello and goodbye song.

Taking Time to Make Progress

Music therapists are encouraged to outline the aims of the work, determined during an assessment period, and an "intervention plan" which sets out the length of sessions and when they will take place (Lawes, 2012; Wigram, 2002). However, there is very little literature addressing the number of therapy sessions that might be needed to achieve meaningful change for tamariki takiwātanga. While it is accepted that programmes often span months or years it can be difficult to predict the amount of therapy needed to achieve adequate progress. Nevertheless, it is important to be able to define and convey the anticipated duration of a programme to potential providers (Wigram, 2002). Following an initial 2–3 session assessment period, a further ten to twelve sessions can provide a clearer picture and enable the therapist to report whether therapy will be long term.

As noted earlier (Chapter 4, Sect. "The Context") research funding for this project allowed tamariki takiwātanga to have weekly sessions, for up to twelve months, but funding could be used flexibly according to needs. Programmes therefore varied in length with one involving 10–20 sessions, five involving 20–30 sessions and four involving 30–40 sessions. At least one dyad was continuing to work together beyond the research period, with families paying privately for the music therapy. Commentators acknowledged that it was important to take time to build a therapeutic relationship, and that "for music therapy to be helpful, regular sessions need to be held over many months" (Hilda). "Building relationships and rapport even one-to-one takes time and is not something that can be rushed" (Vivian). In James's case, for example "while the first session was very impressive and the musical communication was well captured, the growing therapeutic relationship becomes evident in the ninth session" (Vivian). Ben's aunt drew attention to his "very shy nature" saying "it takes a while for him to develop trust and warm up to people he does not know. I have to acknowledge the music therapist for taking the time to build that trust with Ben."

> It can be quite hard engaging with autistic children as many seem to be very much in the 'here and now' and do not seem to have any concern

> about pleasing adults, teachers, or music therapists. So, their attention has to be worked hard for [...] the cases demonstrate that many sessions over a considerable time are usually required to build relationships and develop trust and, ultimately, skills. (Hilda)

Sophia was involved in 29 sessions over a period of eight months. The music therapist was described as "skilful" in the way she followed Sophia's interest without coercion, "giving her the time and space to become comfortable with the context of learning" (Vivian).

"(Sophia) didn't talk to the therapist until the 10th session, (but) by the end of the music therapy programme she was using much more language" (Hilda). "It took time and patience to build Sophia's trust and allow her to build her confidence in using verbal language" (Freyer).

> (This) showed the worth and potential of a long period of regular music therapy and the benefit of taking that time to build a relationship and develop trust and understanding, and for the music therapist to really get to know the child and their interests. (Hilda)

> I could see that Sophia had been learning how to navigate a new relationship and new space using what was available to her. She clearly took her time: testing the boundaries of the new space and the people therein; retreating and observing and then slowly coming out of her shell to respond; in whatever way she was willing. (Sophia's mother)

However, while there seemed to be general agreement among the commentators that music therapy programmes need to involve regular sessions over many months, in this study people who did not know the children did not always agree on whether individuals were making timely progress. For example, in stark contrast to the above comments, Dana suggested Sophia's progress was "relatively slow given the amount of music therapy sessions (29) she had attended." And in Elijah's case, while Vivian argued he made "slow but steady" progress over the ten months he attended therapy, Mike reasoned that given takiwātanga involves an "extraordinary spectrum of challenges and strengths" Elijah made "extremely strong progress." Both of Elijah's parents wished the sessions could have gone for longer, perhaps with a view to helping him interact with other children.

In James' case, the music therapy closed when James indicated he wanted to finish, at a time which also coincided with changes in family circumstances. People who knew him made tentative comments regarding the progress he made over 23 sessions of therapy. For example, his mother wrote "it was an interesting experience [...] I had hoped for more results, but it was worth the try." However, they were curious as to what might have been possible if the sessions had continued, especially beyond the introduction of medication for his hyperactivity which significantly increased his capacity to participate. James' grandmother suggested "half an hour once a week might not have been enough for James - he may have got more out of it if it was longer or more frequent" and a family friend wrote:

> Maybe if these sessions had continued for a bit longer after James started taking medication for hyperactivity, he may have been able to concentrate for longer periods and developed more skills and therefore more pleasure in his music [...] if he could focus for longer periods of time, I definitely think he would have wanted to continue with the sessions. (James Friend)

Nevertheless, commentators who did not know James argued strongly that the 23 sessions of music therapy were beneficial. Mike for example, wrote:

> I still think the music therapy intervention has been extremely helpful [...] the goals that James's mother expressed around managing anxiety and developing verbal communication skills will have been greatly assisted and achieved by this sustained intervention. (Mike)

Lucas' case is interesting too, in terms of making progress over time. His mother observed that he initially seemed to have *more* difficulty managing himself immediately after music therapy sessions and developed more resilience a few days later as he moved towards the next session. However, the short-term patterns of regression and progress between sessions resulted in overall improvement in his ability to regulate his emotions.

> Throughout the year I saw Lucas become more settled, cooperative and improve in self-regulation. Initially, his ability to process much after sessions would rapidly decline after sessions and remain unstable for a couple of days thereafter; until about Friday (His sessions were on Tuesdays). His irritability, sensory tolerance and communication would decrease – then a few days later, a happy and more resilient Lucas would reappear. It was as if he went into regression mode to progress but would come back with massive improvements. Now, a year after the first sessions, I do not notice any regressive or stressed behaviour on music therapy day, only happy reports from Lucas. He looks forward to his time with his music therapist and now it is almost like a recharge for him rather than emotionally taxing. (Lucas, mother)

Regular sessions were therefore very important for Lucas. Similarly, Ruella reported a "disjointed feeling" when evaluating Oliver's case and, noting his "less than ideal" personal circumstances, suggested "regular, predictable routine of music therapy sessions" would be important for "continuity and the ability to build on previous sessions."

Children's individual circumstances naturally impact on whether they can attend regular therapy, their abilities to engage, to progress, and ultimately on how long their programmes will run. Mike wrote that a "prolonged period of therapy was important in terms of growth and development" for Noah. His mother agreed.

> I think the main thing with music therapy, just like anything else that is tried with tamariki takiwātanga is that they are still individuals and so their absorbing of the sessions and how they integrate this into their being going forward isn't always as we expect or as fast as we want it to be. Usually, kids like Noah have more than one thing to deal with and if the other stressors in their life aren't being addressed it will be harder for people around them to see the progress they may be wanting for the child. (Noah's mother)

Perhaps it is ok just to join them in their world, for a while, every now and then.

Welcome to My World

Welcome to my world. Won't you come on in?
Miracles, I guess, still happen now and then.
Step into my heart, leave your cares behind
Welcome to my world, built with you in mind.
Knock and the door will open. Seek and you will find.
Ask and you'll be given, the key to this world of mine.
I'll be waiting here, with my arms unfurled.
Waiting just for you, welcome to my world.

References

Aigen, K. (2014a). Music-centered dimensions of Nordoff-Robbins music therapy. *Music Therapy Perspectives, 32*(1), 18–29. https://doi.org/10.1093/mtp/miu006

Aigen, K. (2014b). *The study of music therapy: Current issues and concepts*. Taylor and Francis.

Bergmann, T. (2016). Music therapy for people with autism spectrum disorder. In J. Edwards (Ed.), *The Oxford handbook of music therapy*. Oxford University Press. https://doi.org/10.1093/oxfordhb/9780199639755.013.3

Bevan-Brown, J. (2021). *Neurodiversity and Christmas tree lights* [Curriculum Document]. Massey University.

Bruscia, K. (2014). *Defining music therapy*. Barcelona Publishers.

Carpente, J. A. (2014). Individual Music-Centered Assessment Profile for Neurodevelopmental Disorders (IMCAP-ND): New developments in music-centered evaluation. *Music Therapy Perspectives, 32*(1), 56–60. https://doi.org/10.1093/mtp/miu005

Geretsegger, M., Elefant, C., Mössler, K. A., & Gold, C. (2014). Music therapy for people with autism spectrum disorder. *The Cochrane Database of Systematic Reviews, 6*(6). https://doi.org/10.1002/14651858.CD004381.pub3

Lawes, M. (2012). Reporting on outcomes: An adaptation of the 'AQR-instrument' used to evaluate music therapy in autism. *Approaches: Music Therapy & Special Music Education, 4*(2), 110–120. http://approaches.primarymusic.gr

Ministry of Education. (2014). *Key competencies*. Te Kete Ipurangi. Ministry of Education. Retrieved 25 August 2020 from https://nzcurriculum.tki.org.nz/Key-competencies

Rickson, D. J., Molyneux, C., Ridley, H., Castelino, A., & Upjohn Beatson, E. B. (2015). Music therapy with people who have autism spectrum disorder—Current practice in New Zealand. *New Zealand Journal of Music Therapy, 13*, 8–32. https://www-proquest-com.helicon.vuw.ac.nz/docview/1897698669?accountid=14782

Rolvsjord, R. (2010). *Resource-oriented music therapy in mental health care*. Barcelona Publishers.

Schumacher, K., & Calvet, C. (2007). The "AQR-instrument" (assessment of the quality of relationship)—An observation instrument to assess the quality of relationship. In T. Wosch & T. Wigram (Eds.), *Microanalysis in music therapy* (pp. 79–91). Jessica Kingsley Publishers.

Thompson, G. A. (2020). A grounded theory of music therapists' approach to goal processes within their clinical practice. *The Arts in Psychotherapy, 70*, 101680. https://doi.org/10.1016/j.aip.2020.101680

Wigram, T. (2002). Indications in music therapy. Evidence from assessment that can identify the expectations of music therapy as a treatment for Autistic Spectrum Disorder (ASD): Meeting the challenge of evidence based practice. *British Journal of Music Therapy, 16*(1), 11–28.

Winkler, R., & Hathcock, J. (1963). Welcome to my world. On *Jim Reeves, A touch of velvet*.

20

The Nature of Music Therapy with Tamariki Takiwātanga in New Zealand (Aotearoa)

Child-Centred, Strengths-Based, Music Therapy Practices

> Each music therapist brought their own personality and way of being and doing things, however I also noticed a lot of commonalities in their approaches. All the therapists (whether they explicitly stated this or not) appeared to share a similar philosophical orientation about music therapy – one where the approach is child-centred, with a focus on active participation in music-making activities. (Ruella)

Commentators valued the therapists "pursuing goals in a naturalistic, child-centred way" (Ruella), and their "understanding of the 'whole child'" (Dana). The case studies "showcased the individualised and adaptive nature of music therapy" (Freyer); and "demonstrated that a truly child-centred and strengths-based approach is extremely important in furthering progress for children" (Mike). Music therapists were observed to "'see past' the communication barriers to create opportunities for the child to explore and express themselves through music" (Dana); to

D. Rickson, *Music Therapy with Autistic Children in Aotearoa, New Zealand*,
https://doi.org/10.1007/978-3-031-05233-0_20

"recognise the child's 'way of being' and to work with her in a manner that suited her needs and personality" (Freyer).

> A striking thing that stood out to me was how client-led the sessions were. Sophia very much had freedom to move about and explore and her music therapist was able to purposefully use this direction to develop and work on Sophia's goals. (Sophia's mother)

The commentators praised the ways in which the children's special interests were utilised (Freyer; Ava's mother; Dana; Mike; Vivian) making the sessions "familiar and enjoyable" for them (Dana). Working with the child's interests created an atmosphere of fun and was seen to be an effective way to build a positive connection and develop trust (Vivian, Freyer) and "thus to elicit more interactions and expressive communication" (Vivian). Hilda noted, for example, that Lucas was typical of many tamariki takiwātanga who are "easily bored yet thrive on one-to-one learning with an attentive adult who draws on their talents while gently challenging them."

Commentators observed that the music therapy environments were "genuinely collaborative" (Freyer) "gentle and fun" (Ava's grandmother) and "without some of the pressures associated with verbal communication" (Freyer), thereby enabling tamariki takiwātanga to feel comfortable and safe. For example:

> Emma was given space to slowly develop trust. She had time and space to express her interests and preferences. As the trust built so did her confidence to interact with humour and to have greater agency in the sessions [...] Taking time over the relationship, and truly seeing the therapy from the child's point of view has been key. (Freyer)

That said, Mike also suggested that "there were some vignettes where it seemed like the child's interests were seen as tangentially relevant to the experience" and that deep focus on children's interests should be core to the practice (Mike). He commented for example that he was conscious that one of the children was Filipino, and this was important "because there are different cultural reactions to ASD especially in non-western cultures." While it was clear that engagement with autism culture was central to the music therapists' work, none drew attention to the ways in which other cultural interests and/or needs might have intersected and influenced the direction of music therapy sessions.

Nevertheless commentators, including Mike, argued that music therapy was effective because it is an "authentic" child-led process. Children can "be themselves" (Ruella, Dana), and make their own choices (Mike). The music therapist is "modelling [...] while allowing children to interact on their own terms" (Freyer) and adjusting their support "according to the person's ability to manage on the day" (Ava's grandmother). Mike suggested that Elijah's case demonstrates that "even in the most challenging and difficult situations, valuable and important learning gains can be made as long as the therapist is willing to modify their practice and expectations on the basis of the child's presentation" (Mike). For example, Anna-Maria "works with Elijah's need to put toys and fingers in his mouth, his joy in swinging, and his pleasure in making sounds" (Hilda). Similarly, Lisa "accepted, and even incorporated into the sessions, (Emma's) need to put her fingers in her ear; to lick, taste and smell objects; to look intently and closely; and to shake her limbs. The music therapy environment (was therefore) safe for her" (Hilda).

> Music therapy is a non-confrontational way of changing behaviours [...] music therapists work with children from where they are, join them, then bring them alongside so in time they can tolerate and build up trust [...] to enact change over time. (Noah's mother)

> As Ava senses she's leading the music and has control over what's sung she relaxes and joins in more [...] she becomes excited as she realises, she has a KEY role in making music. Because she was able to control her own levels of participation, she was more willing to engage even when feeling anxious. (Ava's grandmother)

Most commentators observed that children gain a sense of being in control in music therapy sessions, and that "the clear desire to give the child agency and be led by the child's responses is extremely helpful" (Mike) and "one the real strengths of music therapy" (Freyer). Children were able to "explore boundaries and possibilities in the sessions at their own pace" (Freyer) and were given the freedom to play and to explore "without restrictions" (Dana) and "without judgement" (Liam's Aunt). "Being able to choose" (James's friend), to "take the lead" (Ben's aunt), and to "make their own discoveries" (Freyer) helps tamariki takiwātanga to feel good about themselves. Ben was enabled "to feel important or to feel as if he can do things on his own" (Ben's aunt).

> Noah had the agency to decide how he wanted to engage with music therapy, his opinions were taken into consideration, and the sessions were adapted to accommodate his wishes. His opinions were not only important but could shape the course of the therapy itself. (Freyer)

> I think that other children would find this kind of therapeutic approach quite empowering. Sophia obviously demonstrated a sense of empowerment and confidence and she explored just where her interactions could take her. (Sophia's mother)

The music therapists were observed not only to respect but also to appreciate the children's way of being. They demonstrated that they were genuinely interested in the children (Ben's Aunt) and identified and validated their feelings (Lucas's mother). Mike noticed for example that Anna-Maria, Elijah's music therapist, was "extremely sensitive to context—she recognised that the family home might be a difficult space to work in, took the time to understand and connect with the family context […] (and) understood and shared in the joy of the small gains that Elijah was able to make through therapy" (Mike). And in Oliver's case:

> It is lovely to see read such positive comments about an autistic child as many interactions with the education or health systems are often 'pathologised' and children's behaviours are seen as problematic. The music therapist clearly expressed warmth and understanding of Oliver and his autism. (Hilda)

Music Therapy Methods

The music therapists who contributed data for this study worked with each child's interests, skills, and choices, to create interesting physical and musical environments in which they could engage children in playful music-related interaction (Hilda; Sophia's mother). They were acting intuitively, often deciding what to do in the moment, in response to the child's presentation or initiation, and the activities often involved simultaneous singing, playing and movement, improvised according to the child's needs in the moment. They were improvising a process and so, in the same way that it was difficult to demarcate specific goals for the work, it was hard to delineate the specific music therapy "methods" that were being employed. The following paragraphs therefore outline the *predominant* methods/activities that were identified.

Liam and Jodie were engaged with play songs, singing familiar songs, and the production of a musical artefact, as well as improvisation at the keyboard. Noah and Amy were also engaged in shared musical improvisation, as well as musical games such as "copy me," and musical statues. The musical statues game also involved Noah improvising the music.

In Oliver's case, Karen frequently used familiar songs which she introduced in the moment, firstly choosing a song which had a cultural match to the instrument he was playing, but then introducing songs in subsequent session which built on the "theme" of the first (bees). In a contrasting example, the act of tuning the guitar morphed into a mutual improvisation. Karen's singing was also used in conjunction with finger and hand movements, and Oliver's running and "flying" around the room. Similarly, Lisa's improvised songs, accompanied with guitar and/or incorporating body percussion, also accompanied Emma's movements and "dance." Pamela also developed improvised songs while encouraging Ava to play musical instruments or to vocalise with her. From the examples given, they were the only dyad to engage in songwriting.

Mary's approach was seemingly the most "music-centred" with all the examples focusing on shared improvisation. However, in the third learning story, improvisations also emerge from and/or incorporate snippets of familiar songs. Similarly, Anna-Maria provided five examples of engaging Elijah in shared improvisation. However, she also attempted to engage him using familiar songs, and encouraged him to respond using voice and/or instrument. In one other example she improvised song to support his activity on a swing.

Lianne and Sophia also engaged in shared improvisation. In one example, Lianne encouraged Sophia to play musical instruments to promote dialogic conversation, and in another Sophia "conducted" Lianne's music. In a contrasting example Lianne spontaneously introduced a song—likely to be familiar, but this is not clarified—to reinforce the letters of the alphabet. Annabelle sang a familiar song for Ben, while accompanying herself at piano, and while Ben played guitar. In subsequent examples Ben was leading, conveying a dramatic story, while Annabelle improvised soundtrack for the narrative. In the third example, Ben is singing an adaption of a familiar song, with Annabelle accompanying him.

Finally, Rachael provides an example of "improvising on a theme" (the sea) with Lucas, and others in which the dyad used instruments and voice to explore dynamic communication. She also provides examples of playing familiar music to him, and another of listening as he played music he had learnt by ear. Recording his music was also a feature of their work together.

In summary, music therapists in New Zealand, like their international colleagues, employ a wide range of methods and techniques in their work with tamariki takiwātanga including interactive playing or learning of instruments; vocalisation and singing; song writing and composition; movement and dance; and improvisation. Importantly though, the process within each session, and thus the activities and the ways they are implemented, is improvised according to the needs of each child in the moment.

Music Therapy Procedures

Bruscia (1987) suggests a procedure is a strategy or method which may consist of a series of operations or interactions and may be accomplished using various techniques (p. 16). Commentators noticed that while the music therapists were acting intuitively within an improvised process, they were carefully crafting the session boundaries and the music to ensure that the children felt safe enough to explore and interact. For example, they observed that the predictability that is important to children with ASD was accommodated within the music; within carefully structured activities (often familiar material repeated over time); and within carefully structured sessions and programmes.

> Most of the case studies seemed to describe a mixture of more structured activities (e.g., specific musical games, pre-composed songs, the use of hello and goodbye songs to start and end the sessions) and less structured activities (e.g., telling stories with music, instrumental improvisation, and improvised songs). (Ruella).

> (Music therapy) has the potential to be very effective for children with ASD [...] (who) often have a unique way of thinking and communicating. They can find comforting patterns in unpredictable ways and allowing them to have the agency to affect the structure of therapy sessions helps them to feel safe. (Freyer)

Structure Within Music

Music is made from patterns of sound. Rhythmic patterns emerge according to the length of sounds, and the ways in which they are accented (beat and rhythm). Similarly, patterns of pitch intervals form melodies, and notes played simultaneously (harmony) form patterns when they are repeated over time. Taking a wider perspective, multiple rhythmic patterns (phrases, verses, choruses, and so on) can structure the entire piece. Music therapists are acutely aware of the ways in which they use the elements of music. That is, they can maintain various patterns and structural elements to retain the familiarity of the music, while varying others.

Thus, commentators observed that improvised music can provide familiarity and security, as well as flexibility and freedom. Freyer noted, for example, that "improvisation was used to help create a safe environment [...] (where) children could be themselves and be free to explore music in all its elements [...] without rules and therefore without the need to be perfect" (Freyer). Others observed some of the ways music therapists use the patterns that are inherent in music making to help tamariki takiwātanga feel secure. "Patterns are often an easier way for autistic children to understand than oral information, so this is a clever strategy" (Hilda).

> The creativity and flexibility of the music therapy in supporting Lucas's social and emotional development has been vital [...] Particularly exploring in a world where things were being created and were NOT black and white; right or wrong. Being perfect and the anxiety around that has been a large block to him attempting new learning and things he finds challenging. (Lucas's Teacher)

> The auditory information that music and rhythm provides can be a very useful strategy to help tamariki takiwātanga moderate their emotions and volume while the interactive nature of the therapy allows social skills to develop in an engaging way. (Freyer)

Structured Activities, Sessions, and Programmes

The predictability that is important to tamariki takiwātanga was also accommodated by offering carefully structured activities, activities that were likely to be familiar to them, and/or enabling them to repeat activities that they enjoyed, as well as by carefully structuring sessions and programmes. Music therapy sessions usually begin and end with familiar songs or activities, sometimes "Hello" or "Goodbye" songs, to signal the opening and closing of sessions. The programme of activities might remain relatively constant for some children, and they might be reminded of what has been completed and what is to come, verbally and/or with the utilisation of a visual schedule as in Emma's case. Writing about Sophia's case Hilda observed:

> I liked the way that therapist encouraged a structure for sessions with beginning and packing up songs and routines. That is usually reassuring for an autistic child who is anxious or unsure about predictability. (Hilda)

For Oliver too, "familiar songs and activities were important [...] to help him feel comfortable and safe [...] especially during a time with so many changes for him and his family" (Ruella). Freyer noticed that Oliver's therapist "made excellent use of repetition of activities while varying tone and pace to help Oliver to self-calm when he became over excited." That is, she noticed that Karen was "holding" him with music—particularly tone of voice. She also noticed that Liam "enjoyed repeating interactive activities like the 'wake up' song that became a favourite" (Freyer).

> The structure of music therapy sessions which build on a pattern of familiar repeated routines which are then extended as the sessions develop allows the child to feel secure and more willing to explore reciprocal and imaginative play. (Freyer)

However, as Freyer notes, "the therapy (not only) allows for a combination of familiar routines and structures that are often reassuring (but) is also able to be child-led so that they can feel a sense of control and agency in the direction of the sessions" (Freyer). Moreover, while the use of familiar materials can reduce anxiety and support engagement, the high levels of motivation and responsiveness that tamariki takiwātanga typically and naturally have to music also means that they can be challenged to engage with new and unfamiliar material in the music therapy context.

> While many tamariki takiwātanga will respond to the familiarity of song-based routines, these sessions show how a mixture of improvisation with instruments and games with social rules can help a learner acquire important social skills as well as self-regulate emotions while also feeling they retain an element of control. (Freyer)

> It was good to see a mixture of free play and games in the sessions. Noah has said he does not always enjoy being told what to do so choices are important for him and help him to feel that he has ownership over what he is participating in. (Noah's Teacher)

In initial sessions the music therapists would have been getting to know the children, assessing their responses in the music therapy setting. Hilda noticed that "given some choice (although not too much for those with autism) children will usually find instruments that they like to use and play" (Hilda). In the following example, the music therapist's improvised greetings song would not have been familiar to Emma, but the way in which it was presented enabled her to feel comfortable and a connection to be made between them. More session structure was introduced as the music therapist developed a clearer understanding of Emma's needs.

> Although Emma was fairly reserved in the beginning, she maintained very good eye contact with the music therapist and was content to engage from a slight distance. The music therapist started off the session by singing an improvised song called, 'the hello song' and asking Emma if she was "ready", this was a nice icebreaker as was the slow tempo of the guitar. This approach allowed Emma to participate at her leisure and as she became comfortable, she began to let her guard down (Dana).

"The combination of 'repetition of familiar and comforting routines' and 'the introduction of new components' has the potential to help children to adapt to change in routines" (Freyer). Referring again to James' case, Freyer wrote:

> Children with ASD and anxiety often take a long time to 'warm' to unfamiliar adults which then creates a barrier to develop meaningful connections. Music therapy allows for interaction to happen in what often feels like a spontaneous manner for the child and communication begins without the need for words. [...] The medium of music allowed (James) to have a safe interactive form of communication where he was able to influence the direction (of the therapy) without the pressure of verbal social cues. As the therapeutic relationship developed, James's expressive language increased to the point where he was able to choose the subject for a co-constructed song and make verbal decisions about its content. This shows that using familiar musical constructs in the sessions allowed James to feel safe to express his ideas while giving him an understood routine that could be varied at his direction. Music appeared to become a safe medium for him where he could take risks on his terms. (Freyer)

Music therapy programmes would typically be structured to include a period of assessment, intervention, evaluation, and closure. Managing the period of closure is important because it can be distressing for tamariki takiwātanga when sessions end, especially when they must withdraw from the strong positive relationship that has been established with the therapist. Moreover, since change is difficult for tamariki takiwātanga to manage, particular care needs to be taken with transitions. Hilda and Freyer particularly liked the countdown chart Lianne used for the last four sessions of Sophia's programme "which showed very good planning for an autistic child coming to an end of a long-term programme" (Hilda).

> I really liked that consideration was given to managing the end of the therapeutic relationship, especially as Sophia was starting to acknowledge the therapist by name and developing a bond with her. By using the strength-based focus and tools like the countdown chart the therapist helped to support Sophia with the transition surrounding the final sessions. Many people with ASD struggle with changes to routine so this was an effective way of allowing Sophia to have some ownership in the process. (Freyer)

Ava, Case Vignette

Ava's case "exemplified an interesting tension between providing opportunities for spontaneity and the importance of structure to maximise the impact of therapy" (Mike). Predictable musical structures were used initially to help Ava anticipate what would happen next, thus reducing her anxiety (Ruella). However, Mike felt that Ava may have benefitted from more structure at times, particularly to help her stay on task.

On the other hand, other commentators suggested (1) predictability and familiarity were important features of the *therapist's presence* and (2) the structure and predictability of the music contained her. Ava's creative expressions were contained within various structures provided within music (songwriting techniques) and wider props (such as the blue sheet that represented the sea). Her teacher noticed that "the therapist wove into the song instructions, comments, and narration, cleverly making changes to keep her engaged and to challenge her." And, when a strong working alliance was established and trust had developed, structure was reduced, and Ava was challenged to cope with new experiences. According to Hilda and Dana, the improvisational nature of the music and the overall session was important, and Ava's mother shared that "it was great to see Ava have a creative "outlet'." Music therapy offered Ava "experimental learning opportunities where she could express herself through the medium of music" (Dana).

> This study is an example of how a therapist discovers what the child's interests are and responds to them, weaving them into words and music. Music therapy would not have been as effective if the therapist had a preconceived programme that she had to deliver in a certain way." (Hilda)

Maintaining Boundaries

Behavioural Boundaries

While child-centred music therapy offers a non-judgemental and emotionally supportive therapeutic environment, clear boundaries are maintained to ensure the child feels safe. Dana felt, however, that Noah and James would have benefited from more direct guidance from their music therapists regarding "rules of behaviour," because clear rules can help to make things more predictable for tamariki takiwātanga (Hilda; Dana). Dana suggested "it is important for therapists to establish clear guidelines around acceptable and non-acceptable behaviour. The music therapist must be clear, concise and specific about what is expected" (Dana). Through this lens, Dana thought James' initial sessions were "somewhat disorganised" but "as the sessions progressed there was a lot more structure and his ability to respond improved" (Dana). Hilda agreed:

> The sessions seem(ed) to follow a regular and predictable routine including a hello song which would likely have helped James feel safe rather than anxious [...] there is structure in the sessions which also

> likely helped James and the common autistic need for predictability and patterns. (Hilda).

However, while structure is important, child-centred music therapists aim to provide tamariki takiwātanga with a safe, consistent therapeutic environment where they can experience full acceptance, empathy, and understanding "without the pressures of a classroom learning environment" (Oliver's teacher) and, in Lucas' case, "without really realising that he is in therapy" (Lucas' teacher). Music therapists who have the privilege of working individually with children can help them to experience new ways of relating, and chaos is often part of this process (see "My Reflections on Noah's Case"). In Elijah's case, Anna-Maria's ability to remain calm, flexible, and spontaneous was important in helping him to manage his sensory difficulties and oppositional behaviour. And in Oliver's case Freyer noted that his music therapist needed to be "quite strict" in one of his sessions but was still able to help him manage his behaviour by employing humour.

> I thought it was very well done that (Oliver's music therapist) kept the activities structured while also being responsive to his mood. Those kinds of boundaries can often provide comfort and a sense of safety for tamariki takiwātanga and responding with humour when a mistake happened as it did with the castanets is also a powerful way to manage anxiety. (Freyer)

Psychological Boundaries

In Chapter 9, when discussing Oliver's case, I interrogated Freyer and Mike's contrasting opinions on the moment when Oliver told Karen he loved her, and she responded with "I love you too." Mike also questioned Annabelle's suggestion that she would be Ben's "active and non-judgemental playmate." The therapeutic relationship is of course different from other relationships, so Mike's questions seem important. Music therapists need to develop and maintain boundaries, within which they have certain roles and functions that they need to carry out. They provide a safe space, and a designated time for therapy, and they keep these boundaries as consistent as possible. They listen, empathise, and come to understand tamariki takiwātanga in a non-judgemental way. They are genuinely interested in the children, engage authentically in music and other forms of play, and demonstrate hopeful and positive expectations that the children will experience improved well-being.

All these ingredients help to develop the crucial trusting relationship which underpins the child's ability to interact productively in music therapy. The genuine interaction is very often playful and loving. Oliver's message of love to Karen, and Annabelle's decision to position herself as Ben's playmate, seem very appropriate in their contexts. As noted in Chapter nine, love in the therapeutic relationship can be viewed as a "dynamic, living energy which can be safely experienced because it is therapeutically boundaried [...] a non-possessive love, compassionate love, openness to work with the other as they are, as well as the potential of what they could be" (Charura & Paul, 2015, p. 7).

References

Bruscia, K. (1987). *Improvisational models of music therapy*. Charles C. Thomas.

Charura, D., & Paul, S. (2015). What has love to do with it? In D. Charura & S. Paul (Eds.), *Love and therapy: In relationship* (1st ed.). Routledge. https://doi.org/10.4324/9780429476907

21

Personal Resources

Child Musicality

The musical abilities and interests of tamariki takiwātanga have been reported since Kanner (1943) first diagnosed the condition. It is not surprising then that tamariki takiwātanga in this study were frequently observed to have an interest in or passion for music, as well as movement and/or dance, and some children had particularly strong music skills. This love of music and music making was seen to afford a "gravitational pull" between child and therapist, which drew them in to the therapeutic process and kept the children mostly eager to attend and remain at music therapy. Dana and Hilda argued that "affinity for music and rhythm [...] seems to be a prerequisite for successful music therapy."

Parents noticed children's positive response to music, from infancy. When they were babies, their mothers noticed that James "would settle from crying" if she sang "Don't Worry" by Bob Marley; Lucas would calm when listening to classical music; and Sophia was strongly affected by the emotional qualities in music, sometimes crying silent tears when listening. Parents continued to notice the affordances that music

D. Rickson, *Music Therapy with Autistic Children in Aotearoa, New Zealand*, https://doi.org/10.1007/978-3-031-05233-0_21

provided as the children grew. For example, Elijah's parents shared that "music has always been a way for (him) to communicate."

> I remember that it was thru music that I first made eye contact with him (about age 4). He was on my lap but facing me and then I was singing a song (probably "The Wheels on the Bus") he would hold eye contact with me and interact with me. So, I knew that for a child with autism who usually has trouble interacting with others, music would be a way to penetrate his 'bubble'. (It) allows him to be sociable without becoming anxious. (Elijah's mother)

Commentators reported it was their love of music that supported Noah to "self-manage and to interact," Liam to "gain confidence to interact with others and develop friendships"; and Elijah to tolerate a variety of sounds. Elijah's eyes lit up whenever his music therapist would sing or play the piano for him (Elijah's mother). Liam came from a musical family and appeared to be "naturally musical." He was described as "an amazing singer" who displayed a "good sense of rhythm" (Dana). Sophia was reportedly "musically talented" for her age (Dana), and Lucas was readily engaged in music to the extent that his teacher argued he was participating in sessions "without really realising that he is in therapy." For Ava, whose siblings learnt musical instruments "music therapy provided her with a way to have her own special music time" (Ruella) and her keen interest in music led to "increased involvement and enjoyment" as well as "calmness and persistence" (Ava's teacher). She seemed particularly excited by the guitar, and had her recorder proudly displayed in her room.

Commentators therefore also suggested that ongoing engagement in music activities would enrich children's lives. For example, Hilda noted that Lucas has a talent for music which could be developed and that learning an instrument and being able to play for pleasure, without taking formal examinations, could increase his confidence further. Similarly, Dana argued that "Ava will continue to grow holistically if she is encouraged to engage in music at every opportunity." Dana also suggested Sophia appeared to have "much more to offer in terms of musical aptitude," seemed "reluctant to reveal her true musical potential." She "has the potential to be an accomplished musician [...] Using music as a vehicle will certainly lift her confidence and encourage her to socialise with people other than her immediate circle" (Dana).

Vivian observed that some tamariki takiwātanga can process musical information when other cognitive tasks are difficult for them. The affinity that tamariki takiwātanga have with music could be associated with the predictability of rhythmic, melodic, and harmonic patterns often inherent in music. However, the potential for music to influence emotionality, empathy, and affective regulation is also relevant and evidenced in music therapy practice (Bergmann, 2016). Moreover, while children may demonstrate interest and/or talent for music, the music therapists' support was considered crucial in maximising, and supporting the children to engage with, musical opportunities. For example, while Ben demonstrated a love of music, he also felt strongly that songs needed to be sung "correctly," so care needed to be taken to develop his ability to be musically flexible. Elijah's music therapist "demonstrated sensitivity, skill, and experience" (Mike) taking care to present music at an appropriate volume which reduced the potential for him to become overwhelmed by the auditory stimuli (Dana). Dana even suggested she had "reservations about 'music' being the main component of music therapy" noting "the music therapist plays a major role in nurturing a child to utilise music as a therapeutic intervention."

Music Therapists' Expertise

Throughout the descriptive evaluations there were many references to the music therapists being highly skilled and versatile practitioners. Commentators variously suggested that "the skill of the music therapist is key in this intervention" (Freyer); "many bows exist in a music therapist's kete (kit) to work with children with autism" (Vivian); and "the success of the therapy depends on the music therapists' skill-set" (Dana).

> We must be mindful that all children are different [...] I think the music therapist will determine whether a music therapy session will be a success

> or a failure because of what they bring to the session and how they support the child to engage. (Dana)

Hilda felt it was "pleasing to see these skilled therapists apparently enjoying working with and liking these children" and Freyer that it was a "privilege" to view the work of this "group of very talented practitioners" (Freyer). Commentators noticed that the therapists worked intuitively and sensitively, with perseverance and good humour. They variously described them as being appropriately gentle, calm, patient, supportive, energetic, enthusiastic, and spontaneous; and observed they drew on considerable ingenuity, insight, creativity, and excellent music skills in their work. For example, Amy gave gentle suggestions rather than instructions (Freyer); Rachael "calmly de-escalated a potentially stressful situation" (Dana); Lianne worked with "great perseverance and clinical precision" (Freyer); while Anna-Maria demonstrated "sensitivity, skill and experience" (Freyer). Further,

> (Annabelle) created an environment where she was able to draw upon her expertise to create a range of learning opportunities for Ben while nurturing his musical creativity. (She) was consistent in all her sessions, showed enthusiasm, was upbeat, and was engaged with him throughout. (Dana)

Commentators valued the music therapists' abilities to draw on the strengths and interests of the children, and their dedication to finding out "what action, instrument, music or song engages them" (Hilda). They also valued the music therapists' willingness to incorporate other modalities or sensory experiences into their sessions, to meet the children's needs. However, they were particularly impressed with the music therapists' abilities to improvise and to build relationships, especially as it occurred through non-verbal, mostly musical, communication.

For example, Sophia's mother observed that Lianne used instruments "in different ways to reflect the moods and happenings as she and Sophia interacted" and Ava's mother was "fascinated" by Pamela's ability to "make it sound like Ava was playing the recorder or harmonica in tune when it was really her skilled background accompaniment!" Vivian highlighted the versatility of the therapists "not only their skills to play a number of musical instruments, but more importantly their ability to adapt to every situation depending on the response of the child" (Vivian). They were responding to children in the moment, "reading the situation and improvising as the situation demanded to obtain better engagement from the child" (Vivian).

However, commentators also observed that the music therapists' spontaneity and flexibility was grounded in careful planning. They were noted to have a good understanding of tamariki takiwātanga broadly, as well as developing knowledge of the individuals they were working with. For example, Vivian wrote "it was evident that Jodie had a sound understanding of working with children on the autism spectrum in general and a sound knowledge of the social difficulties Liam was experiencing" and Pamela was "excellent – she really understood Ava and worked with what Ava would offer, but also managed to 'tease' out more from her than we expected" (Vivian). The music therapists' abilities to model social behaviours for children in natural ways within their sessions (Freyer) and their "careful planning and really knowing and understanding the individual child and seeing the world from the child's point of view" were considered "key in the success of this intervention" (Mike).

The invitation for commentators to make suggestions about what might have been done differently, resulted in some constructive criticism of the work of individual therapists. Firstly, as noted above, Lisa was a new graduate and as such was encouraged to continue learning about children with ASD. Secondly, referring to James' case, Dana wrote she "would've liked to have seen more structure, a wide repertoire of musical activities, (and) more enthusiasm on the part of the therapist." Dana also "had a sense that Amy struggled to manage Noah's behaviour or wasn't sure how to manage his behaviour." Finally, Vivian and Freyer wondered whether the music therapists might have given the children more time to respond to them. "When children with ASD are in a state of arousal they sometimes take a lot longer to process their responses" (Freyer).

> At times it felt that there were questions asked in quick succession, and a long pause for the child to process the information would have been

> helpful [...] therapists may have a range of expertise and experience in working with children with autism. They too are likely to be on a learning curve as they work with these children. (Vivian)

Collaboration and Consultation

Commentators also recognised that the music therapists' knowledge of the children's strengths and the challenges they faced was gained through careful collaboration with families and other team members. Interestingly, Vivian thought Lisa "seemed very experienced" because she was "very aware of the curriculum key competencies", and "able to make links between them and the skills that were the focus in the sessions." Yet Lisa was a new graduate, who was drawing inspiration and support from Emma's school team.

> At first the sessions were tricky as both Emma and Lisa were uncertain of what to expect. Over time Lisa came to understand that with Emma it was a matter of "going with her flow". [...] I was impressed with Lisa's dedication to improving the sessions. (Emma's Teacher)

Commentators therefore reinforced the importance of music therapists maintaining ongoing and regular communication with other people who interact with the children they are working with.

> Music therapy certainly has the potential to help children over-come behaviour concerns, anxiety and other underlying issues that may cause distress. However, the music therapist must work in closely with others particularly parents and classroom staff including teacher-aides because those closest to the child are the best source of information. (Dana).

Knowing how a child is managing on a particular day can inform not only what might be offered to the child in terms of supports and challenges, but also how the child's responses might be interpreted and evaluated. For example, in response to one of the video clips, Noah's teacher was able to add meaning to his responses by interpreting them in the context of the "bad day" he was having before arriving at music therapy.

Dana emphasised the importance of gaining information about a child from those closest to them. She felt, for example, that Oliver would have had a behaviour management plan that should have been discussed with Karen as part of the music therapy referral process.

> There have been some quite significant changes that have happened in Oliver's life which may have contributed to his unwillingness to participate in some sessions. Therefore, it's important to acquire all the relevant information prior to actively starting a session [...] I would've liked to have seen a lot more dialogue between mum and the music therapist about his behaviour, to the point where she might call the music therapist to let her know if he has had a good/bad day prior to the music sessions beginning. (Dana)

It can be helpful to know what health and education programmes the children are involved in; how other members understand the child; and what strategies are being employed to help them manage. Dana argued that "a team of skilled professionals including the music therapist" must be involved "to ensure (work) is carried out respectfully and professionally." Writing about Lucas' case, Freyer reinforced the need for a collaborative team approach.

> This case study provided excellent background information about Lucas and his family. It really captured some of the challenges that ASD presents for him as well as reflecting on what some of his triggers and soothing strategies might be. This emphasises the importance of understanding a learner in the context of their wider environment including family and school, to be able to measure his progress and development. (Freyer)

As noted above, Lisa was a recent graduate, new to working with children who have autism, and her interactions with the child's teacher and family were crucial in her coming to understand what she needed to do.

> (Lisa) was very open to receiving advice, and help, from the team [...] and shared her feelings of uncertainty in knowing what to do [...] I suggested

> that she visit another music therapist so she could get an idea of what the sessions might look like." (Emma's Teacher)

The sharing of information needs to be reciprocal; family and other team members also benefit from learning about how the child manages in a music therapy setting. When people can witness a music therapy session, they can develop a greater appreciation for the child's strengths and abilities. Freyer observed "music therapy helps support families and care givers by allowing them to see their child interact in unexpected ways as well as providing strategies to be built on at home." She and Ruella both felt that James might have benefited from having his skills highlighted in other contexts, perhaps by sharing music therapy artefacts.

> It was so wonderful to see James initiating and creating a song about his cat in the last learning story. It showed his creativity, playfulness, self-expression, and confidence in using music and verbal language and I started to think about how this could be taken beyond the music therapy room. I wonder how James might feel about sharing his song creations with his family and friends. (Ruella)

It can be validating for parents to see their children in an environment where they feel comfortable, and where they can emulate the positive behaviours that they demonstrate at home. When she saw Lucas calmy unroll himself from his sensory blanket and proceed to help Rachael pack up, Lucas' mum wrote, "his disposition at that point confirms his overall disposition outside of music therapy – particularly at home – where when his sensory needs are met, and validated, Lucas can continue with transitions, routine, instructions, and is more confident to use initiative" (Lucas' mother). Learning from the music therapy process can also help teachers to "get to know (a child) on a deeper level, with evidence based not just on a 'teacher's hunch'" (Lucas's Teacher). "Moving the therapy into the school space was the highlight of Elijah's therapeutic intervention. (It gave) his teachers and peers the opportunity to see what he was capable of" (Vivian).

While the music therapists in this study did not report that they were specifically aiming to resource other team members to work with a child, commentators recognised the potential for this to be an important part of the work. "Including the parent as part of the therapy sessions was indeed a very good move on the part of the therapist, as it also gives the parent ideas to follow up at home" (Vivian). Resourcing others could be as simple as sharing information so that "the skills children display in music therapy can help provide the collaborative team with information that can be used to support a child in other contexts" (Freyer). It could involve, for example, using the book shared during the music session back in the classroom (Ava's case, Vivian); or developing the technique of praising the desired behaviour in class (Lucas' case, Freyer).

> I was delighted to read about the breakthroughs that took place where Lucas felt confident enough to express his emotions [...] the way his therapist gave him the phrase of 'we can't know everything' as a learning tool could have been very effective to help him release some of the anxiety he feels, around making mistakes. (Freyer)

On the other hand, collaboration could involve more complex skill-sharing to support the child's generalisation of developing or newly acquired abilities to home or classroom. For example, they might be supported to "transfer fine motor development from using fingers on the piano keyboard to assistive technology for writing"; draw on "a music cue [...] to promote calm in other contexts [...]; and "generalise use of quiet voice into a classroom environment" (Freyer). Further:

> I thought the session with the kazoo was an effective example of the music therapist using Sophia's interest in wind instruments to encourage her to use her words and (it) had me wondering about how this could be applied to other tamariki takiwātanga, many of whom need to use assistive technology of different kinds to facilitate communication. (Freyer)

Music therapists would typically aspire to be members of a child's multidisciplinary team and in many cases would be involved in the development and/or implementation of aspects of their Individual Education Plan (IEP). Freyer argued that one of the strengths of music therapy was that "it can be used by schools to help facilitate IEP goals" (Freyer). Similarly, Ava's teacher and Elijah's father were keen for the music therapist to work with the school team, and to contribute to Individual Education Plans.

> (In future it might be helpful) to involve the teacher aid, or classroom teacher, or even the Special Education Needs Coordinator (SENCO) of the school where the child is enrolled and maybe even the other therapists (like speech therapist) so the team working with the child is in the loop. (Elijah's Father)

In contrast, Mike suggested that it might not necessarily be helpful for music therapists to be involved in the IEP process. In Noah's case, for example, he wondered whether "a separation between the education process and therapy might have been helpful" because "it seemed like the IEP was focused on 'success'" (Mike). And in Lucas' case while music therapy and classroom goals were said to be clearly well linked, the importance of therapy, i.e., taking a therapeutic *approach* to learning and development was clearly articulated by Lucas' teacher.

> The creativity and flexibility of the music therapist in supporting Lucas's social and emotional development has been vital. In coming at his issues from a different place to school learning, Rachael got past the barriers which Lucas put up around him for his own sense of safety. (Lucas' Teacher)

References

Bergmann, T. (2016). Music therapy for people with autism spectrum disorder. In J. Edwards (Ed.), *The Oxford handbook of music therapy*. Oxford University Press. https://doi.org/10.1093/oxfordhb/9780199639755.013.3

Kanner, L. (1943). Early infantile autism. *Journal of Paediatrics, 25*, 211–217.

22

Music Therapy Places and Spaces

Psychological and Physical Spaces

The venues for the music therapy sessions described in these case studies were varied and included rooms in family homes where parents were present, schools, a therapist's home, and a music therapy centre. While familiar predictable environments with few distractions were noted to be important for tamariki takiwātanga, other factors such as availability of instruments, family circumstances, timing of sessions, and the desire to include other children in sessions also influenced where and when sessions took place. Balancing all these factors can be difficult. For example, Ava had her sessions at home because this was a reassuring environment for her, yet sessions had to be held after school, which "can be problematic for some tamariki takiwātanga, as negotiating a school day can leave them exhausted and uncooperative" (Hilda). Nevertheless, Hilda also put the counterargument that "very anxious children often prefer the familiar including a mother present (particularly at first), while that is unlikely in the school setting […] (so) home can be a good venue if there is sufficient space and quiet" (Hilda). Further, if the environment is suitable from an acoustic perspective, "a neutral environment such as a

D. Rickson, *Music Therapy with Autistic Children in Aotearoa, New Zealand*, https://doi.org/10.1007/978-3-031-05233-0_22

room in a community centre rather than home or school can be positive for building the professional therapist and child relationship" (Hilda).

Spaces need to be big enough to enable the music therapist and participant/s to move and be creative, without seeming overwhelming and uncontained. While his teacher felt Noah's sessions were held in "a safe environment without the pressures of a classroom" Dana and Ruella both felt that it would have been helpful if Noah's therapy was held in a bigger space than the school withdrawal room could provide. He was "energetic (and) needed space to burn off some of the bottled-up energy and to allow for his creativity to flow" (Dana). Mike also questioned whether the room was appropriate because of the psychological connotations of it being a "withdrawal" room for potentially "negative aversive activities" (Mike).

> The withdrawal room was rather small for three people and a range of instruments. [...] (However) I understand that music therapists often do not get much choice in where they can hold their sessions, particularly in schools where space can be at a premium. (Ruella)

Considering the acoustic and visual elements of the environment is of course crucial when working with tamariki takiwātanga, to help them to tolerate and organise sensory input and maintain an appropriate level of alertness. Ruella was concerned to hear a baby in the background while listening to one of Ava's sessions and thought this would be good reason to change the venue. She also noted that Noah seemed to be distracted by several items in the "withdrawal" room which introduced additional challenges to the sessions.

> Additionally, the music-making could potentially get quite loud. In such a confined space, I could imagine that the noise from this could be difficult for everyone to manage, and especially challenging for somebody with different sensory sensitivities. (Ruella)

The physical space for Elijah's therapy changed during the year. Sessions initially began at home, but the needs of the family led to it being moved to school relatively early in the process. Music therapists naturally also need to be aware of risks to physical safety, and to choose or manage the environment accordingly. In Elijah's case, for example, when the therapist placed her percussion instruments on a piece of material on the floor, Elijah immediately came over and began to skid across the floor with the material under his feet. Freyer suggested a mat would not only have been safer but might also have helped Elijah to focus on the musical instruments and the music, rather than the sensory input of the from the movement of the material underfoot (Freyer). The management of risks always involves balancing those risks with potential benefits. In this case the therapy was held in a room large enough to contain a swing. Mike suggested Anna-Maria's recognition that the family home might be a difficult space to work in, was extremely important.

Access to music instruments can be an important factor in deciding where the therapy might take place. Music therapy venues, where appropriate music equipment can be set up before sessions, can look "inviting and engrossing" (Hilda). Hilda went on to note:

> Permanent venues have the luxury of pianos and drum kits while an itinerant therapist is limited by what she can carry and the space available. […] (However), sometimes a smaller selection of fewer instruments can actually be less stressful for tamariki takiwātanga as choice can be overwhelming. (Hilda)

Finally, while music therapists appreciate opportunities to video record sessions for evaluation purposes, it is not always appropriate to do so. In two of ten cases in this series, it was not possible to video, and in some of the other cases the therapy process may have been influenced by the presence of the camera.

> Liam appeared to be quite conscious of the camera […] which had the potential to distract him from the activity. It did not appear to have a negative impact for Liam but might for another child so a more covert camera set up might be an advantage. (Freyer)

Individual or Group Sessions

The choice of venue for music therapy sessions is of course influenced by the need for individual or group sessions. Emma's initial music therapy goal was "relating to others," and early sessions included classmates, but Emma's team agreed that individual music therapy "to increase and develop interpersonal communication and interaction in a one-to-one relationship" would be likely to be beneficial. Thus, she was "withdrawn" for music therapy sessions which took place in a small classroom away from other children, where she reportedly felt secure. Freyer applauded this collaborative decision.

> Careful consideration was given to finding the right environment for this therapy to take place [...] It was good to see that the collaborative team who work with her were involved in goal setting and adapting the space and session format moving from a group setting to a specific space that allowed one on one interaction. Consideration was given to the importance of not only the physical environment, but also the tools Emma needed for her emotional safety and regulation. (Freyer).

The decision to include other children in a music therapy session is typically based on the needs of the child, balanced with available physical resources. Therapists need to make sometimes difficult decisions regarding whether to involve peers, in or out of the classroom, or family members, in or out of the home, in music therapy sessions (for further discussion see Sect. "Relationships with Peers," p. 254; and Sect. "Inclusion," p. 313). As Noah's mother notes, the decisions that are made can have a significant impact on a child's ability or willingness to engage with the therapy.

> (When Noah) was able to have a friend from class join in on the sessions it made a real difference, and he was able to connect better with the therapy. He had spent quite a bit of time isolated or taken away from the class when things were going wrong for him [...] (so) over time as he became more integrated back in the classroom and was interacting with the other children, he was more reluctant to participate (in music therapy). (But) when he got to have other children from class join him his

> protest about having to do music therapy just about disappeared. (Noah's mother)

Noah was the only one of the ten children in this study who regularly had music therapy with peers, even though other children reportedly had difficulty "engaging with and relating to peers" and "playing alongside peers"; and needed help to "play." Instead of developing peer or group music therapy programmes, it seems that the music therapists made decisions to develop skills that would *underpin* the children's ability to interact with their peers. "From the children's perspective, the one-to-one interactions provided an opportunity in which they could be less anxious and able to self-regulate without much distraction" (Vivian).

Interviewees in our exploratory study (Rickson et al., 2015b) recognised that group work can present significant challenges in responding to the needs of individual tamariki takiwātanga, especially in terms of timing, pacing, and adapting music, and that group sessions tend to be more structured. Several reasons were outlined to explain why children might benefit from individual sessions before joining group work, including if they experienced auditory sensitivity, were very easily distracted, or needed to develop more awareness of self and other (p. 18). Further, while the music therapists in our previous study emphasised the potential to "'link' music therapy to other aspects of participants' lives by having peers in the music session, taking artefacts from the music room to the classroom, and ensuring the music that is familiar is used across contexts" (p. 22) they did not describe working within classrooms. Rather, they "valued the music therapy session as an opportunity to give children and their team members a 'break'" (Rickson et al., 2015a, p. 52).

In the current study, while some commentators "hinted" at negative implications of withdrawing children from the classroom for therapy, they seemed to agree that the children they were observing benefitted from individual or small group work and that this was a step towards inclusion.

> The video clips provide good snapshots of Noah extremely comfortable in turn taking and working alongside his more boisterous peer. Together with the music therapists' comment that he was initially reluctant to

> leave the classroom, this augurs well for Noah to be totally included in a classroom programme. (Vivian)

> Amy has developed an interesting and safe but developing therapeutic space for Noah where his verbal, physical coordination, negotiation, self-regulation, musical and social skills can be developed within an inclusive school setting. (Hilda)

Nevertheless, it is perhaps surprising, given that New Zealand has one of the most inclusive education systems in the world (Mitchell, 2016), that none of the work described in this study took place in a classroom. An obvious explanation is that the research funding enabled ten music therapists to work with *individual* children who had not experienced music therapy before. Nevertheless, music therapists were advised that the research funding could be used flexibly according to tamariki takiwātanga' needs, and work could have taken place within the regular classroom if that was a team's wish. In the one case where peers were involved, several children were withdrawn from the classroom, which raises questions about whether tamariki takiwātanga *and* their peers might feel exposed and/or excluded from the mainstream classroom, or in contrast, privileged to be selected for a rewarding activity. Hilda proffers the view that including peers in small group work "normalises" tamariki takiwātanga's experiences.

> (Introducing a partner to music therapy) serves to provide practice for learning skills such as turn taking and socialisation. But it (also) helps make the music therapy sessions something desirable and less exclusionary for the rest of the class. The partners in these four sessions in this study look and sound as if they are enjoying the experience very much. It also shows that there are no real differences between some 6-year-olds in a MT session whether they are autistic or not. (Hilda)

Inclusion

The discussion about "collaboration and consultation" (on "Collaboration and Consultation") as well as the paragraphs above highlight the need for music therapists to carefully consider their practice in the light of the philosophy of inclusion. McFerran and Silverman (2018) note that there is considerable difference internationally in the ways students with ASD are educated within mainstream schools, special schools, and schools which are independent of the education sector; and, across contexts, the values and priorities of the policymakers, managers, educators, and families vary highly. I therefore offer the following discussion of music therapy practice as it relates to the New Zealand situation, while recognising that some of the information may be unfamiliar to some readers.

The goal of inclusive education is to provide rich learning opportunities for all learners—grounded in values of equity, participation, community, sustainability, and respect for diversity. It involves redefining of the purpose of education, and demands a transformation of schools, ultimately to ensure that children and staff have good social and emotional health, and the community has an overall sense of well-being. Educators in New Zealand have been challenged to adapt, modify, or develop curriculums and assessment regimes to ensure they are accessible to all children including those with disabilities (Mitchell, 2016).

There are many schools in New Zealand where all children, including those with significant disabilities, are fully engaged with the curriculum and other school activities (Morton et al., 2019). However, many teachers misunderstand and remain apprehensive about inclusive education because they see it as an ideological rather than a practical idea. And, if they do not have the necessary knowledge and skills to meet the needs of diverse students, they are likely to lack confidence, seek alternative placements outside the classroom, and pass responsibility for disabled students on to teachers' aides (Kearney, 2013), and therapists. Children continue to be removed from classrooms for individual teaching—often delivered by teachers' aides—and for various forms of therapy, including music therapy. Emma's teacher, for example, was delighted to have an additional team member with the time and expertise to work with her outside the classroom.

So often in schools like ours the first thing to go when the budget is tight is music, the arts and movement programmes, and these are all

> programmes our children love and benefit the most from. To have a therapist working with our children one to one is crucial to their learning and development [...] If all children with autism had the opportunity to work with a music therapist, I would be a very happy teacher. Personally, I love music and work hard to incorporate it into my learning programmes. I have been lucky to learn from others, but I have limited expertise and time due to having to teach a full curriculum and deal with many of the other challenges our children have. I know that very few teachers have the skills to use music with their students beyond the basics of singing and YouTube videos! Music therapy for children with autism, in my opinion, is a must! (Emma's Teacher)

The current study confirms that teachers, parents, and children themselves, value music therapy because it can offer the child a "little oasis" away from the challenges of the classroom; provide an opportunity for them to participate in meaningful activity which will contribute to their learning, development and/or overall well-being. While Emma's teacher's response is understandable, and might even give music therapists a boost, it is important to remember that when children are withdrawn for music therapy, they are highlighted as being "different," exposed, and potentially marginalised. And withdrawing children for music education, by a therapist, is not only absolving teachers from their responsibilities, but is an inappropriate use of resources. Moreover, when children are withdrawn for therapy, music therapists also face the dilemma of deciding with the team whether other children will accompany and work with the child, who that might be, and how the programme will be framed. Noah's teacher asked him to choose the children who would go to music with him and requested permission from the peers' families for this to happen, but it was unclear what the anticipated benefits were for the neurotypical children.

> In hindsight, I would have chosen the children myself. Two are closer friends of Noah's, whereas the child he chose is a classmate that is not a close friend. However, they hadn't had any issues between them in the past and I thought it would be good to open Noah up to new relationships. (Noah's Teacher)

The question of whether to withdraw children from their regular classrooms for music therapy, in the context of an inclusive education system, can therefore create significant predicaments for music therapists. There is often an expectation in schools that teachers and therapists will embrace the prevailing ethos of the school and learn from more experienced staff—a "passing the baton" approach which means everyone is acculturated to existing processes (Dharan, 2013). It is understandable that music therapists who are keen to gain or maintain employment might "fall in line" with what is expected not only because it is easier, but also because we will be appreciated for it. Music therapy researchers have found that we need to feel connected to, and validated by, other professionals (Warren & Rickson, 2016) and that our collaboration with school teams can be impeded by fear of losing our professional identity (Arns & Thompson, 2019).

Another reason to protect the status quo is that a special education system might be easier for music therapists to engage with, professionally and fiscally. Special schools provide us with a "captive" population and, in New Zealand they have typically managed their own funding. This has meant that they have had more opportunity to directly employ music therapists to be part of their allied health teams, and the more homogenous population makes group/classroom music therapy easier to rationalise. In contrast, inclusive schools often do not, and philosophically should not, have funding for children with "special" needs. It is therefore harder for families to access music therapy.

> I was desperate for my daughter to be accepted into this research project. I had heard about the amazing things music therapy could do for children with special needs and really wanted to see if my child would benefit. The biggest obstacle in the past had been the cost of therapy. (Ava's mother)

> My concern is that children from low socio-economic areas might be excluded from experiencing the benefits of music therapy if the sessions are unaffordable. Many children from low socio-economic areas are naturally musical and would benefit from music therapy sessions to consolidate their musical talent. (Dana)

Moreover, if children are decentred from the "problem" why do they need therapy? Surely the work needs to focus on systems that create or contribute to the problem. On the other hand, criticism of professional discourse and the withdrawal approach does not mean professionals are not needed in schools, and it is not meant to suggest tamariki takiwātanga don't ever need medical care and therapy support (Hassanein, 2015). Music therapists often work with children who have extreme difficulty communicating, and who may exhibit dangerous behaviours such as self-injury. It is easier to argue that for these children symptom amelioration is crucial, and/or individual therapy is necessary. However, inclusion is about tamariki takiwātanga developing a sense of belonging and having equal opportunities to participate in school activities. When we continue to provide music therapy to individuals or small groups in schools, we are highlighting the children's "difference" and the difficulties they have managing in the classroom environment. This in turn protects the status quo, justifying and strengthening the idea that "expert" intervention is in a child's best interest (Hassanein, 2015).

So, what is the relevance of music therapy in inclusive education contexts? Music therapists are challenged to think about how, when, and why support might be provided. Supporting teachers to understand and experience genuinely inclusive activities is a good place to start. When musicking, children are engaged in activities that are meaningful and purposeful and can facilitate their happiness, connectedness, and creativity (McFerran & Rickson, 2014). A cyclic process can result, with music leading to the development of positive relationships with peers and teachers which in turn results in children experiencing support and acceptance and feeling connected to school. Musicking communities are therefore likely to be more inclusive communities (McFerran & Rickson, 2014). And, when children with disabilities are fully included their peers learn about how different individuals make their way in the world, and teachers learn new skills which are useful for all children (Morton et al., 2019).

Learning stories too can become a vehicle for inclusion, as creating them encourages teachers to focus on the child's abilities rather than their "dis"ability. In Ava's case the stories of Ava in music enabled her teacher to see the potential for further collaboration towards inclusion. She was keen for Pamela to continue working with the school, to contribute to Ava's Individual Education Plan (IEP), and to provide advice and direction to staff about how they might use music to address goals in the classroom.

> I see the value of this, particularly calming Ava down and reducing her anxiety in the context of what can be a busy and noisy school environment. I see this opening the doors for her to interact with others through music. (Ava's Teacher)

Despite the challenges, many teachers and therapists do wish to work in mutually empowering ways with learners. Katrina McFerran and I have provided a practical model for building more inclusive and empowering music cultures in schools which embrace the values of "mutuality," "empowerment," "respect," and "commitment" (Rickson & McFerran, 2014). We suggest music therapists can employ resource-oriented and participatory approaches to enhance the well-being of children and staff generally, and we advocate for music therapists to collaborate with all willing participants in schools including school leaders, teachers as well as students to empower them to develop inclusive and sustainable music programs.

Inclusion involves understanding diversity and challenging the hegemony of the "norm"—not only how we understand what is "normal" about bodies and minds, but also what we consider to be "normal" attitudes and practices. Until we challenge our own assumptions, we cannot begin to engage in genuine collaborations, or to understand what empowerment might mean for the people we work with. This means that we need to be actively reflexive; and if we work in schools, to consider how our own beliefs, attitudes, and knowledge frameworks align with inclusive philosophy, as well as how they might align with the beliefs and attitudes of school communities. And we need to be prepared to be unsettled by what we discover. It can be painful to learn how our own actions are creating or contributing to the problems we experience.

We also need to have the skills and confidence to critique the philosophies and practices of schools that have deeply ingrained cultures if necessary. We cannot leave the responsibility for building more inclusive societies to others. Just as societies are rethinking the role and design of schools, we need to be proactive in rethinking roles for music therapists within inclusive schools. If we are to work in inclusive education settings, we need to collaborate with children, families, educators, other therapists, and wider communities, to consciously disrupt marginalising processes in schools. Luke Annesley suggested in 2014 that part of the job of therapists in schools is to hold on to an alternative viewpoint, to be advocates for a different agenda, and to help the school with its holistic responsibilities (Annesley, 2014). He said, as "outsiders" we can stand up for what we believe, no matter how unpopular or risky those beliefs might be. And when we challenge assumptions, we might find that understanding and actions change too. Music therapy training institutions therefore have a responsibility to ensure that students and graduates have the skills to advocate for and to carry out, collaborative work in regular classrooms, or wider school environments.

However, it is important to acknowledge that changing cultures takes time. Commentators in this study have highlighted the value of children experiencing the "little oases" that music therapy can provide when classrooms are overwhelming for them. It is important that music therapists provide opportunities for children to participate in meaningful activity which will contribute to their learning and development when teachers are not able to provide such opportunities. And it is important that all children have access to music. However, I would encourage us to remember that music therapists have unique skills to support inclusive music making in schools, and to support the development of inclusive schools—because sharing music enables diverse people to experience a profound togetherness that is difficult to achieve in other ways. The small steps we are making towards inclusive music making in schools are to be valued, because we are gradually contributing to alternative regimes of truth that will lead to more inclusive policies and practices across the board.

References

Annesley, L. (2014). The music therapist in school as outsider. *British Journal of Music Therapy, 28*(2), 36–43.

Arns, B., & Thompson, G. A. (2019). Music therapy teaming and learning: How transdisciplinary experience shapes practice in a specialist school for students with autism. *Australian Journal of Music Therapy, 30*, 31–52.

Dharan, V. (2013). Understanding diversity: Moving beginning teachers beyond receiving the baton. In *Inclusive education: Perspectives on professional practice* (pp. 52–65). Dunmore Publishing Ltd.

Hassanein, E. (2015). *Inclusion*. Sense. https://doi.org/10.1007/978-94-6209-923-4

Kearney, A. (2013). Barriers to inclusive education: The identification and elimination of exclusion from and within school. In *Inclusive education: Perspectives on professional practice* (pp. 40–51). Dunmore Publishing Ltd.

McFerran, K. S., & Rickson, D. J. (2014). Community music therapy in schools: Realigning with the needs of contemporary students, staff and systems. *International Journal of Community Music, 7*(1), 75–92. https://doi.org/10.1386/ijcm.7.1.75_1

McFerran, K. S., & Silverman, M. J. (2018). *A guide to designing research questions for beginning music therapy researchers*. The American Music Therapy Association, Inc.

Mitchell, D. (2016). Inclusive education strategies in New Zealand, a leader in inclusive education. *Eesti Haridusteaduste Ajakiri, 4*(2), 19–29. https://doi.org/10.12697/eha.2016.4.2.02a

Morton, M., McIlroy, A.-M., & Guerin, A. (2019). Sociocultural perspectives on curriculum, pedagogy and assessment: Implications for participation, belonging and building inclusive schools and classrooms. In M. J. Schuelka, C. J. Johnstone, G. Thomas, & A. J. Artiles (Eds.), *The sage handbook of inclusion and diversity in education*. Sage.

Rickson, D. J., & McFerran, K. S. (2014). *Creating music cultures in the schools: A perspective from community music therapy*.

Rickson, D. J., Molyneux, C., Ridley, H., Castelino, A., & Upjohn-Beatson, E. (2015a). *Music therapy for children who have autism spectrum disorder ASD: Exploring the potential for research in New Zealand using a mixed methods design*. Victoria University of Wellington.

Rickson, D. J., Molyneux, C., Ridley, H., Castelino, A., & Upjohn Beatson, E. B. (2015b). Music therapy with people who have autism spectrum disorder—Current practice in New Zealand. *New Zealand Journal of Music Therapy, 13*, 8–32. https://www-proquest-com.helicon.vuw.ac.nz/docview/1897698669?accountid=14782

Warren, P., & Rickson, D. (2016). What factors shape a music therapist? An investigation of music therapists' professional identity over time in New Zealand. *The New Zealand Journal of Music Therapy, 14*, 55–81.

23

Evaluating and Reporting

Narrative Assessment as a Tool for Reporting Progress

The Value of Rich, Descriptive Data

Commentators made many positive references to the rich and detailed stories, and it was clear from their feedback that they were able to get a strong sense and appreciation for the therapeutic processes that were occurring over time. For instance, Freyer noted that the stories gave her "in-depth analysis of what appeared to be a very successful intervention," that she could "imagine what the child might be like in person," and that she learned a great deal about the adaptive nature and potential of music therapy for tamariki takiwātanga. Commenting specifically on Emma's case, she wrote "the transcripts of the sessions outline in detail the small indications that Emma is gaining confidence." Others suggested the stories provided "insight into various approaches that a music therapist can use" (Vivian) and offered "a good introduction" to music therapy (Hilary). Hilda, who has experience of takiwātanga in her family, wrote:

D. Rickson, *Music Therapy with Autistic Children in Aotearoa, New Zealand*, https://doi.org/10.1007/978-3-031-05233-0_23

> Although I have met dozens of children and adults with autism and their parents over the last few decades, I did not know much about music therapy when I started this evaluation exercise. These diverse learning stories and Narrative Assessments have been fascinating and educational for me as I have learnt how music therapists work, and how goals are developed which are appropriate to the child as well as align with the New Zealand curriculum [...] This would be very useful for parents wanting to know how music therapy works. (Hilda)

Rich description illustrated with video and/or audio examples enabled the music therapists not only to demonstrate, and celebrate, the subtle but crucially important gains that tamariki takiwātanga can make across a variety of domains (Freyer), but also to convey some of the emotional quality of the work, and to engender emotion in observers (see "Including Children's Voices"). Hilda appreciated the narrative in Oliver's case which "clearly expressed a warmth and understanding of the child and his autism"; and in Emma's case "described Emma in positive terms as a cheerful child who enjoys activities, rather than as a tragic autistic child (as might be the case for other 'interventions')" (Hilda). In another example, Sophia's grandmother shared, "I can picture most of the expressions, eye contact avoidances, kazoo-talking and other things described in the report, and I feel so excited to see growth for Sophia, through this music therapy journey" (Sophia's grandmother).

Adherence to "Learning Story" and "Narrative Assessment" Guidelines

The therapists typically (1) structured each learning story with some background, the narrative, and comment regarding the therapeutic significance and focus areas for ongoing goals; and (2) laid them out clearly and related them to identified key competencies. Commentators variously described "succinct," "well-presented" case studies with "clear purpose," detailed background notes, IEP goals clearly outlined at the start and next steps clearly identified throughout; "excellent background information about the child's communication styles and interests"; strategies informed by the literature; and pictures of the different instruments that were used in therapy sessions. Hilda wrote, "I like how after each session the therapist reviews and evaluates and asks – where to next? (and) little notes such as a reminder that feeling safe helps relationship building." Commentators also appreciated reading about music therapists' philosophical stance, and their reflections on the work. "By articulating her philosophy, the music therapist sets the context for the interactions, which is more about "active music-making," rather than verbal exchanges in the music sessions between the client and the therapist" (Vivian).

It is clear then that the learning stories "speak for themselves" to a certain extent, and that the description not only provides evidence of children's progress, but also affords insight into the music therapists' values and beliefs. On the other hand, in some cases commentators felt further information would have enhanced the case studies. There were instances when they thought the learning stories were quite brief, could have been more detailed, contained greater analysis or reflection, and/or been more clearly linked to each other and/or the music therapy goals and key competencies. Examples include:

> While the first story showed that Noah could be alongside another student, although seemingly oblivious of the other's presence, the second learning story was an excellent example of spontaneous sharing and turn-taking. Some narrative around what may have contributed to this level of engagement would have assisted the reader. For example, was it the familiarity of the peer since they had prior contact in social situations, or increased comfort level of the context and place of therapy? (Vivian)

> The way Oliver's case study was presented felt a little disjointed – each learning story seemed to stand alone without much flow to the next one. […] Perhaps this disjointed feeling was reflective of the music therapy experience overall, as the therapist mentioned there was a break of 2.5 months between sessions at one point, and a sudden and unexpected ending to music therapy with the family moving away. (Ruella)

It is important to note however, that the music therapists were asked, for research purposes, not to provide their summary of the therapy, in the belief that the learning stories would speak for themselves. While it was clearly necessary to provide context for the work, the case studies varied in how much information was woven around each learning story.

The Inclusion of Video Examples

The inclusion of video examples certainly enhanced the learning stories, "provided valuable additional detail to support understanding of the learning that was taking place" (Ruella) and enabled commentators to "see for themselves" what was going on in the therapy room, as this reflection from Ava's teacher demonstrates.

> Using both recorder playing and using her voice in this session, Ava readily switched between the two. Echoing the therapist's sound pattern was fun and Ava at times did this with full gusto, e.g., holding onto the last note and tilting her head up. When the therapist switched the vocalisation sound to 'zoo zoo zoo' it certainly grabbed her attention back again. For Ava the change was fun, and she was playing with her voice. When echoing the phrases, she often looked at the therapist. What was interesting in this session was that Ava didn't use words, instead, the communication was the recorder and voice phrases. She knows she can do this and enjoys the experience with some confidence. (Ava's Teacher)

However, two of the case studies did not include video examples, and in other cases children would disappear from camera view for a time. Commentators understood that for some children the presence of a camera was too distracting. Obviously, without video it was harder for commentators to assess the progress children were making. Nevertheless, where the description was rich, and/or audio was included, it seemed they were still able to obtain a strong sense of the music therapy process.

> I found Sophia's case study interesting to read and I enjoyed learning about the development of her relationship with Lianne. The sessions were described in excellent detail and even without video or audio evidence it was easy to imagine how Sophia might have been testing the noise tolerance of her 'audience' in her early sessions and it was encouraging to read about her understanding about imitation play emerging from the start. (Freyer)

Some appreciated the inclusion of audio instead, while others found it disappointing not to have video. Freyer suggested "while it would have been interesting to have seen additional videos, it was clear that Noah did respond to the presence of the camera and so the alternative of an audio recording was very well done." Hilda found the videos "much more useful for evaluation than the audio clips," and others seemed to agree. Ruella wrote for example that the highlight of Elijah's case study for her was when he said his own name for the first time. Imagining that it would have been very exciting for his mother to witness, she wrote "I was a little disappointed that there was no video clip to show this as I would have liked to see it too!" (Ruella).

> I like to see what the children are doing with movement and attention [...] Audio clips reveal musical and verbal interactions but for me music therapy is much more than that. But I understand that there are sometimes practical and ethical issues of videoing children [...] There is so much more going on in these sessions than mere sound making, as the videos reveal [...] They illustrate music as a relationship which is lovely to see. (Hilda)

Given how highly valued the video and audio material was, it is disappointing the complexities of ethical processes prohibit the inclusion of examples with this text.

Narrative Assessment as a Tool for Reporting Progress

However, even when video examples are included it can be difficult to demonstrate "progress" if intended outcomes are not clear. Video material often needs to be accompanied by rich description to provide context for the interactions. While there was variation among the ten cases reported for this study, some commentators felt they needed further information to enhance their understanding of the tamariki takiwātanga's goals and outcomes.

> What would have also been useful to document was (Elijah's) progress in social skills, one of the goals of the therapy. Also, what was the duration of the therapy and how would the skills targeted in the music session be extended to his whole school and home contexts. Perhaps adding another focused intervention such as social stories alongside the music sessions would enable greater gains. (Vivian)

As argued in Chapter 19, music therapists need to be able to clearly communicate the purpose of the therapy to team members, using professional language. Commentators made occasional comments about lack of writing clarity (e.g., Vivian, in Noah's case) and the overall style of writing (e.g., Mike, in Oliver's case). In the latter case, even though the music therapist's practice was clearly child-centred, "the goals of the therapy were not fully expressed in a 'child-centred' way" (Mike) and it was unclear how the practice related to the original goals for therapy (Vivian). Mike and Vivian noted that Oliver's case study focused strongly on Karen's interventions and reflections, rather than on Oliver's responses. "There were good insights from the therapist in terms of what was meaningful learning for Oliver [...] but one could not get a sense of the purpose of the sessions linking back to the original goals for the intervention" (Vivian).

Mike wondered whether Karen had misunderstood the request for "Narrative Assessment" and, like Vivian, argued that clearer connection to curriculum goals, and far more extensive planning, was needed in this case. In Lucas' case, Vivian also questioned the role of verbal interaction in music therapy and challenged the music therapist to consider whether other approaches, or combination of approaches, might have better outcomes.

> There were some profound learning moments described (in Lucas' case), but I was not able to make the causal link to the therapy per se. More seemed to come from the dialogues between the therapist and Lucas, and partly because Lucas is extremely articulate. This case study demonstrates that music therapy is equally a powerful intervention even for those in the high end of the spectrum, but these students can have better outcomes, when combined with more cognitive therapeutic interventions, as the music therapist has tried to do in places. (Vivian)

James' case provides a good example of the potential for readers to interpret or understand the same material differently, according to their own background, context, or focus. James's aunt stated that music therapy did not appear to have helped his learning or development, yet others were impressed with his developing confidence. Dana felt that his sessions might have held more structure, while Mike was "particularly impressed with what James and Mary did with their time together." Dana, Ruella, and Freyer were convinced that the attunement and synchronisation that occurred in music making was crucial in his relationship development, while his grandmother felt "it had little to do with the music and more to do with time spent together". So, particularly in James' case but also in others, it would have been helpful to have feedback from the children themselves. James' music therapist asked him to complete evaluation forms, which Mike felt was "an appropriate way to receive his feedback," but these, or comments from these, were not included with the case study.

Commentators highlighted other instances where more information would have been helpful. Ruella wanted more information about "how Emma interacted in the group setting […] and what led to the decision to focus on individual sessions." And in Ben's case Mike was interested in the therapist suggesting they would be "an active and non-judgemental playmate."

> Initially I was uncomfortable with this description, and I feel as I watched the videos, I got more of a sense of what the music therapist was meaning… all I would suggest, is that the therapist be really clear about the nature of the relationship. (Mike)

Freyer suggested it would have also been interesting to have had evidence of the children's presentation outside of music sessions, particularly when they were demonstrating challenging behaviour, for baseline or comparative purposes. Similarly, commentators also suggested that it would have been helpful to have more information regarding whether/how children's learning and development generalised to other contexts to "better highlight the value of the therapy," perhaps later in the process or after therapy had finished.

Feelings Matter

Importantly it seems that in almost all cases the commentators were able to "sense" the quality of the children's musical engagement, and the work "resonated" with them. Resonance is a term that is often used in music therapy clinical practice to describe the subjective and objective interactions of music, client, and therapist (Lindvang et al., 2018). As Matthiesen et al. (2018) note, resonance is a wonderful metaphor for being affected as a human being; when one person is "moved," and another is caused to be "moved." As qualitative researchers, we seek to be moved by the phenomena we are investigating, and we endeavour to produce reports that resonate with our readers, to clarify and deepen their understandings. Commentators experienced a range of positive feelings while viewing the case reports, including admiration, confidence, delight, enjoyment, excitement, pride, satisfaction, and surprise. They described cases as "heart-warming" "special," "moving," and emotionally rewarding, and expressed "gratitude" for the music therapists' work. Regarding Elijah's case Mike wrote:

> It was an extraordinary privilege to watch this work. I feel that this relationship has been extremely beneficial to Elijah's progress, and I am feeling a strong sense of the joy that Elijah's family must have been feeling when he made that progress. (Mike)

Ben's mother shared "I am filled with aroha (love) watching my son," and his aunt was similarly moved, describing feeling "happy" and "a sense of relief" after watching the videos. In Ava's case Freyer wrote, "Ava's story gave me lots of reasons to smile, she is an engaging young woman, and it was delightful to see her confidence and sense of humour shine through as the sessions progressed." Likewise, she found it "delightful to see Liam dancing with such joy, yet obviously listening to what was going on" (Freyer), while his aunt "laughed out loud" seeing him interact with the video camera. James's mother and a family friend also described smiling while watching James respond to Mary. Hilda, who didn't know him, said "it is so nice to see an autistic child smiling and enjoying what they are doing" (Hilda). Ben's series of stories were also deemed to be "such a pleasure to watch" (Freyer) and "thoroughly enjoyed" (Dana).

Lucas' mother suggested viewing her son at music therapy "filled her with confidence" and his teacher shared "I feel proud of him. Lucas's social and emotion growth in 2018 was huge. It is great to look back and remember how far he has come and how these sessions have helped him" (Lucas's Teacher). Sophia's mother and grandmother were similarly proud of her efforts at music therapy.

> My personal reactions and feelings to this story are surprise, delight, pride and gratitude. Signing up to music therapy for Sophia, I really did not know what to expect. I did wonder how playing instruments would assist her in developing her ability and confidence to speak, interact and initiate play with her peers… (So) I am surprised to see how much she has grown and developed in these music therapy sessions and at the purposefulness of each interaction and play in the sessions to help Sophia to develop. […] I am (also) grateful at how much easier this therapy and its values were for us to incorporate into our lives at home. It was such a natural approach, and totally changed our parenting style and mind-set around rigid and repetitive exercises for our daughter. I am grateful for this work, which has helped Sophia so much. (Sophia's mother)

> I feel very proud of my granddaughter as I read through her report. I can picture most of the expressions, eye contact avoidances, gazoo-talking and other things described in the report. And I feel so excited to see growth for Sophia, through this music therapy journey […]. While I am mindful that each child will respond differently to music therapy, I absolutely recommend it for other children. (Sophia's grandmother)

It is clear then that music therapists in this study were able to convey the music therapy process in ways that resonated with the commentators. That is the case materials provoked "sympathetic vibrations," helped them to "understand," to "nod" as they recognise the children in this new context (van Manen, 1990, p. 27), and to see the music therapy processes as valid. The commentators in turn were able to describe their experience of "understanding," as well as their personal feelings and reactions, in ways that resonated with me, and hopefully you—the reader.

On the other hand, it is likely that the resonance diminished, like a ripple effect, as the interaction widened. That is, music therapists and children who were in the room will have had different and potentially stronger experiences of the music, than commentators witnessing video recordings. Similarly, the commentators' accounts of their witnessing will be qualitatively different, and perhaps, weaker, than their experiences. Moreover, it can be extremely difficult, if not impossible, for observers to know what is occurring when highly attuned participants are engaged in a synchronous musicking experience. Commenting on James' case, Dana noted "It was difficult to ascertain whether the activity was turn-taking or if James was leading."

Including Children's Voices

It is now well-known that it is best practice to involve those directly impacted by a therapy in evaluating and reporting on the impact of the work. This is strongly reinforced by (Low, 2021) who interviewed four autistic adults about their experiences in Nordoff-Robbins Music Therapy (see "Music Therapy Research Focusing on Adolescents and Adults") and Jeong and Darroch (2021) who, as music therapist and autistic participant, co-wrote an article about their experiences of working together in music therapy. As Low argues, these publications "not only affirm that autistic participants have valuable insight in their music therapy experiences, but also give music therapists and other autism-related healthcare professions and researchers new, patient-centered considerations when working with the autistic community" (p. 98).

It was disappointing then that the learning stories did not include childrens' voices. As noted above, James was able to participate in self-review of the sessions and to indicate when he wanted his sessions to stop, but his voice—and others—were missing from the case studies. Freyer was keen to hear directly from Liam and James. "It would have been interesting to have learned why James wanted the therapy to end. I understand family circumstances were also a factor, but his perspective would have been helpful if he was willing to share it" (Freyer). Importantly, in this research context, additional clarification of the meaning of the work came from the solicited data—comments contributed by people who knew the children. This in turn provides a strong argument for routinely including parent or caregiver's voice, as well as child's voice, in learning stories.

Music Therapists' Learning and Development

It is important that the process of reporting is helpful not only for readers of the reports, but also for the therapists. The music therapists involved in this study found the Narrative Assessment process a helpful way to reflect and report on the music therapy process. Mary wrote, for example, "as James's therapist it has been very motivating for me to be sharing these stories of James's success in music therapy. These stories also help me to reflect on the way I work with clients." An advantage of Narrative Assessment is that it recognises learners for what they can do, regardless of the primary focus of the learning, which in turn increases teachers', parents', therapists', and other team members' awareness of learners' strengths. It recognises that learners' progressions are not predictive and predictable, and that progress is often evident with the benefit of hindsight (Ministry of Education, 2009).

Narrative Assessment is therefore useful for therapists employing individualised developmental and improvisational approaches in their work because the learning stories are strung together *retrospectively* from recorded observations and reflections, thereby enabling them capture what has been meaningful in a coherent progressive way. Molyneux and colleagues note that descriptive evaluation pays attention to "the whole child, their communication, intentions, interactions, verbal and non-verbal gestures, affect and emotions, musical patterns, themes and preferences" (Molyneux et al., 2012, p. 37). Some of the most beautiful "moments" in music therapy stand alone; those aspects of music therapy practice are intangible; and occasionally children are unable, or it is not the right time for them to "progress" (Molyneux et al., 2012).

Generalisability and Sustainability of Gains

Generalisability and sustainability are important concepts in therapy. As Hilda argued, music therapy might be considered "a little oasis of one-on-one therapy that is enjoyable and sensory in a positive way without any problematic peers or puzzling school routines" which could be valued for its own sake. On the other hand, music therapists working with tamariki takiwātanga, their colleagues, and the tamariki's whānau, generally anticipate that music therapy will support the children's learning, development, and/or overall well-being, and would aim for the gains they make to be sustained and generalised to other contexts. For example, it is likely that both Oliver's mother and his music therapist would aim for him to develop more independence over time (i.e., for him to be able to work with a music therapist, teacher, or other support person without the need to return to his mother for support); and/or to actively involve his mother in music therapy sessions with the aim of enhancing her knowledge and skills to use music therapeutically with Oliver in the home environment.

Narrative Assessment lends itself well to understanding whether generalisation has occurred because it invites the perspective or voices not only of the teacher, or in this case the music therapist, but also of the child and/or their family or whānau. The process of music therapy involves mutual sharing of information with others, so it was possible for music therapists to include the perspectives of others in their case stories. In this instance, however, the learning stories and overall Narrative Assessments (case studies) did *not* contain comments from other people; and the six commentators who did not have knowledge of the children also did not have access to the families' or educators' comments on the cases. Vivian was therefore eager to see some examples of how the children transferred their learning to home and/or school.

For example, she would have liked some information "on how James' ability to be less anxious and more spontaneous transferred to his school and home setting"; "how much Emma's goals, [...] such as turn-taking, initiating, and responding to peers, would occur in her everyday educational context"; and whether Ben's "transfer of learning to classroom setting and with his peers could have been observed and documented."

> As the long-term goal for any student with autism is social communication, I wondered if another student/peer could have been introduced halfway through the yearlong sessions, to enable Ben to practice and generalise his learning.[…] (More broadly) It was heartening to see parents involved and half yearly reviews undertaken for prolonged music therapy programmes, but more of how the learning was generalised is needed to strengthen our arguments for advocating music therapy as an important intervention for children and young people with autism. (Vivian)

Similarly, Dana suggested "it wasn't clear if the music therapy sessions had a lasting effect on the children once programmes ended or if the sessions were only effective in the moment" (Dana).

> I think music therapy has the potential to help a good majority of children. I would question whether the intended focus for music therapy intervention is sustainable as a behaviour or anxiety management strategy. For instance, if behaviour is well managed during the therapy session, does the child tend to regress once the session has concluded or are strategies established to ensure the behaviour doesn't resurface? (Dana)

Further, while praising the music therapy in the clinic setting, Vivian also questioned how the learning demonstrated in music therapy was reinforced and/or extended in home and school contexts in Sophia's case.

> If one were to evaluate the success of the therapy sessions per se, then the music therapist comes out with flying colours for her achievement. However, unless the learnings are transferred to real life contexts, and the reciprocal interactions with her peers show improvement, the benefits of such a child-centred approach, will be less useful. […] How was it encouraged in the school? How did it link with her interactions with peers? Perhaps there were many interventions in place in relation to the curriculum, but since they were not a feature of the case study, it was hard to see the benefits of the music therapy in a more holistic form. (Vivian)

Freyer, however, had a very different opinion.

> Overall, this was an in-depth analysis of what appeared to be a very successful intervention for Sophia. I especially liked the work that was done towards the end of the course of therapy to help build her confidence and take her newly acquired skills into other areas of her life. Towards the end of the therapy Sophia was showing increased eye contact and reciprocal play and there was evidence to suggest that she was beginning to generalise some of those skills. (Freyer)

Ava's case provides an interesting example too since many of the expert commentators noted that music was important to Ava and her family, and they wondered about how the music therapy might support her to continue to be involved in music activity. Outcomes within the music therapy sessions were encouraging. "Overall, this was such a positive case study to view" (Freyer) and "in the context of these sessions, as demonstrated by the text and videos, there has been progression towards the goals" (Hilda). On the other hand, commentators who didn't know her wondered about "how the skills Ava was acquiring in the therapy sessions might be generalised in other family activities where music is present" (Freyer); whether her "interest and skill with music for expression and responding to the world around her would continue" (Hilda); how family might be "involved in extending the skills (she) demonstrated in the music therapy sessions" (Vivian); and the "ways in which her school staff were involved to build upon the learning from music therapy" (Vivian).

> While one can get a sense of Ava being more relaxed and willing to experiment (towards the end of the therapy), there was less information to confirm if the goals of decreasing her anxiety during unexpected changes and if her vocal self-expression was generalised to other situations. (Vivian)

Ava's mother perceived that her generalisation of music skills had been relatively limited, and Ava's teacher was eager for the music therapist, Pamela, to be involved in ongoing education planning, to further both Ava's reduction in anxiety and her ability to engage with others in music.

> Ava developed a love for performance during the year which we've never really seen before. This wasn't really translated outside of music therapy – but within the lesson several times she encouraged us to listen to her. (Ava's mother)

It is likely that the music therapists did not provide information on the ways in which tamariki might have transferred or generalised the skills they demonstrated in sessions, because it would have been easier to capture the meaningful examples that were written up as learning stories, in the music therapy setting. While this might be disappointing on one level, the research design allowed "familiar" commentators to add another layer of understanding by interpreting the case studies in the light of what they knew of their child in other contexts. And from their responses, it is possible to suggest that in six of the cases (Liam, Noah, Elijah, Lucas, Sophia, and Emma) tamariki takiwātanga were able to generalise some development and/or learning to home and/or school.

Liam's grandmother, for example, suggested there was a noticeable change in Liam during the year. She argued that music therapy not only provided him with confidence to sing a solo at his school concert but also helped to "minimise his autistic traits enabling him to start to develop some friendships at school." Noah's mother shared that he had been to two birthday parties of boys who participated in music therapy and noted that, overall, he was "socially connecting at a better level."

Elijah's mother and father provided important evidence of his increased eye contact, interest in music, and conversational babbling continuing to develop at home. Further his caregiver was convinced that Elijah was more responsive to others who talked or played with him, that "he is more inclined to interact with people he is not familiar with and to develop relationships further with those he already is connected to." Indirect feedback from teachers and teacher aides at school suggested that Elijah was more able to sit alongside other children in class too.

> When Elijah started music therapy in January 2017, he hardly had eye contact with anybody other than me, my husband and his sister. He also hardly had any verbal communication. But when the sessions ended, he had been making long eye contacts with his therapist. It was such a big

> social development for him. I have also noted improvement in his interaction with other children as well as adults in his school. He also began making musical sounds like humming his own tunes, even humming along some classical music we play at home. He has also said his name while playing the drums. Towards the end of the school year, he also said "Mom" when a teacher was talking to the class after reading a book and saying, "Was it the granny or the mom?" (Elijah's mother)

Lucas' mother and teacher were both adamant that music therapy had supported his abilities to communicate his feelings, manage his anxiety, try a variety of activities, and play with other children at school.

> If Lucas had not received music therapy last year, I do not think he would be in the same place emotionally and able to self-regulate as well as he can now. Through this work he has also begun to understand that his actions can also affect other people's emotions and reactions. It has made such a massive improvement in his life and our family life in general, that we have continued on, funding the sessions privately. (Lucas's mother)

> Lucas is becoming a self-regulated member of the class who people want to interact with and be around. His anxieties are still there but are greatly reduced and under control. [...] As the year progressed, Lucas became more willing and able to be part of activities and gatherings he does not want to do. This included changing activities and getting ready to go home at the end of the day. He is no longer leaving the classroom without any explanation and is returning to class after breaks with less supervision. [...] He had repeatedly said he wants friends but did not know how to begin being part of their world and allowing them to be part of his. In class and at times in the playground he is now able to play with other children with a lot less adult support. Turn taking has been an area where I have particularly noticed an improvement. (Lucas, Teacher)

Sophia's family had also observed some changes outside of music therapy—with Sophia interacting with peers more, not needing to be in control so much at home and gaining confidence in using verbal language with new people. Moreover, her mother wrote that the incorporation of music therapy values and techniques "totally changed their parenting style." They took on what they felt was a "much easier," "more natural approach" than the rigid, repetitive, training they had been adhering to.

Finally, Emma's mother argued that Emma had less need to put things in her mouth or fingers in her ears, was more able to make choices, and had developed an increased sense of agency—all developments that she attributed, at least in part, to music therapy. Her teacher too argued that "over time it was obvious Emma was making gains."

> Lisa was very proactive in utilising Emma's talker during sessions, and we added some relevant items [...] specifically for these sessions. However, we found that she also refers to these at home as a request for Mum to sing the songs of her choosing, which has increased (our) interactions with Emma at home. Emma has also worked out she can request these songs to be played on the TV, which has expanded her choices of entertainment at home. (Emma's mother)

Several of the case studies linked outcomes to the New Zealand Curriculum Key Competencies, "which showed that there was intent that skills learnt in the therapeutic sessions would be transferred to school settings" (Vivian). However, when music therapists are working on mutual goals alongside other professionals, it can be difficult—and seems unnecessary—to attribute specific gains to one intervention. As Noah's mother suggests, generalisability and sustainability are impacted by multiple variables.

> Personally, I feel that the music sessions were beneficial for Noah, and they did contribute alongside other things at school and home to help him with the ASD, Anxiety and ADHD he has. I think the changes were a bit more subtle than expected with not a lot of change at home. I also think as he has been struggling with dyslexia as well that this was an added stressor for him this year that made him more mentally tired. (Noah's mother)

Commentators also suggested that even if generalisation is not evident, the "oasis" that music therapy can provide (Hilda) might be important in helping children to maintain their stability and to manage everyday stress. For example, Freyer was saddened that Oliver's programme came to an unexpected ending as she felt the therapeutic relationship that he had established with Karen would have supported him as he began to face "additional disruptions in his already unsettled world." Similarly, Ben's aunt felt that the development of the therapeutic relationship and the opportunities that music therapy provided for self-expression were more than enough to validate the provision of music therapy for Ben and others.

> If Ben grew to like/trust a therapist and to have the confidence to express him freely through doing music therapy, then is that not something in it-self? [...] I would say that music therapy would be a great tool to not only help other children on the autism spectrum but help all children because it will be a ground where they can be free, build their confidence and express themselves." (Ben's Aunt)

When children have a love for or skills in music yet are unable to access typical music activities or lessons because of their learning support needs, it is not only logical but essential that they are provided with opportunities to access music supported by a qualified music therapist in the interim.

> I do hope Lucas has ongoing music therapy and eventually music lessons. He has talent and a good ear, and it could lead to skills. (But do not make him do examinations). Hopefully Lucas will get confidence from the ability to play an instrument and it could be something he will be able to pursue intensely and individually. Playing an instrument is a skill with status that gives him pleasure. (Hilda)

References

Jeong, A. A. Y., & Darroch, B. (2021). Using letter boards in client-centred music therapy: "Autistics can teach if some are ready to listen." *New Zealand Journal of Music Therapy, 19*, 34–53.

Lindvang, C., Nygaard Pedersen, I., Ole Bonde, L., Lindahl Jacobsen, S., Ridder, H. M., Daniels Beck, B., Gattino, G., Hannibal, N., Holck, U., & Anderson-Ingstrup, J. (2018). Collaborative resonant writing and musical improvisation to explore the concept of resonance. *Qualitative Studies, 5*(1), 4–23. https://tidsskrift.dk/qual/article/view/105455/154259

Low, M. Y. (2021). *Experiences of autistic clients in Nordoff-Robbins music therapy: An interpretive phenomenological analysis*. Drexel University.

Matthiesen, N., Elmholdt, K., Wegener, C., & Meier, N. (2018). Editorial: Resonance in a hurried world. *Qualitative Studies, 5*(1), 1–3. https://tidsskrift.dk/qual/article/view/105454/154258

Ministry of Education. (2009). *Narrative assessment: A guide for teachers*. Learning Media. http://www.throughdifferenteyes.org.nz/a_guide_for_teachers

Molyneux, C., Koo, N.-H., Piggot-Irvine, E., Talmage, A., Travaglia, R., & Willis, M. (2012). Doing it together: Collaborative research on goal-setting and review in a music therapy centre. *New Zealand Journal of Music Therapy, 10*, 6–38. https://www.proquest.com/scholarly-journals/doing-together-collaborative-research-on-goal/docview/1270322224/se-2?accountid=14782

van Manen, M. (1990). *Researching lived experience*. New York State University.

24

Epilogue

Best Practice Guidelines

As noted in the introduction, the intention of this book is not to tell readers how to work with tamariki takiwātanga, or to *prove* that music therapy works. However, commentators have painted a rich picture of music therapy practice in New Zealand, which can be considered alongside government documents outlining best practices for supporting tamariki takiwātanga. Firstly, the New Zealand Autism Spectrum Guideline (Ministries of Health and Education, 2016) provides recommendations and statements of "best practice" for the care and treatment of takiwātanga. Secondly, the New Zealand Government has just announced the formation of a new Ministry for Disabled People, to come into existence in July 2022, and, as part of this transformation, will be emphasising the Enabling Good Lives (EGL) approach (Ministries of Health, Education, & Social Development, 2021) which has already been trialled in parts of the country.

Enabling Good Lives aims to provide supports for disabled people that are tailored to individuals' needs and goals (person-centred); builds and strengthens relationships between them and their whānau and

D. Rickson, *Music Therapy with Autistic Children in Aotearoa, New Zealand*, https://doi.org/10.1007/978-3-031-05233-0_24

communities (relationship building); and is simple to use and flexible (easy to use). It aims to ensure disabled people have control of their lives (self-determination); that their contributions are recognised and respected (mana enhancing); they have access to mainstream services before disability services (mainstream first); and are supported to live ordinary lives (ordinary life outcomes). The approach emphasises the need for early investment in families and whānau to promote aspirations and build community supports (beginning early). In a somewhat similar vein, New Zealand Autism Spectrum Guideline, the "guideline" as I will refer to it from here, suggests all behavioural interventions for tamariki takiwātanga should involve person-centred planning, functional assessment, positive multifaceted intervention strategies, and focus on environment, ecological validity, systems-level intervention, and meaningful outcomes (Ministries of Health and Education, 2016, p. 137). Interestingly, while commentators were not asked to report on the ways in which the music therapy practices might align with the guideline, some spontaneously did so.

Music Therapy Is a Child-Centred, Strengths-Based Practice

Commentators in this study consistently praised the child-centred and strengths-based nature of music therapy. They commended its naturalistic and holistic nature, describing it as an "authentic," "respectful," process. They observed, among other things, that music therapists create "genuinely collaborative" environments; "work with children in ways that suit their needs and personalities"; and give them "time and space to express interests and preferences" (Freyer). Lucas' teacher wrote that the implications of this approach were "enormous."

> I have observed that music therapy gives an opportunity for students to come at social and emotional issues from a non-threatening different direction to other schooling. Linking into the creative for many students is extremely beneficial. It takes away the barrier that words and numbers can be for some students. (Lucas' Teacher)

The guideline urges that the child or young person's interests be incorporated into programmes whenever possible (p. 17) and suggests that they should have access to meaningful activity tailored to their needs and interests (p. 21). They strongly recommend positive behavioural supports which focus on what the child can do, rather than on their difficulties. In this study, observers noticed that the high level of interest that tamariki takiwātanga had in music afforded a "gravitational pull" which drew them in to the music therapy process. However, while Takiwātanga may be attracted to music it is the music therapists' careful crafting of the sessions and the music that maximises the children's engagement and promotes their participation. The commentators viewed the music therapists as highly skilled practitioners who facilitated sessions in sensitive, respectful, and supportive ways. This is important because, as the guideline suggests, "knowledge and understanding of ASD are crucial for the success of any therapeutic encounter" (p. 142).

> (When evaluating the cases) I have looked at whether these autistic children are doing an activity which treats them with respect and dignity and provides an enjoyable and appropriate but safely challenging learning opportunity. From the information provided I have found this to be the situation in all cases. I have now become a convert to music therapy for children with autism. (Hilda)

Music Therapy Promotes Self-determination

In the child-centred music therapy environment tamariki takiwātanga were able to "be themselves" and to lead the direction of the sessions. Commentators suggested the music therapists' responsive, non-confrontational approach could be highly liberating and a powerful tool in promoting children's agency. Moreover, while the children were seen to be engaged in activities that would support their learning and development, they were also observed to be less anxious, and to be having fun. The guideline suggests takiwātanga will respond to individualised programs that are engaging and encourage development and skills for independent living while minimising stress. Because they were less anxious, the tamariki takiwātanga described in this study were more able to attend and listen, to interact, and to express their own needs and preferences. The music therapists imbued a sense of safety by carefully preparing the environment, and providing familiarity and predictability both within the music, and within carefully structured activities, sessions and programmes, and environments, as needed. Hello and goodbye songs, for example, helped to prepare the children for transitions. "Preparing for and supporting children and young people through transitions, both between activities and different settings, are important to minimise stress and anxiety" (Ministries of Health and Education, 2016, p. 119).

It was disappointing that the children did not contribute directly to the music therapy reporting process, not only because doing so would likely have been empowering but also because it is important that therapists and researchers include the perspectives of those they are working with. Unfortunately, there are few self-reports describing the experiences of autistic people in music therapy (LaGasse, 2017). It was certainly possible for the voices of the children, as well as their families, and educators to be included in the learning stories. The music therapists and children were not primary participants in the research, and were encouraged negotiate processes with relevant people, to do what they would typically do in their context. Thus, the music therapists were given the responsibility to determine what would ultimately be included in the case materials they submitted to the research project.

Consent was obtained from each child's music therapist, parent or guardian, and the child themselves, for the case study material to be used for research purposes. Children were informed, among other things, that I was writing a story about music therapy for tamariki takiwātanga. I wrote "I would like to write about you, and the things you do at music, in my story. If you say ok, (your music therapist) will give me a copy of the stories they have written about you at music." I anticipated that for some children, their participation in music therapy would include their input into programme evaluation. With hindsight, I believe it would have been better to write "If you say ok, (your music therapist) will give me a copy of the stories they, and maybe you, have written about your music sessions." This is important, because all children have a right to participate in matters that concern them, and this right applies widely and to all children (UN Committee on the Rights of the Child [CRC], 2009). They must be supported to participate, and their views must be taken seriously.

The word participation is used to describe "ongoing processes, which include information-sharing and dialogue between children and adults based on mutual respect, and in which children can learn how their views and those of adults are taken into account and shape the outcome of such processes" (UN Committee on the Rights of the Child [CRC], 2009, p. 3). Various levels of participation are possible depending on the child's capabilities. Children are supported to participate when they are encouraged to think for themselves, to share ideas, make decisions, develop a sense of agency, and achieve their goals. It is a process that can involve a wide range of experiences ranging from being present to taking part, while supporting children to develop awareness of their abilities, to upskill, and to gain increasing confidence.

Music Therapy Focuses on Relationship Building

In this study, commentators consistently highlighted the importance of the trusting, secure therapeutic relationships that were formed between the therapist and tamariki. The relationship was reportedly a "key element to the success of the therapy" (Ruella), a "bond (that) naturally leads to better engagement and more communication" (Emma's mother). The "attunement" and "synchronisation" that occurred as part of the musical relationship contributed significantly to the establishment of rapport, and music therapy was therefore considered a valuable alternative to verbal therapies. Interestingly the guideline states that approaches that rely on the development of a therapeutic alliance are unlikely to be successful, arguing that Cognitive Behaviour Therapy (CBT) may be more promising (p. 142). Yet the therapeutic relationship—involving empathy, warmth, and acceptance—is now accepted as the most important factor in therapy (Cabaniss et al., 2017; Charura & Paul, 2015) and has been found to be an important predictor of the development of social skills, as well as language, in music therapy with tamariki takiwātanga (Mössler et al., 2017). It is therefore likely that opportunities for non-verbal relating through musicking crucially differentiate music therapy from talk therapies. Music was seen to be motivating and engaging, prompting tamariki takiwātanga's communication, whether they typically used verbal language or not. This is also important because focusing on the establishment of more effective communication strategies is said to be "the most successful means of reducing difficult or disruptive behaviours" for tamariki takiwātanga (Ministries of Health and Education, 2016, p. 140).

Music Therapy Leads to Meaningful Outcomes

The guideline suggests children and young people should receive carefully planned and systematic instruction tailored to their individual needs and abilities (p. 17) and that spontaneous communication, socialisation, and play goals should be a priority educative outcome (p. 17). In music therapy, tamariki takiwātanga were engaged in playful, expressive, creative interactive exchanges, which supported their developing communication and social skills.

> Children with ASD who have educational programmes that effectively target appropriate pro-social and positive skills (communication, social interaction, cognitive, adaptive behaviour and sensorimotor skills) are less likely to develop problem behaviours […] Increasing engagement in activities, providing choices, and using preferred materials and topics are effective prevention strategies for young children. (Ministries of Health and Education, 2016, p. 118)

The gains made in regulation, communication and socialisation through music therapy were considered meaningful for the tamariki takiwātanga. The goals were clearly linked to the children's Individual Education Plan (IEP), or with curriculum guidelines such as the Key Competencies (Ministry of Education, 2014), and while they may have been broad, commentators who knew a child agreed that they were appropriate. However, while outcomes were meaningful in many respects, Mike suggested that the music therapists might have given more consideration to the children and family's cultural needs. The guideline states that the cultural perspectives of the family and whānau should be respected and evident in services and resources (p. 14) and while it was clear that engagement with and respect for autism culture was central to the music therapists' work, none drew attention to the ways in which the children or families' other intersectional cultural interests and/or needs might have been addressed, utilised, and/or valued in music therapy sessions. In Chapter three, I suggest practitioner understanding of the cultural background of music therapy participants is crucial, giving Bevan-Brown & Moldovanu's (2016) example that child-centred approaches may be uncomfortable for parents with Asian backgrounds because they expect programs to be structured and involve the systematic repetitious practice of skills. New Zealand music therapists might therefore pay more attention to the cultural backgrounds of their participants, and/or highlight in the case studies how they addressed this.

However, the respectful and person-centred practices described and valued by commentators in this study suggest that their work was likely to be culturally safe because they cultivated reciprocity, respect, and collaboration; nurtured trust-based relationships in which parents would likely feel safe to talk about their beliefs and the interventions and treatments they were already using; and had the potential to problem solve and resolve conflict (Bevan-Brown & Moldovanu, 2016). The guideline suggests outcome measures can include report of improvements by families and whānau and others (p. 121), assessments should include observations across a variety of settings and activities (p. 92), and professionals, people with ASD, family, whānau, and carers should evaluate treatment approaches before and during implementation (p. 140). Learning stories can provide a useful tool for evaluating music therapy processes, because they encourage the incorporation of observations or feedback from family and/or other team members.

Should Tamariki Takiwātanga Be in Therapy for Ever?

The number and length of sessions that children attend as part of a research project does not necessarily reflect typical practice. For example, ten studies in Geretsegger et al.'s (2014) Cochrane review involved daily treatment for 1–2 weeks, while the other five involved weekly sessions for periods ranging from five weeks to seven months. Further, following their systematic review of the literature relating to the therapeutic use of music with takiwātanga, De Vries et al. (2015) suggested that sessions should be 30–60 min in length, four to five times per week (p. 234). This is likely to be extremely impractical unless therapists are working with the children in a concentrated setting, such as a school. In contrast, a survey involving 328 members of AMTA found only 14% provided individual sessions to autistic people five or more times per week, while the average frequency of individual or group sessions was once per week, mostly lasting 30 min. Programme duration averaged 1–3 years. Music therapists need to vary lengths of sessions according to children's abilities to regulate (Accordino et al., 2007; Carpente, 2011; Oldfield, 2006) and further research is still needed to understand how frequency of sessions and length of time in music therapy impact on outcomes (Kaplan & Steele, 2005).

When children and their families are gaining the levels of pleasure described on "Feelings Matter", music therapy teams can have difficulty making the decision that programmes should stop. The commentators in this study were aware that it takes time to build a therapeutic relationship, and that for music therapy to be helpful, regular sessions need to be held over many months. It therefore seems logical that many programmes will be long-term, while there is evidence that music therapy is supporting the child's learning, development, and/or well-being. The problem with this is that unless wider communities become autism-friendly, children will continue to be in therapy for long periods. There comes a time when it is likely to be more beneficial for the therapist to support others in the community to musick with, or teach music to, the child. In brief, the music therapists' role in working with individuals is to work their way, carefully, out of a job!

Moving Towards Mainstream Services and "Ordinary Lives"

"Good interventions result in adding elements to the child's life that improve the richness or effectiveness of living and learning" (Ministries of Health and Education, 2016, p. 121) and having "regular, timetabled 'down time'" can provide children with an opportunity to have a break from social expectations and busy environments, and reduce stress (p. 119). The high level of value that families and team members bestowed on the individual music therapy programmes described in this study is therefore highly meaningful. As Hilda argued, "music therapy can provide a little oasis of positive one-on-one therapy that is enjoyable without the need to manage peer relationships or puzzling school routines." However, in New Zealand there is an emphasis on inclusive education which aims for children to be actively involved in meaningful play and learning with and alongside their peers. The guideline therefore also suggests "the learning of new skills should take place in the child or young person's usual environment, i.e., with their usual carers and teachers, and with access to peers who do not have ASD" (p. 17). Further, it is stated that "priority for professional learning and development should be given to those who provide a specialist or consultancy service and support and education to others" (p. 190).

> Family-centred treatment approaches result in greater generalisation and maintenance of skills. Development of management strategies that can be implemented consistently but do not demand extensive sacrifice in terms of time, money or other aspects of family life seem most likely to offer benefits for all involved (Ministries of Health and Education, 2016, p. 140).

While some of the cases in this series had outcomes linked to the Key Competencies, demonstrating "intent that skills learnt in the therapeutic sessions would be transferred to school settings" (Vivian), few of the studies involved peers and/or family members and none focused specifically on providing direct support to the family or team members living or working with tamariki takiwātanga. Nevertheless, input from family members and teachers suggests that many skills developed in music therapy were able to be sustained and generalised to other contexts. Moreover, Sophie's family found it easy to incorporate music therapy values and techniques into their daily lives and argued that this led to a radical and positive change in their parenting style.

On the other hand, music therapy can be provided individually, in groups, and in homes and classrooms. Music therapists can support children to achieve "greater participation in their school or community setting" (Ministries of Health and Education, 2016, p. 121), by working directly with families (Thompson, 2012) or school communities (Rickson & McFerran, 2014). While there are several good reasons why the best option might be to offer individual music therapy, music therapists in New Zealand might also be encouraged to consider how they can develop more inclusive practices.

Is Music Therapy an Evidence-Based Practice?

Music therapists are frequently called upon to produce "evidence" that the services they offer are "effective" yet face significant dilemmas in designing research to meet the traditional demands of evidence-based practice with tamariki takiwātanga (Rickson et al., 2016). Randomised controlled trials (RCTs), which have by convention been considered the "gold standard" of evidence, might yield important information about the effectiveness of a carefully defined treatment, yet provide little understanding of processes, and are notoriously difficult to design. McLeod (2010) argues for example, that person-centred therapy defines a set of boundary conditions for a range of possible interactions from which a variety of outcomes are possible, and that it is therefore meaningless to talk about causality in this context. "In any interactional therapy, there will automatically be variations both from child to child, and session to session, and research has to be planned accordingly rather than modifying the intervention to meet research criteria" (Oldfield, 2020, p. 109).

Nevertheless, it *is* possible and interesting to observe an individual's engagement in complex interactive processes, and the outcomes they achieve (Borgnakke, 2017; McLeod, 2010). Moreover, qualitative synthesis approaches, such as the cross-case analysis employed in this study, enable researchers to speak beyond the individual case, to generate new interpretation or theory, and to uncover "how" and "why" an intervention might be helpful for an individual or group of people, rather than uncovering "what works" (Borgnakke, 2017; Noblit, 1988; Pilkington, 2018). It is also possible to develop an understanding of "what works, in which situations, and for whom," and therefore to talk of "multiple contextualised truths," that is of findings that might be considered "*a* truth" in context, rather than "*the* truth" in general (Solesbury, 2002). I wanted music therapists to be able to practice in natural ways, not to modify what they were doing to suit the research. And I wanted the commentators to "see for themselves," as much as possible, what happens in music therapy, and then to report on how they understood it. The multiple case study design has highlighted the rich variations within and between cases that Oldfield (2020) refers to, while enabling commentators to convey a sense of what the therapy is like for both client and therapist (McLeod, 2010).

The application of meta-ethnography to primary data rather than published studies allows for the retention of context and "thick description" (Pilkington, 2018). The benefits of generating multiple case reports for a single project are therefore clear. Typically, however, it can be difficult to obtain clinical case reports for research purposes because of the ethical issues involved in reusing data for a purpose other than originally specified; and difficulty obtaining somewhat homogeneous cases. A strength of the current project then is that despite the obvious diversity of practice, the ten case reports were drawn from a common research project, supported by cross-project guidelines. Moreover, in this study cases were broadly homogenous; involving ten children living in New Zealand who were by chance in a similar age group. None of the children had music therapy previously, and they were all offered up to one year of therapy over the same period, with their local therapist. The children and therapists came together in a natural way and were encouraged to engage in usual practice, thus allowing for diversity within cases and promoting ecological validity. The music therapists all produced rich detailed description of practice which was, in eight of the cases, accompanied by video examples which enabled the work to "speak" directly to the commentators. Moreover, each case report was interpreted by the same team of six autism experts, as well as several people who knew the child. Inductive analysis of the evaluations allowed for the elicitation of unforeseen concepts. James' case emerged as an "exception" or "outlier" which could be used to enhance understanding (Pilkington, 2018). I am confident then that the findings will help readers to understand "how" and "why" child-centred music therapy works for tamariki takiwātanga in the New Zealand context.

The importance of "how" and "why" questions, and the value of systematic reviews of qualitative studies as a way of informing policy and practice, is being increasingly recognised by international organisations, including the Cochrane Collaboration (Borgnakke, 2017). Policy makers and practitioners are becoming increasingly aware of the limitations of using systematic reviews of randomised controlled trials as the exclusive evidence base for informing practice (Kinn et al., 2013). Moreover, medical practices are gradually changing to allow more patient and client autonomy; including the voices of end-users in research processes are becoming increasingly important; and expert opinion plays an important role in many areas of paediatrics, including the planning of child healthcare services.

> Evidence-based practice (EBP), a cornerstone of professional practice currently in New Zealand (Aotearoa), has undergone a paradigmatic shift in the past decade. It has if anything moved away from the narrow reliance on 'gold standard' RCT studies. Both educational as well as medical practitioners now rely on not only using research-based evidence, but also necessarily include the knowledge and experiences of practitioners, families and where possible, the voices of children and young people. (Vivian)

Comments from Dana and Vivian suggested they were at times viewing the work through more of a medical or educational lens because they anticipated more "measurable" developmental or academic outcomes. Target behaviours are often viewed as inadequate when music therapists work intuitively and flexibly (Pater et al., 2019), preferring to "see where (the work) takes us" (Rickson et al., 2015b, p. 17). Our 2015 interviewees communicated that it was not easy to measure improvement because "progress can look different for various people, be slow, hard to pinpoint, and difficult to quantify; and it can be difficult to communicate what a little progress can mean in a child's life" (p. 25).

Regardless of one's epistemological lens, with high numbers of children diagnosed with ASD continuing to rise there is an increasing need for research that supports management and/or promotes understanding of the condition. Baron-Cohen (2017) argues that parents need to be able to access early interventions for their children, just as parents of all children make choices of how to promote their child's potential, but "this is different to the default assumption that autism is a disorder that needs to be eradicated, prevented or cured" (Baron-Cohen, 2017, p. 746). Nevertheless, it is likely that a turn from the medical model will pose a threat to services that support takiwātanga, in some instances (Evans, 2018). In some countries including the USA, programmes are more likely to be funded if there is quantifiable evidence to suggest positive outcomes (McFerran & Silverman, 2018; Rickson et al., 2016). However, in New Zealand where new policies are focused on giving disabled people and their families increasing control and choice over their everyday activities, and ensuring their voices are embedded at all levels of decision-making, there are likely to be significant opportunities for service growth. Moreover,

> I think there is an opportunity for music therapists to engage with the growing range of "lived experience literature" from people on the spectrum ourselves which outlines the positive impacts on our lives. I think this would give an additional body of evidence from which to draw from. (Mike)

Implications for Practice

Overall, I believe this study has produced two important findings. Firstly, the commentators appear to have developed understandings of music therapy which align well with what music therapists are trying to achieve (Rickson, 2021) and secondly their reports suggest that music therapy practice aligns well with best practice guidelines for work with tamariki takiwātanga in New Zealand.

> Firstly, I would like to say how much I enjoyed and was privileged to see the variety of practice and progress that I did. The New Zealand Autism Spectrum Disorder Guideline (2016) provides a series of recommendations around how interventions should be developed and practiced. The recommendations include starting early, with programmes that are individualised, engaging, and highly supportive, and which prioritise spontaneous socialisation and play goals. Programmes should be supplemented by informal assessments, and the child's interests should be incorporated whenever possible (ASD Guideline Summary, 2016, p. 12). The best practice which I saw here showed all these elements in large measure. By doing this, they achieved results which were highly meaningful to the child and their whanau as well as being curriculum based [...] some of the best practice I saw affected me very deeply in positive ways. (Mike)

> The National Autism Centre (NAC) is the epicentre for identifying EBP in the field of autism. They state that robust evidence must be informed by professional judgment and data-based decision making; values and preferences of families, including the student on the autism spectrum whenever feasible; and capacity to accurately implement interventions. The case studies (in this research) have taken all the above points into consideration, where the therapy has been requested by families and the therapists' interventions are based on their gathering and monitoring of students' progress. (Vivian)

Reports that music therapy is one of parents' most preferred interventions for tamariki takiwātanga in New Zealand (Dharan, 2015; Kasilingam et al., 2019) were reinforced by the strong appreciation expressed in this study. The integration of knowledge and understandings from family members, caregivers, friends, teachers, and other autism experts provides further support for the use of music therapy with tamariki takiwātanga. However, Kasilingam and colleagues found a large discrepancy between the parents' desire for music therapy for their child, and their ability to access the service in this country. This is disappointing, when "the values, knowledge, preferences of the family and whānau should be respected and evident in services and resources" (Ministries of Health and Education, 2016, p. 14) and family and service users are encouraged to have "direct involvement in planning and implementation of service provision" (p. 15).

There can be substantial gaps between the strategies espoused in guidelines, families feeling supported, and children accessing quality and comprehensive services (Nanclares-Nogues et al., 2010). Moreover, while parental interest in music therapy has been high, up until this year the New Zealand Autism Guideline (Ministries of Health and Education, 2016) gave little support to music therapy, calling for more evidence regarding its effectiveness. However, the document is a "living guideline" which means that when new and significant research comes to hand, topics can be updated. It is exciting, and perhaps not surprising given the increasing international literature base, that a very recent supplementary paper produced for the guideline concludes that "music therapy can enhance social communication skills and should be considered for children and young people on the autism spectrum" (Broadstock, 2021, p. xii).

Conclusion

In this research I have invited people who have significant interest in the well-being of tamariki takiwātanga to look closely at the practice of music therapy and to comment on what they observed. Commentators summarised that music therapy can support tamariki takiwātanga to regulate emotions, to express themselves in a variety of ways, and therefore to develop communication and socialisation skills. The child-centred nature of music therapy, the development of authentic and respectful therapeutic relationships, the children's inherent interest in music, and the music therapists' expertise which involved careful balancing of freedom and structure within sessions enabled all the children to feel comfortable to engage in play, try out new ideas, take leadership and communicate with others in a variety of ways. Thus, music therapy is highlighted as a situated relational encounter (Ansdell, 2014) in which the tamariki takiwātanga, music therapists, their musicking, and the environments, reciprocally influenced the encounters and outcomes. Given the already high levels of interest in music therapy (Kasilingam et al., 2019) and the high levels of appreciation expressed in this study, training institutions, music therapists, and providers might anticipate an exponential rise in demand for haumanu ā-puoro to support tamariki takiwātanga in New Zealand (Aotearoa). May music therapy lift their wings so they might soar.

References

Accordino, R., Comer, R., & Heller, W. B. (2007, January–March). Searching for music's potential: A critical examination of research on music therapy with individuals with autism. *Research in Autism Spectrum Disorders, 1*(1), 101–115. https://doi.org/10.1016/j.rasd.2006.08.002

Ansdell, G. (2014). *How music helps in music therapy and everyday life*. Ashgate.

Baron-Cohen, S. (2017). Editorial perspective: Neurodiversity—A revolutionary concept for autism and psychiatry. *Journal of Childhood Psychology and Psychiatry, 58*, 744–747. https://doi-org.helicon.vuw.ac.nz/10.1111/jcpp.12703

Bevan-Brown, J., & Moldovanu, A. (2016). The role of culture in the perception, assessment, diagnosis, treatment and education of children and young people with autism spectrum disorder. In J. Bevan-Brown & V. M. Dharan (Eds.), *Autism spectrum disorder in Aotearoa New Zealand: Promising practices and interesting issues* (pp. 155–168). NZCER Press.

Borgnakke, K. (2017). Meta-ethnography and systematic reviews—Linked to the evidence movement and caught in a dilemma. *Ethnography and Education: Meta-Ethnographic Synthesis in Education: Challenges, Aims and Possibilities, 12*(2), 194–210. https://doi.org/10.1080/17457823.2016.1253027

Broadstock, M. (2021). *New Zealand autism spectrum disorder guideline's supplementary paper on the effectiveness of music therapy*. Ministries of Health and Education. https://www.health.govt.nz/publication/new-zealand-autism-spectrum-disorder-guidelines-supplementary-paper-effectiveness-music-therapy

Cabaniss, D. L., Cherry, S., Douglas, C. J., & Schwartz, A. R. (2017). *Psychodynamic psychotherapy: A clinical manual* (2nd ed.). John Wiley & Sons Inc.

Carpente, J. A. (2011). Addressing core features of autism: Integrating Nordoff-Robbins music therapy within the developmental, individual-difference, relationship-based (DIR®)/Floortime™ model. In A. Meadows (Ed.), *Developments in music therapy practice: Case study perspectives* (pp. 124–135). Barcelona.

Charura, D., & Paul, S. (2015). What has love to do with it? In D. Charura & S. Paul (Eds.), *Love and therapy: In relationship* (1st ed.). Routledge. https://doi.org/10.4324/9780429476907

De Vries, D., Beck, T., Stacey, B., Winslow, K., & Meines, K. (2015). Music as a therapeutic intervention with autism: A systematic review of the literature. *Therapeutic Recreation Journal, 49*(3), 220. https://js.sagamorepub.com/trj/article/view/6085

Dharan, V. (2015, July 22–23). *Hearing from the experts: Parents' knowledge of what works for their children.* Altogether Autism Conference, Auckland, New Zealand.

Evans, B. (2018). *The Autism paradox: How an autism diagnosis became both a clinical label and an identity: A stigma to be challenged and a status to be embraced.* Aeon. Retrieved November 24, 2018 from https://aeon.co/essays/the-intriguing-history-of-the-autism-diagnosis

Geretsegger, M., Elefant, C., Mössler, K. A., & Gold, C. (2014). Music therapy for people with autism spectrum disorder. *The Cochrane Database of Systematic Reviews*. https://doi.org/10.1002/14651858.CD004381.pub3.

Kaplan, R. S., & Steele, A. L. (2005). An analysis of music therapy programme Goals and outcomes for clients with diagnoses on the autism spectrum. *Journal of Music Therapy, 42*(1), 2–19. https://doi.org/10.1093/jmt/42.1.2

Kasilingam, N., Waddington, H., & Van Der Meer, L. (2019). Early intervention for children with autism spectrum disorder in New Zealand: What children get and what parents want. *International Journal of Disability, Development, and Education, 68*(4), 521–537. https://doi.org/10.1080/1034912X.2019.1696949

Kinn, L. G., Holgersen, H., Ekeland, T. J., & Davidson, L. (2013). Metasynthesis and bricolage: An artistic exercise of creating a collage of meaning. *Qualitative Health Research, 23*, 1285–1292. https://doi.org/10.1177/1049732313502127

LaGasse, A. B. (2017). Social outcomes in children with autism spectrum disorder: A review of music therapy outcomes. *Patient Related Outcome Measures, 8*, 23–32. https://doi.org/10.2147/PROM.S106267

McFerran, K. S., & Silverman, M. J. (2018). *A guide to designing research questions for beginning music therapy researchers*. The American Music Therapy Association, Inc.

McLeod, J. (2010). *Case study research in counselling and psychotherapy*. Sage.

Ministries of Health and Education. (2016). *New Zealand autism spectrum disorder guideline* (2nd ed.). Ministry of Health. https://www.health.govt.nz/publication/new-zealand-autism-spectrum-disorder-guideline

Ministry of Education. (2014). *Key competencies*. Te Kete Ipurangi, Ministry of Eudcation. Retrieved August 25, 2020 from https://nzcurriculum.tki.org.nz/Key-competencies

Ministries of Health, Education, & Social Development. (2021). *Enabling good lives*. Ministries of Health, Education, & Social Development. Retrieved November 10 from https://www.enablinggoodlives.co.nz/

Mössler, K., Gold, C., Aßmus, J., Schumacher, K., Calvet, C., Reimer, S., Iversen, G., & Schmid, W. (2017). The therapeutic relationship as predictor of change in music therapy with young children with autism spectrum disorder. *Journal of Autism and Developmental Disorders, 49*(7), 2795–2809. https://doi.org/10.1007/s10803-017-3306-y

Nanclares-Nogues, V., Lin, E., Rolland, C., & Msall, M. E. (2010). Enhancing multidisciplinary community supports for minority preschool children with autistic spectrum disorders: Promoting family centered and evidence based practices. *International Public Health Journal, 2*(1, Special Issue), 69–82.

Noblit, G. W. (1988). *Meta-ethnography synthesizing qualitative studies*. Sage.

Oldfield, A. (2006). *Interactive music therapy: A positive approach*. Jessica Kingsley.

Oldfield, A. (2020). Book Review. In P. Kern & M. Humpal (Eds.), Early childhood music therapy and autism spectrum disorder. *British Journal of Music Therapy, 34*(2), 108–120.

Pater, M., de Graaf, P., & van Yperen, T. (2019). Working elements of music therapy for children and young people with autism. *Open Journal of Medical Psychology, 08*(04), 78–96. https://doi.org/10.4236/ojmp.2019.84008

Pilkington, H. (2018). Employing meta-ethnography in the analysis of qualitative data sets on youth activism: A new tool for transnational research projects? *Qualitative Research, 18*(1), 108–130. https://doi.org/10.1177/1468794117707805

Rickson, D. J. (2021). Family members' and other experts' perceptions of music therapy with children on the autism spectrum in New Zealand: Findings from multiple case studies. *The Arts in Psychotherapy, 75*, 101833. https://doi.org/10.1016/j.aip.2021.101833

Rickson, D. J., Castelino, A., Molyneux, C., Ridley, H., & Upjohn-Beatson, E. (2016). What evidence? Designing a mixed methods study to investigate music therapy with children who have autism spectrum disorder (ASD), in New Zealand Contexts. *The Arts in Psychotherapy, 50*, 119–125. https://doi.org/10.1016/j.aip.2016.07.002

Rickson, D. J., Molyneux, C., Ridley, H., Castelino, A., & Upjohn Beatson, E. B. (2015b). Music therapy with people who have autism spectrum disorder—Current practice in New Zealand. *New Zealand Journal of Music Therapy, 13*, 8–32. https://www-proquest-com.helicon.vuw.ac.nz/docview/1897698669?accountid=14782

Rickson, D. J., & McFerran, K. S. (2014). *Creating music cultures in the schools: A perspective from community music therapy*. Barcelona.

Solesbury, W. (2002). The ascendancy of evidence. *Planning Theory & Practice, 3*(1), 90–96. https://doi.org/10.1080/14649350220117834

Thompson, G. A. (2012). Family-centered music therapy in the home environment: Promoting interpersonal engagement between children with autism spectrum disorder and their parents. *Music Therapy Perspectives, 30*(2), 109–116. http://ezproxy.massey.ac.nz/login?url=http://search.ebscohost.com/login.aspx?direct=true&db=ccm&AN=2012088717&site=eds-live&scope=site

UN Committee on the Rights of the Child (CRC). (2009). *General comment No. 12: The right of the child to be heard*. https://www.refworld.org/docid/4ae562c52.html

References

Accordino, R., Comer, R., & Heller, W. B. (2007, January–March). Searching for music's potential: A critical examination of research on music therapy with individuals with autism. *Research in Autism Spectrum Disorders, 1*(1), 101–115. https://doi.org/10.1016/j.rasd.2006.08.002

Aigen, K. (2014a). Music-centered dimensions of Nordoff-Robbins music therapy. *Music Therapy Perspectives, 32*(1), 18–29. https://doi.org/10.1093/mtp/miu006

Aigen, K. (2014b). *The study of music therapy: Current issues and concepts*. Taylor and Francis.

Aigen, K. (2015). A critique of evidence-based practice in music therapy. *Music Therapy Perspectives, 33*(1), 12–24. https://doi.org/10.1093/mtp/miv013

Alagoz, M., Kherad, N., Gavaz, M., & Yuksel, A. (2019). New genetic approaches for early diagnosis and treatment of autism spectrum disorders. *Review Journal of Autism and Developmental Disorders, 6*(4), 367–380. https://doi.org/10.1007/s40489-019-00167-w

Allgood, N. (2005). Parents' perceptions of family-based group music therapy for children with autism spectrum disorders. *Music Therapy Perspectives, 23*(2), 92–99. https://doi.org/10.1093/mtp/23.2.92

Alvin, J. (1978). *Music therapy for the autistic child*. Oxford University Press.

D. Rickson, *Music Therapy with Autistic Children in Aotearoa, New Zealand*, https://doi.org/10.1007/978-3-031-05233-0

American Psychiatric Association. (2013). *Diagnostic criteria from DSM-V*. American Psychiatric Association.

Anastasiou, D., & Kauffman, J. M. (2012, May 1). Disability as cultural difference: Implications for special education. *Remedial and Special Education, 33*(3), 139–149. http://dx.doi.org/10.1177/0741932510383163

Anderson-Lopez, K., & Lopez, R. (2017). Remember me. In *Coco (Original Motion Picture Soundtrack)*. Walt Disney.

Annesley, L. (2014). The music therapist in school as outsider. *British Journal of Music Therapy, 28*(2), 36–43. https://doi.org/10.1177/135945751402800207

Ansdell, G. (2014). *How music helps in music therapy and everyday life*. Ashgate.

Ansdell, G. (2020). *Shining some (gentle) light on ecological validity in music therapy research*. 2020 Online World Congress of Music Therapy, University of Pretoria.

Ansel, A., Rosenzweig, J. P., Zisman, P. D., Melamed, M., & Gesundheit, B. (2017). Variation in gene express ion in autism spectrum disorders: An extensive review of transcriptomic studies. *Frontiers in Neuroscience, 10*, 601. https://doi.org/10.3389/fnins.2016.00601

Antezana, L., Scarpa, A., Valdespino, A., Albright, J., & Richey, J. A. (2017). Rural trends in diagnosis and services for autism spectrum disorder. *Frontiers in Psychology, 8*, 590–590. https://doi.org/10.3389/fpsyg.2017.00590

Arns, B., & Thompson, G. A. (2019). Music therapy teaming and learning: How transdisciplinary experience shapes practice in a specialist school for students with autism. *Australian Journal of Music Therapy, 30*, 31–52.

Bailey, B., & Arciuli, J. (2020). Indigenous Australians with autism: A scoping review. *Autism, 24*(5), 1031–1046. https://doi.org/10.1177/1362361319894829

Bakan, M. B. (2014). Ethnomusicological perspectives on autism, neurodiversity, and music therapy. In *Voices: A world forum for music therapy* (Vol. 14, No. 3). https://doi.org/10.15845/voices.v14i3.799

Bakan, M. B. (2015). "Don't go changing to try and please me": Combating essentialism through ethnography in the ethnomusicology of autism. *Ethnomusicology, 59*(1), 116–144. https://doi.org/10.5406/ethnomusicology.59.1.0116

Bakan, M. B. (2018). *Speaking for ourselves*. Oxford University Press. https://doi.org/10.1093/oso/9780190855833.003.0005

Baker, F., Wigram, T., Stott, D., & McFerran, K. S. (2009). Therapeutic songwriting in music therapy, Part II: Comparing the literature with practice across diverse clinical populations. *Nordic Journal of Music Therapy, 18*(1), 32–56. https://doi.org/10.1080/08098130802496373

Baron-Cohen, S. (2017). Editorial perspective: Neurodiversity—A revolutionary concept for autism and psychiatry. *Journal of Childhood Psychology and Psychiatry, 58*, 744–747. https://doi-org.helicon.vuw.ac.nz/10.1111/jcpp.12703

Berger, D. S. (2002). *Music therapy, sensory integration and the autistic child*. Jessica Kingsley.

Berger, R. (2015). Now I see it, now I don't: Researcher's position and reflexivity in qualitative research. *Qualitative Research, 15*(2), 219–234. https://doi.org/10.1177/1468794112468475

Bergmann, T. (2016). Music therapy for people with autism spectrum disorder. In J. Edwards (Ed.), *The Oxford handbook of music therapy*. Oxford University Press. https://doi.org/10.1093/oxfordhb/9780199639755.013.3

Bevan-Brown, J. (2004). *Maori perspectives of autistic spectrum disorder: Report to the Ministry of Education*. Ministry of Education.

Bevan-Brown, J. (2013). Including people with disabilities: An indigenous perspective. *International Journal of Inclusive Education, 17*(6), 571–583. https://doi.org/10.1080/13603116.2012.694483

Bevan-Brown, J. (2021). *Neurodiversity and christmas tree lights* [Curriculum Document]. Massey University.

Bevan-Brown, J., & Moldovanu, A. (2016). The role of culture in the perception, assessment, diagnosis, treatment and education of children and young people with autism spectrum disorder. In J. Bevan-Brown & V. M. Dharan (Eds.), *Autism spectrum disorder in Aotearoa New Zealand: Promising practices and interesting issues* (pp. 155–168). NZCER Press.

Bhaskar, R. (1989). *Reclaiming reality: A critical introduction to contemporary philosophy*. Verso.

Bieleninik, L., Geretsegger, M., Mossler, K., Drusmus, J. A., Thompson, G., Gattino, G., Elefant, C., Gottfried, T., Igliozzi, R., Muratori, F., Suvini, F., Kim, J., Crawford, M. J., Odell Miller, H., Oldfield, A., Casey, O., Finnemann, J., Carpente, J. A., Park, A.-L., … Gold, C. (2017). Effects of improvisational music therapy vs enhances standard care on symptom severity amount children with autism spectrum disorder. The TIME-A randomized clinical trial. *Journal of the American Medical Association, 318*(6), 525–535. https://doi.org/10.1001/jama.2017.9478

Blauth, L. (2017). Improving mental health in families with autistic children: Benefits of using video feedback in parent counselling sessions offered alongside music therapy. *Health Psychology Report, 2*(2), 138–150. https://doi.org/10.5114/hpr.2017.63558

Borgnakke, K. (2017). Meta-ethnography and systematic reviews—Linked to the evidence movement and caught in a dilemma. *Ethnography and Education: Meta-Ethnographic Synthesis in Education: Challenges, Aims and Possibilities, 12*(2), 194–210. https://doi.org/10.1080/17457823.2016.1253027

Boso, M., Emanuele, E., Minazzi, V., Abbamonte, M., & Politi, P. (2007, September). Effect of long-term interactive music therapy on behavior profile and musical skills in young adults with severe autism. *Journal of Alternative & Complementary Medicine, 13*(7), 709–712.

Boucher, H., & Ryan, C. A. (2011). Performance stress and the very young musician. *Journal of Research in Music Education, 58*(4), 329–345. https://doi.org/10.1177/0022429410386965

Bowden, N., Thabrew, H., Kokaua, J., Audas, R., Milne, B., Smiler, K., Stace, H., Taylor, B., & Gibb, S. (2020). Autism spectrum disorder/Takiwātanga: An integrated data infrastructure-based approach to autism spectrum disorder research in New Zealand. *Autism: The International Journal of Research and Practice, 24*(8), 2213–2227. https://doi.org/10.1177/1362361320939329

Boxill, E. H., & Chase, K. M. (2006). *Music therapy for developmental disabilities* (2nd ed.). Pro-Ed.

Bradt, J., Burns, D. S., & Creswell, J. W. (2013, June 20). Mixed methods research in music therapy research. *Journal of Music Therapy, 50*(2), 123–148. https://doi.org/10.1093/jmt/50.2.123

Brandt, A., Slevc, L. R., & Gebrian, M. (2019). The role of musical development in early language acquisition. In D. A. Hodges & M. Thaut (Eds.), *The Oxford handbook of music and the brain* (pp. 567–597). Oxford University Press. https://doi.org/10.1093/oxfordhb/9780198804123.013.23

Braun, V., & Clarke, V. (2006, April). Using thematic analysis in psychology. *Qualitative Research in Psychology, 3*(2), 77–101. http://dx.doi.org/10.1191/1478088706qp063oa

Broadstock, M. (2021). *New Zealand autism spectrum disorder guideline's supplementary paper on the effectiveness of music therapy*. Ministries of Health and Education. https://www.health.govt.nz/publication/new-zealand-autism-spectrum-disorder-guidelines-supplementary-paper-effectiveness-music-therapy

Broder-Fingert, S., Feinberg, E., & Silverstein, M. (2017). Music therapy for children with autism spectrum disorder. *Journal of the American Medical Association, 318*(6), 523–524. https://doi.org/10.1001/jama.2017.9477

Brondino, N., Fusar-Poli, L., Rocchetti, M., Provenzani, U., Barale, F., & Politi, P. (2015). Complementary and alternative therapies for autism spectrum disorder. *Evidence-Based Complementary and Alternative Medicine, 2015*, 258531–258589. https://doi.org/10.1155/2015/258589

Brownell, M. D. (2002, Sum). Musically adapted social stories to modify behaviors in students with autism: Four case studies. *Journal of Music Therapy, 39*(2), 117–144. https://doi.org/10.1093/jmt/39.2.117

Bruscia, K. (1987). *Improvisational models of music therapy*. Charles C. Thomas.

Bruscia, K. (2014). *Defining music therapy*. Barcelona.

Burleson, B. R. (2009). The nature of interpersonal communication. In C. R. Berger, M. E. Roloff, & D. R. Ewoldsen (Eds.), *The handbook of communication science* (2 ed., pp. 145–164). Sage. https://doi.org/10.4135/9781412982818

Bury, S. M., Jellett, R., Spoor, J. R., & Hedley, D. (2020). "It defines who I am" or "It's something I have": What language do [autistic] Australian adults [on the autism spectrum] prefer? *Journal of Autism and Developmental Disorders*. https://doi.org/10.1007/s10803-020-04425-3

Cabaniss, D. L., Cherry, S., Douglas, C. J., & Schwartz, A. R. (2017). *Psychodynamic psychotherapy: A clinical manual* (2nd ed.). John Wiley & Sons Inc.

Cage, E., & Troxell-Whitman, Z. (2019). Understanding the reasons, contexts and costs of camouflaging for autistic adults. *Journal of Autism & Developmental Disorders, 49*(5), 1899–1911. https://doi.org/10.1007/s10803-018-03878-x

Campbell, C. (2008). Further towards an affirmation model. In T. Campbell, F. Fontes, L. Hemingway, A. Soorenian, & C. Till (Eds.), *Disability studies: Emerging insights and perspectives*. The Disability Press.

Cappella, J. N. (1987). Interpersonal communication: Definition and fundamental questions. In C. R. Berger & S. H. Chaffee (Eds.), *Handbook of communication science* (pp. 184–238). Sage.

Carpente, J. A. (2011). Addressing core features of autism: Integrating Nordoff-Robbins music therapy within the developmental, individual-difference, relationship-based (DIR®)/Floortime™ model. In A. Meadows (Ed.), *Developments in music therapy practice: Case study perspectives* (pp. 124–135). Barcelona.

Carpente, J. A. (2014). Individual music-centered assessment profile for neurodevelopmental disorders (IMCAP-ND): New developments in music-centered evaluation. *Music Therapy Perspectives, 32*(1), 56–60. https://doi.org/10.1093/mtp/miu005

Carpente, J. A. (2017). Investigating the effectiveness of a developmental, individual difference, relationship-based (DIR) improvisational music therapy program on social communication for children with autism spectrum disorder. *Music Therapy Perspectives, 35* (2), 160–174. https://doi.org/10.1093/mtp/miw013

Carpente, J. A., & LaGasse, A. B. (2015). Music therapy for children with autism spectrum disorder. In B. L. Wheeler (Ed.), *Music therapy handbook* (pp. 290–301). The Guilford Press.

Charura, D., & Paul, S. (2015). What has love to do with it? In D. Charura & S. Paul (Eds.), *Love and therapy: In relationship* (1st ed.). Routledge. https://doi.org/10.4324/9780429476907

Chevallier, C., Kohls, G., Troiani, V., Brodkin, E. S., & Schultz, R. T. (2012). The social motivation theory of autism. *Trends in Cognitive Sciences, 16*(4), 231–239. https://doi.org/10.1016/j.tics.2012.02.007

Church, C., Alisanski, S., & Amanullah, S. (2000). The social, behavioral, and academic experiences of children with Asperger syndrome. *Focus on Autism and Other Developmental Disabilities, 15*(1), 12–20. https://doi.org/10.1177/108835760001500102

Clarke, V., & Braun, V. (2013). *Successful qualitative research: A practical guide for beginners.* Sage.

Coffey, A. (2003). Ethnography and self: Reflections and representations. In T. May (Ed.), *Qualitative research in action* (pp. 313–331). Sage.

Crawford, M. J., Gold, C., Odell-Miller, H., Thana, L., Faber, S., Assmus, J., Bieleninik, Ł, Geretsegger, M., Grant, C., Maratos, A., Sandford, S., Claringbold, A., McConachie, H., Maskey, M., Mössler, K. A., Ramchandani, P., & Hassiotis, A. (2017). International multicentre randomised controlled trial of improvisational music therapy for children with autism spectrum disorder: TIME-A study. *Health Technology Assessment (Winchester, England), 21*(59), 1–40. https://doi.org/10.3310/hta21590

Creswell, J. W., Klassen, A. C., Plano Clark, V. L., & Clegg Smith, K. (2011). *Best practices for mixed methods research in the health sciences.* Office of Behavioral and Social Sciences Research, National Institute of Health.

De Jaegher, H. (2013). Embodiment and sense-making in autism. *Frontiers in Integrative Neuroscience, 7*, 15. http://dx.doi.org/10.3389/fnint.2013.00015

De Vries, D., Beck, T., Stacey, B., Winslow, K., & Meines, K. (2015). Music as a therapeutic intervention with autism: A systematic review of the literature. *Therapeutic Recreation Journal, 49*(3), 220. https://js.sagamorepub.com/trj/article/view/6085

Dharan, V. (2013). Understanding diversity: Moving beginning teachers beyond receiving the baton. In *Inclusive education: Perspectives on professional practice* (pp. 52–65). Dunmore Publishing Ltd.

Dharan, V. (2015, July 22–23). *Hearing from the experts: Parents' knowledge of what works for their children.* Altogether Autism Conference, Auckland, New Zealand.

Dissanayake, E. (2012). The earliest narratives were musical. *Research Studies in Music Education, 34*(1), 3–14. https://doi.org/10.1177/1321103X12448148

Donnellan, A. M., Hill, D. A., & Leary, M. R. (2012). Rethinking autism: Implications of sensory and movement differences for understanding and support. *Frontiers in Integrative Neuroscience, 6*, 124–124. https://doi.org/10.3389/fnint.2012.00124

Dromi, E., Rum, Y., & Florian, J. G. (2018). Communication, language, and speech in young children with autism spectrum disorder (ASD). In A. Bar-On, D. Ravid, & E. Dattner (Eds.), *Handbook of communication disorders* (pp. 811–828). De Gruyter Mouton. https://doi.org/10.1515/9781614514909

Drysdale, H., & van der Meer, L. (2020). Rates of autism spectrum disorder diagnoses for children and adolescents in the Hutt Valley Region of New Zealand between 2012 and 2016. *Research in Autism Spectrum Disorders, 73*, 101547. https://doi.org/10.1016/j.rasd.2020.101547

Dunn, W. (2007). Supporting children to participate successfully in everyday life by using sensory processing knowledge. *Infants and Young Children, 20*(2), 84–101. https://doi.org/10.1097/01.IYC.0000264477.05076.5d

Dyches, T. T., Wilder, L. K., Sudweeks, R. R., Obiakor, F. E., & Algozzine, B. (2004). Multicultural issues in autism. *Journal of Autism and Developmental Disorders, 34*(2), 211–222. https://doi.org/10.1023/B:JADD.0000022611.80478.73

Edwards, J. (2014). The role of the music therapist in promoting parent-infant attachment/Favoriser l'attachement parent-enfant: Rôle du musicothérapeute. *Canadian Journal of Music Therapy, 20*(1), 38–48. https://doi.org/10.1037/0003-066x.46.4.333

Edwards, J. (2016). Approaches and models of music therapy. In J. Edwards (Ed.), *The Oxford handbook of music therapy* (1st ed., pp. 418–427). Oxford University Press. https://doi.org/10.1093/oxfordhb/9780199639755.001.0001

Eggleston, M. J. F., Thabrew, H., Frampton, C. M. A., Eggleston, K. H. F., & Hennig, S. C. (2019). Obtaining an autism spectrum disorder diagnosis and supports: New Zealand parents' experiences. *Research in Autism Spectrum Disorders, 62*, 18–25. https://doi.org/10.1016/j.rasd.2019.02.004

Elliott, R. (2002). Hermeneutic single-case efficacy design. *Psychotherapy Research, 12*(1), 1–21. https://doi.org/10.1080/713869614

Epstein, S., Elefant, C., & Thompson, G. (2020). Music therapists' perceptions of the therapeutic potentials using music when working with verbal children on the autism spectrum: A qualitative analysis. *The Journal of Music Therapy, 57*(1), 66–90. https://doi.org/10.1093/jmt/thz017

Evans, B. (2018). *The Autism paradox: How an autism diagnosis became both a clinical label and an identity: A stigma to be challenged and a status to be embraced.* Aeon. Retrieved November 24, 2018 from https://aeon.co/essays/the-intriguing-history-of-the-autism-diagnosis

Farmer, S. (no date). *How music has helped me along*. Asperger/Autism Network. Retrieved September 17, 2021 from https://www.aane.org/music-helped-along/

Finnigan, E., & Starr, E. (2010). Increasing social responsiveness in a child with autism. *Autism, 14*(4), 321–348. https://doi.org/10.1177/1362361309357747

Forsingdal, S., St John, W., Miller, V., Harvey, A., & Wearne, P. (2014). Goal setting with mothers in child development services. *Child Care Health and Development, 40*(4), 587–596. https://doi.org/10.1111/cch.12075

Freeman, L., Caserta, M., Lund, D., Rossa, S., Dowdy, A., & Partenheimer, A. (2006, March 1). Music thanatology: Prescriptive harp music as palliative care for the dying patient. *American Journal of Hospice and Palliative Medicine, 23*(2), 100–104. https://doi.org/10.1177/104990910602300206

Funabiki, Y., Murai, T., & Toichi, M. (2012). Cortical activation during attention to sound in autism spectrum disorders. *Research in Developmental Disabilities, 33*(2), 518–524. https://doi.org/10.1016/j.ridd.2011.10.016

Garcia, E. M. (2020). Covering the politics of neurodiversity: And myself. In S. K. Kapp (Ed.), *Autistic community and the neurodiversity movement: Stories from the frontline* (pp. 233–241). Springer Singapore. https://doi.org/10.1007/978-981-13-8437-0_17

Gattino, G. S., Riesgoa, R. D. S, Longo, D., Leite, J. C. L., & Faccini, L. S. (2011). Effects of relational music therapy on communication of children with autism: A randomized controlled study. *Nordic Journal of Music Therapy, 20*(2), 142–154. https://doi.org/10.1080/08098131.2011.566933

Geretsegger, M., Elefant, C., Mössler, K. A., & Gold, C. (2014). Music therapy for people with autism spectrum disorder. *The Cochrane Database of Systematic Reviews*. https://doi.org/10.1002/14651858.CD004381.pub3.

Geretsegger, M., Holck, U., Carpente, J. A., Elefant, C., Kim, J., & Gold, C. (2015). Common characteristics of improvisational approaches in music therapy for children with autism spectrum disorder: Developing treatment guidelines. *Journal of Music Therapy, 52*(2), 258–281. https://doi.org/10.1093/jmt/thv005

Gillespie, L. (2015, July). It takes two: The role of co-regulation in building self-regulation skills. *Young Children, 70*(3), 94–96.

Ginn, N. C., Clionsky, L. N., Eyberg, S. M., Warner-Metzger, C., & Abner, J.-P. (2017). Child-directed interaction training for young children with autism spectrum disorders: Parent and child outcomes. *Journal of Clinical Child & Adolescent Psychology, 46*(1), 101–109. https://doi.org/10.1080/15374416.2015.1015135

Given, L. M. (2008). Secondary participants. In L. M. Given (Ed.), *The Sage encyclopedia of qualitative research methods* (pp. 805–809). Sage. https://dx.doi.org/10.4135/9781412963909

Gray, C. A., & Garand, J. D. (1993). Social stories: Improving responses of students with autism with accurate social information. *Focus on Autistic Behavior, 8*(1), 1–10. https://doi.org/10.1177/108835769300800101

Greenspan, S. I., & Wieder, S. (2006). *Engaging autism: The floortime approach to helping children relate*. Da Capo Press.

Hardy, M., & LaGasse, A. B. (2018). Music therapy for persons with autism spectrum disorder. In A. Knight, A. B. LaGasse, & A. A. Clair (Eds.), *Music therapy: An introduction to the profession* (pp. 185–202). The American Music Therapy Association Inc.

Hardy, M. W., & Lagasse, A. B. (2013). Rhythm, movement, and autism: Using rhythmic rehabilitation research as a model for autism. *Frontiers in Integrative Neuroscience, 7*, 19–19. https://doi.org/10.3389/fnint.2013.00019

Hassanein, E. (2015). *Inclusion.* Sense. https://doi.org/10.1007/978-94-6209-923-4

Heaton, P. (2004). Interval and contour processing in autism. *Journal of Autism and Developmental Disorders, 35*(6), 787–793. https://doi.org/10.1007/s10803-005-0024-7

Hemingway, L. (2008). Introduction: Emerging insights and perspectives within disability studies. In T. Campbell, F. Fontes, L. Hemingway, A. Soorenian, & C. Till (Eds.), *Disability studies: Emerging insights and perspectives*. The Disability Press.

Hernandez-Ruiz, E. (2018). Music therapy and Early Start Denver Model to teach social communication strategies to parents of preschoolers with ASD: A feasibility study. *Music Therapy Perspectives, 36*(1), 26–39. https://doi.org/10.1093/mtp/mix018

Hillier, A., Greher, G., Poto, N., & Dougherty, M. (2011, March 1, 2012). Positive outcomes following participation in a music intervention for adolescents and young adults on the autism spectrum. *Psychology of Music, 40*(2), 201–215. https://doi.org/10.1177/0305735610386837

Holck, U. (2004). Interaction themes in music therapy: Definition and delimitation. *Nordic Journal of Music Therapy, 13*(1), 3–19.

Jaarsma, P., & Welin, S. (2012). Autism as a natural human variation: Reflections on the claims of the neurodiversity movement. *Health Care Analysis, 20*(1), 20–30. https://doi.org/10.1007/s10728-011-0169-9

Jack, N., Thompson, G., Hogan, B., Tamplin, J., Eager, R., & Arns, B. (2016). *My profession, my voice: Results of the Australian Music Therapy Association's 2016 workforce census*. https://www.austmta.org.au/resources

James, R., Sigafoos, J., Green, V., Lancioni, G., O'Reilly, M., Lang, R., Davis, T., Carnett, A., Achmadi, D., Gevarter, C., & Marschik, P. (2015). Music therapy for individuals with autism spectrum disorder: A systematic review. *Review Journal of Autism and Developmental Disorders, 2*(1), 39–54. https://doi.org/10.1007/s40489-014-0035-4

Janzen, T. B., & Thaut, M. H. (2018). Rethinking the role of music in the neurodevelopment of autism spectrum disorder. *Music and Science, 1*, 1–18. https://doi.org/10.1177/2059204318769639

Jeong, A. A. Y., & Darroch, B. (2021). Using letter boards in client-centred music therapy: "Autistics can teach if some are ready to listen." *New Zealand Journal of Music Therapy, 19*, 34–53.

Johnson, R. B., Onwuegbuzie, A. J., & Turner, L. A. (2007). Toward a definition of mixed methods research. *Journal of Mixed Methods Research, 1*(2), 112–133. https://doi.org/10.1177/1558689806298224

Jones, S., Akram, M., Murphy, N., Myers, P., & Vickers, N. (2018). *Community attitudes & behaviours towards autism; and experiences of autistic people and their families: General awareness, knowledge and understanding of autism and social isolation.* AMAZE website http://www.onethingforautism.com.au/wp-content/uploads/2018/05/Autism-research-report-General-awareness-knowledge-and-understanding-of-autism-and-social-isolation-1.pdf

Kanner, L. (1943). Early infantile autism. *Journal of Paediatrics, 25*, 211–217.

Kaplan, R. S., & Steele, A. L. (2005). An analysis of music therapy programme Goals and outcomes for clients with diagnoses on the autism spectrum. *Journal of Music Therapy, 42*(1), 2–19. https://doi.org/10.1093/jmt/42.1.2

Kapp, S. K. (2020). Introduction. In S. K. Kapp (Ed.), *Autistic community and the neurodiversity movement: Stories from the frontline* (pp. 1–19). Springer Singapore. https://doi.org/10.1007/978-981-13-8437-0_1

Kapp, S. K., Gillespie-Lynch, K., Sherman, L. E., & Hutman, T. (2013, January). Deficit, difference, or both? Autism and neurodiversity. *Developmental Psychology, 49*(1), 59–71. http://dx.doi.org/10.1037/a0028353

Kasilingam, N., Waddington, H., & Van Der Meer, L. (2019). Early intervention for children with autism spectrum disorder in New Zealand: What children get and what parents want. *International Journal of Disability, Development, and Education, 68*(4), 521–537. https://doi.org/10.1080/1034912X.2019.1696949

Kawakami, S., Uono, S., Otsuka, S., Yoshimura, S., Zhao, S., & Toichi, M. (2020). Atypical multisensory integration and the temporal binding window in autism spectrum disorder. *Journal of Autism and Developmental Disorders, 50*(11), 3944–3956. https://doi.org/10.1007/s10803-020-04452-0

Kearney, A. (2013). Barriers to inclusive education: The identification and elimination of exclusion from and within school. In *Inclusive education: Perspectives on professional practice* (pp. 40–51). Dunmore Publishing Ltd.

Kenny, C. B. (1989). *The field of play: A guide for the theory and practice of music therapy.* Ridgeview.

Kenny, L., Hattersley, C., Molins, B., Buckley, C., Povey, C., & Pellicano, E. (2016). Which terms should be used to describe autism? Perspectives from the UK autism community. *Autism: The International Journal of Research and Practice, 20*(4), 442–462. https://doi.org/10.1177/1362361315588200

Kern, P. (2018). Evidence-based practice in music therapy: Identifying effective interventions for children with Autism Spectrum Disorder. In P. Kern & M. Humpal (Eds.), *Early childhood music therapy and autism spectrum disorder: Supporting children and their families* (2nd ed., pp. 35–49). Jessica Kingsley.

Kern, P., & Aldridge, D. (2006). Using embedded music therapy interventions to support outdoor play of young children with autism in an inclusive community-based child care program. *Journal of Music Therapy, 43*(4), U1-294. https://doi.org/10.1093/jmt/43.4.270

Kern, P., & Humpal, M. E. (2012). *Early childhood music therapy and autism spectrum disorders: Developing potential in young children and their families* (edited by Petra Kern and Marcia Humpal; foreword by David Aldridge). Jessica Kingsley.

Kern, P., Rivera, N. R., Chandler, A., & Humpal, M. (2013, Win). Music Therapy services for individuals with autism spectrum disorder: A survey of clinical practices and training needs. *Journal of Music Therapy, 50*(4), 274–303. https://doi.org/10.1093/jmt/50.4.274

Kern, P., & Tague, D. (2017). Music therapy practice status and trends worldwide: An international survey study. *Music Therapy Perspectives, 54*(3), 255–286. https://doi.org/10.1093/jmt/thx011

Kern, P., Wakeford, L., & Aldridge, D. (2007). Improving the performance of a young child with autism during self-care tasks using embedded song interventions: A case study. *Music Therapy Perspectives, 25*(1), 43–51. https://doi.org/10.1093/mtp/25.1.43

Kern, P., Wolery, M., & Aldridge, D. (2007). Use of songs to promote independence in morning greeting routines for young children with autism. *Journal of Autism & Developmental Disorders, 37*(7), 1264–1271. https://doi.org/10.1007/s10803-006-0272-1

Khundrakpam, B. S., Lewis, J. D., Kostopoulos, P., Carbonell, F., & Evans, A. (2017). Cortical thickness abnormalities in autism spectrum disorders through late childhood, adolescence, and adulthood: A large-scale MRI study. *Cerebral Cortex, 27*, 1721–1731. https://doi.org/10.1093/cercor/bhx038

Kim, J., Wigram, T., & Gold, C. (2008). The effects of improvisational music therapy on joint attention behaviors in autistic children: A randomized controlled study. *Journal of Autism and Developmental Disorders, 38*(9), 1758–1766. https://doi.org/10.1007/s10803-008-0566-6

Kim, J., Wigram, T., & Gold, C. (2009). Emotional, motivational and interpersonal responsiveness of children with autism in improvisational music therapy. *Autism, 13*(4), 389–409. https://doi.org/10.1177/1362361309105660

Kim, Y. S., Leventhal, B. L., Koh, Y.-J., Fombonne, E., Laska, E., Lim, E.-C., Cheon, K.-A., Kim, S.-J., Kim, Y.-K., Lee, H., Song, D.-H., & Grinker, R. R. (2011, September 1). Prevalence of autism spectrum disorders in a total population sample. *American Journal of Psychiatry, 168*(9), 904–912. https://doi.org/10.1176/appi.ajp.2011.10101532

Kinn, L. G., Holgersen, H., Ekeland, T. J., & Davidson, L. (2013). Metasynthesis and bricolage: An artistic exercise of creating a collage of meaning. *Qualitative Health Research, 23*, 1285–1292. https://doi.org/10.1177/1049732313502127

Knight, A., LaGasse, B., & Clair, A.-A. (Eds.). (2018). *Music therapy: An introduction to the profession*. American Music Therapy Association.

Krosnick, J. A., & Pasek, J. (2010). *Optimizing survey questionnaire design in political science: Insights from psychology*. Oxford University Press. https://doi.org/10.1093/oxfordhb/9780199235476.003.0003

LaGasse, A. B. (2014). Effects of a music therapy group intervention on enhancing social skills in children with autism. *The Journal of Music Therapy, 51*(3), 250–275. https://doi.org/10.1093/jmt/thu012

LaGasse, A. B. (2017). Social outcomes in children with autism spectrum disorder: A review of music therapy outcomes. *Patient Related Outcome Measures, 8*, 23–32. https://doi.org/10.2147/PROM.S106267

Lai, G., Pantazatos, S. P., Schneider, H., & Hirsch, J. (2012, March). Neural systems for speech and song in autism. *Brain, 135*, 961–975. https://doi.org/10.1093/brain/awr335

Lai, M.-C., Lombardo, M. V., Pasco, G., Ruigrok, A. N. V., Wheelwright, S. J., Sadek, S. A., Chakrabarti, B., & Baron-Cohen, S. (2011). A behavioral comparison of male and female adults with high functioning autism spectrum conditions. *PLoS ONE, 6*(6), e20835–e20835. https://doi.org/10.1371/journal.pone.0020835

Lambert, M. J., & Barley, D. E. (2001). Research summary on the therapeutic relationship and psychotherapy outcome. *Psychotherapy Theory Research & Practice, 38*(4), 357–361. https://doi.org/10.1037/0033-3204.38.4.357

Lang, R., Hancock, T. B., & Singh, N. N. (2016). Overview of early intensive behavioral intervention for children with autism. In R. Lang, T. B. Hancock, & N. N. Singh (Eds.), *Early intervention for young children with autism spectrum disorder* (pp. 1–14). Springer International Publishing. https://doi.org/10.1007/978-3-319-30925-5_1

Lawes, M. (2012). Reporting on outcomes: An adaptation of the 'AQR-instrument' used to evaluate music therapy in autism. *Approaches: Music Therapy & Special Music Education, 4*(2), 110–120. http://approaches.primarymusic.gr

Levitin, D. J. (2013). Neural correlates of musical behaviors a brief overview. *Music Therapy Perspectives, 31*(1), 15–24. https://doi.org/10.1093/mtp/31.1.15

Leza, J. (2020). Neuroqueering music therapy: Observations on the current state of neurodiversity in music therapy practice. In D. Milton (Ed.), *The neurodiversity reader* (pp. 210–225). Pavilion.

Lim, H. A. (2009, September). Use of music to improve speech production in children with autism spectrum disorders: Theoretical orientation. *Music Therapy Perspectives, 27*(2), 103–114. https://doi.org/10.1093/mtp/27.2.103

Lim, H. A. (2010). Effect of "developmental speech and language training through music" on speech production in children with autism spectrum disorders. *Journal of Music Therapy, 47*(1), 2–26. https://doi.org/10.1093/jmt/47.1.2

Lim, H. A., & Draper, E. (2011, Win). The effects of music therapy incorporated with applied behavior analysis verbal behavior approach for children with autism spectrum disorders. *Journal of Music Therapy, 48*(4), 532–550. https://doi.org/10.1093/jmt/48.4.532

Lindvang, C., Nygaard Pedersen, I., Ole Bonde, L., Lindahl Jacobsen, S., Ridder, H. M., Daniels Beck, B., Gattino, G., Hannibal, N., Holck, U., & Anderson-Ingstrup, J. (2018). Collaborative resonant writing and musical improvisation to explore the concept of resonance. *Qualitative Studies, 5*(1), 4–23. https://tidsskrift.dk/qual/article/view/105455/154259

Loveland, K. A. (2004). *Social-emotional impairment and self-regulation in autism spectrum disorders*. Oxford University Press. https://doi.org/10.1093/acprof:oso/9780198528845.003.0014

Low, M. Y. (2021). *Experiences of autistic clients in Nordoff-Robbins music therapy: An interpretive phenomenological analysis*. Drexel University.

Lunkenheimer, E., Kemp, C. J., Lucas-Thompson, R. G., Cole, P. M., & Albrecht, E. C. (2017). Assessing biobehavioural self-regulation and coregulation in early childhood: The parent-child challenge task. *Infant and Child Development, 26*(1), e1965. https://doi.org/10.1002/icd.1965

Luyster, R., Kadlec, M., Carter, A., & Tager-Flusberg, H. (2008, September). Language assessment and development in toddlers with autism spectrum disorders. *Journal of Autism & Developmental Disorders, 38*(8), 1426–1438. https://doi.org/10.1007/s10803-007-0510-1

Malaeulu, D. (2020). We're blessed to have a son with autism. *E-tangata (Web site): A Māori and Pasifika Sunday magazine*. https://e-tangata.co.nz/reflections/were-blessed-to-have-a-son-with-autism/

Malloch, S., & Trevarthen, C. (2009). *Communicative musicality: Exploring the basis of human companionship*. Oxford University Press.

Markworth, L. (2014). Without words: Music as communication for children with autism. *Qualitative Inquiries in Music Therapy, 9*, 1–42.

Marom, M. K., Gilboa, A., & Bodner, E. (2018). Musical features and interactional functions of echolalia in children with autism within the music therapy dyad. *Nordic Journal of Music Therapy, 27*(3), 175–196. https://doi.org/10.1080/08098131.2017.1403948

Marquez-Garcia, A. V., Magnuson, J., Morris, J., Iarocci, G., Doesburg, S., & Moreno, S. (2021). Music therapy in autism spectrum disorder: A systematic review. *Review Journal of Autism and Developmental Disorders*. https://doi.org/10.1007/s40489-021-00246-x

Matthiesen, N., Elmholdt, K., Wegener, C., & Meier, N. (2018). Editorial: Resonance in a hurried world. *Qualitative Studies, 5*(1), 1–3. https://tidsskrift.dk/qual/article/view/105454/154258

Mazefsky, C. A., & White, S. W. (2014). Emotion regulation: Concepts & practice in autism spectrum disorder. *Child and Adolescent Psychiatric Clinics of North America, 23*(1), 15–24. https://doi.org/10.1016/j.chc.2013.07.002

Mazefsky, C. A. P. D., Herrington, J. P. D., Siegel, M. M. D., Scarpa, A. P. D., Maddox, B. B. M. S., Scahill, L. M. S. N. P. D., & White, S. W. P. D. (2013). The role of emotion regulation in autism spectrum disorder. *Journal of the American Academy of Child and Adolescent Psychiatry, 52*(7), 679–688. https://doi.org/10.1016/j.jaac.2013.05.006

McFerran, K. S., & Rickson, D. J. (2014). Community music therapy in schools: Realigning with the needs of contemporary students, staff and systems. *International Journal of Community Music, 7*(1), 75–92. https://doi.org/10.1386/ijcm.7.1.75_1

McFerran, K. S., & Silverman, M. J. (2018). *A guide to designing research questions for beginning music therapy researchers*. The American Music Therapy Association, Inc.

McLeod, J. (2010). *Case study research in counselling and psychotherapy*. Sage.

Milton, D. E. (2012). On the ontological status of autism: The 'double empathy problem.' *Disability & Society, 27*(6), 883–887. https://doi.org/10.1080/09687599.2012.710008

Ministries of Health and Education. (2016). *New Zealand autism spectrum disorder guideline* (2nd ed.). Ministry of Health. https://www.health.govt.nz/publication/new-zealand-autism-spectrum-disorder-guideline

Ministries of Health, Education, & Social Development. (2021). *Enabling good lives*. Ministries of Health, Education, & Social Development. Retrieved November 10 from https://www.enablinggoodlives.co.nz/

Ministry of Education. (2009a). *Narrative assessment: A guide for teachers*. Learning Media. http://www.throughdifferenteyes.org.nz/a_guide_for_teachers

Ministry of Education. (2009b). *Special education guidelines*. http://www.minedu.govt.nz/NZEducation/EducationPolicies/SpecialEducation

Ministry of Education. (2014). *Key competencies*. Te Kete Ipurangi, Ministry of Eudcation. Retrieved August 25, 2020 from https://nzcurriculum.tki.org.nz/Key-competencies

Ministry of Health. (2019). *New Zealand health survey*. Ministry of Health. Retrieved December 9, 2021 from https://www.health.govt.nz/nz-health-statistics/national-collections-and-surveys/surveys/new-zealand-health-survey

Mitchell, D. (2016). Inclusive education strategies in New Zealand, a leader in inclusive education. *Eesti Haridusteaduste Ajakiri, 4*(2), 19–29. https://doi.org/10.12697/eha.2016.4.2.02a

Molnar-Szakacs, I., & Heaton, P. (2012). Music: A unique window into the world of autism: Molnar-Szakacs & Heaton. *Annals of the New York Academy of Sciences, 1252*(1), 318–324. https://doi.org/10.1111/j.1749-6632.2012.06465.x

Molyneux, C., Koo, N.-H., Piggot-Irvine, E., Talmage, A., Travaglia, R., & Willis, M. (2012). Doing it together: Collaborative research on goal-setting and review in a music therapy centre. *New Zealand Journal of Music Therapy, 10*, 6–38. https://www.proquest.com/scholarly-journals/doing-together-collaborative-research-on-goal/docview/1270322224/se-2?accountid=14782

Morris, P. O., Hope, E., Foulsham, T., & Mills, J. P. (2021). Dance, rhythm, and autism spectrum disorder: An explorative study. *The Arts in Psychotherapy, 73*, 101755. https://doi.org/10.1016/j.aip.2020.101755

Morton, M., McIlroy, A.-M., & Guerin, A. (2019). Sociocultural perspectives on curriculum, pedagogy and assessment: Implications for participation, belonging and building inclusive schools and classrooms. In M. J. Schuelka, C. J. Johnstone, G. Thomas, & A. J. Artiles (Eds.), *The sage handbook of inclusion and diversity in education*. Sage.

Mossler, K., Gilbertson, S., Kruger, V., & Schmid, W. (2013). Converging reflections on music therapy with children and adolescents: A collaborative seminar on diverse areas of music therapy practice and research. In *Voices: A world forum for music therapy* (Vol. 13, No. 2). https://doi.org/10.15845/voices.v13i2.721

Mössler, K., Gold, C., Aßmus, J., Schumacher, K., Calvet, C., Reimer, S., Iversen, G., & Schmid, W. (2017). The therapeutic relationship as predictor of change in music therapy with young children with autism spectrum disorder. *Journal of Autism and Developmental Disorders, 49*(7), 2795–2809. https://doi.org/10.1007/s10803-017-3306-y

Mössler, K., Schmid, W., Aßmus, J., Fusar-Poli, L., & Gold, C. (2020). Attunement in music therapy for young children with autism: Revisiting qualities of relationship as mechanisms of change. *Journal of Autism and Developmental Disorders, 50*(11), 3921–3934. https://doi.org/10.1007/s10803-020-04448-w

Nanclares-Nogues, V., Lin, E., Rolland, C., & Msall, M. E. (2010). Enhancing multidisciplinary community supports for minority preschool children with autistic spectrum disorders: Promoting family centered and evidence based practices. *International Public Health Journal, 2*(1, Special Issue), 69–82.

Neelands, J. (2009). Acting together: Ensemble as a democratic process in art and life. *Research in Drama Education, 14*(2), 173–189. https://doi.org/10.1080/13569780902868713

Ne'eman, A. (2021). When disability is defined by behavior, outcome measures should not promote "passing." *AMA Journal of Ethics, 23*(7), 569–575. https://doi.org/10.1001/amajethics.2021.569

Neuhaus, E. (2020). *Emotion dysregulation in autism spectrum disorder* (1st ed.). Oxford University Press. https://doi.org/10.1093/oxfordhb/9780190689285.013.20

New Zealand Guidelines Group. (2010). *What does ASD look like? A guide to help identify autism spectrum disorder*. Ministries of Health and Education. https://www.health.govt.nz/system/files/documents/publications/what-does-asd-look-like.pdf

Nind, M., & Powell, S. (2000). Intensive interaction and autism: Some theoretical concerns. *Children & Society, 14*(2), 98–109. http://helicon.vuw.ac.nz/login?url=http://search.ebscohost.com/login.aspx?direct=true&db=a2h&AN=12063702&site=ehost-live

Noblit, G. W. (1988). *Meta-ethnography synthesizing qualitative studies*. Sage.

Nordoff, P., & Robbins, C. (1971). *Therapy in music for handicapped children*. St. Martin's Press.

Nordoff, P., & Robbins, C. (2007). *Creative music therapy* (2nd ed.). John Day.

Nordoff, P., Robbins, C., & Marcus, D. (2007). *Creative music therapy: A guide to fostering clinical musicianship with CD (audio)*. Barcelona.

Nugent, J. (2019). Music therapy with children with autistic spectrum conditions and their fmilies. In H. Dunn, E. Coombes, E. Maclean, H. Mottram, & J. Nugent (Eds.), *Music therapy and autism across the lifespan: A spectrum of approaches* (pp. 179–196). Jessica Kingsley.

Ockelford, A. (2000). Music in the education of children with severe or profound learning difficulties: Issues in current U.K. Provision, a new conceptual framework, and proposals for research. *Psychology of Music, 28*(2), 197–217. https://doi.org/10.1177/0305735600282009

Ockelford, A. (2012). *Songs without words: Exploring how music can serve as a proxy language in social interaction with autistic children.* Oxford University Press. https://doi.org/10.1093/acprof:oso/9780199586974.003.0021

Ockelford, A. (2019). The neuroscience of children on the autism spectrum with exceptional musical abilities. In D. A. Hodges & M. Thaut (Eds.), *The Oxford handbook of music and the brain* (pp. 671–695). Oxford University Press. https://doi.org/10.1093/oxfordhb/9780198804123.013.31

Oldfield, A. (2006). *Interactive music therapy: A positive approach.* Jessica Kingsley.

Oldfield, A. (2018). Humour, play, movement and kazoos: Drama in music therapy with children and families. In A. Oldfield & M. Carr (Eds.), *Collaborations within and between dramatherapy and music therapy* (pp. 113–128). Jessica Kingsley.

Oldfield, A. (2020). Book Review. In P. Kern & M. Humpal (Eds.), Early childhood music therapy and autism spectrum disorder. *British Journal of Music Therapy, 34*(2), 108–120.

Oldfield, A., Blauth, L., Finnemann, J., & Casey, O. (2019). Clinical trials: Are music therapists deluding themselves? In H. Dunn, E. Coombes, E. Maclean, H. Mottram, & J. Nugent (Eds.), *Music therapy and autism across the lifespan: A spectrum of approaches* (pp. 35–56). Jessica Kingsley.

Oldfield, A., & Franke, C. (2005). Improvised songs and stories in music therapy diagnostic assessments at a unit for child and family psychiatry: A music therapist's and a psychotherapist's perspective. In F. A. Baker & T. Wigram (Eds.), *Songwriting: Methods, techniques and clinical applications for music therapy clinicians, educators and students* (pp. 24–44). Jessica Kinsley.

Oosthuizen, H. (2019). The potential of paradox: Chaos and order and interdependent resources within short-term music therapy groups with young offenders in South Africa. *Qualitative Inquiries in Music Therapy, 14*(1), 1–39.

Opai, K. (2020). *From autism to takiwātanga:* ASfAR 2020 Conference, Wellington, New Zealand.

Osborne, L. A., McHugh, L., Saunders, J., & Reed, P. (2008, July). Parenting stress reduces the effectiveness of early teaching interventions for autistic spectrum disorders. *Journal of Autism & Developmental Disorders, 38*(6), 1092–1103. https://doi.org/10.1007/s10803-007-0497-7

Pasiali, V. (2004). The use of prescriptive therapeutic songs in a home-based environment to promote social skills acquisition by children with autism: Three case studies. *Music Therapy Perspectives, 22*(1), 11–20. https://doi.org/10.1093/mtp/22.1.11

Pasiali, V. (2018). Approaches to music therapy. In A. Knight, B. LaGasse, & A. A. Clair (Eds.), *Music therapy: An introduction to the profession* (pp. 139–159). The American Music Therapy Association Inc.

Pasiali, V., LaGasse, A. B., & Penn, S. L. (2014). The effect of musical attention control training (MACT) on attention skills of adolescents with neurodevelopmental delays: A pilot study. *The Journal of Music Therapy, 51*(4), 333–354. https://doi.org/10.1093/jmt/thu030

Pater, M., de Graaf, P., & van Yperen, T. (2019). Working elements of music therapy for children and young people with autism. *Open Journal of Medical Psychology, 08*(04), 78–96. https://doi.org/10.4236/ojmp.2019.84008

Patterson, S. Y., Elder, L., Gulsrud, A., & Kasari, C. (2014, July). The association between parental interaction style and children's joint engagement in families with toddlers with autism. *Autism, 18*(5), 511–518. https://doi.org/10.1177/1362361313483595

Paul, A., Sharda, M., Menon, S., Arora, I., Kansal, N., Arora, K., & Singh, N. C. (2015). The effect of sung speech on socio-communicative responsiveness in children with autism spectrum disorders. *Frontiers in Human Neuroscience, 9*, 555–555. https://doi.org/10.3389/fnhum.2015.00555

Penner, F. (2011). *Animal Boogie*. Barefoot Books.

Peterson, C. (2014). Theory of mind understanding and empathic behavior in children with autism spectrum disorders. *International Journal of Developmental Neuroscience, 39*, 16–21. https://doi.org/10.1016/j.ijdevneu.2014.05.002

Peyton, B. (2018). *Rampage.* Warner Brothers.

Pickard, B., Thompson, G., Metell, M., Roginsky, E., & Elefant, C. (2020). It's not what's done, but why it's done': Music therapists' understanding of normalisation, maximisation and the neurodiversity movement. In *Voices: A world forum for music therapy* (Vol. 20, No. 3, p. 19).

Pilkington, H. (2018). Employing meta-ethnography in the analysis of qualitative data sets on youth activism: A new tool for transnational research projects? *Qualitative Research, 18*(1), 108–130. https://doi.org/10.1177/1468794117707805

Porter, S. (2007). Validity, trustworthiness and rigour: Reasserting realism in qualitative research. *Journal of Advanced Nursing, 60*(1), 79–86. https://doi.org/10.1111/j.1365-2648.2007.04360.x

Porter, S., McConnell, T., McLaughlin, K., Lynn, F., Cardwell, C., Braiden, H. J., Boylan, J., Holmes, V., Rogan, S., Clinician, L., Diamond, K., Allen, J., Reilly, C., Davidson, F., McDowell, C., Boyd, R., Oldfield, A., Mullowney, M., Downes, C., … Heale, A. (2017). Music therapy for children and adolescents with behavioural and emotional problems: A randomised controlled trial. *Journal of Child Psychology and Psychiatry, 58*(5), 586–594. https://doi.org/10.1111/jcpp.12656

Preis, J., Amon, R., Silbert Robinette, D., & Rozegar, A. (2016). Does music matter? The effects of background music on verbal expression and engagement in children with autism spectrum disorders. *Music Therapy Perspectives, 34*(1), 106–115. https://doi.org/10.1093/mtp/miu044

Prizant, B. M., Wetherby, A. M., Rubin, E., Laurent, A. C., & Rydell, P. J. (2006, November 3, 2007). *The SCERTS model in practice: Program planning and intervention.* Retrieved November 3, 2007 from http://www.scerts.com/frequently_asked_questions.htm.

Probst, B. (2015). The eye regards itself: Benefits and challenges of reflexivity in qualitative social work research. *Social Work Research, 39*(1), 37–48. https://doi.org/10.1093/swr/svu028

Probst, B., & Berenson, L. (2014). The double arrow: How qualitative social work researchers use reflexivity. *Qualitative Social Work (QSW): Research and Practice, 13*(6), 813–827. https://doi.org/10.1177/1473325013506248

Rabeyron, T., Robledo del Canto, J.-P., Carasco, E., Bisson, V., Bodeau, N., Vrait, F.-X., Berna, F., & Bonnot, O. (2020). A randomized controlled trial of 25 sessions comparing music therapy and music listening for children with autism spectrum disorder. *Psychiatry Research, 293*, 113377. https://doi.org/10.1016/j.psychres.2020.113377

Reschke-Hernandez, A. E. (2011). History of music therapy treatment interventions for children with autism. *Journal of Music Therapy, 48*(2), 169–207. https://doi.org/10.1093/jmt/48.2.169

Reynolds, M. (1957). Morningtown ride. In *Hide & seekers* [1964 Album]. W&G Records.

Rickson, D. J. (2012). Music therapy school consultation: A unique practice. *Nordic Journal of Music Therapy, 21*(3), 268–285. https://doi.org/10.1080/08098131.2012.654474

Rickson, D. J. (2021). Family members' and other experts' perceptions of music therapy with children on the autism spectrum in New Zealand: Findings from multiple case studies. *The Arts in Psychotherapy, 75*, 101833. https://doi.org/10.1016/j.aip.2021.101833

Rickson, D. J., Castelino, A., Molyneux, C., Ridley, H., & Upjohn-Beatson, E. (2016). What evidence? Designing a mixed methods study to investigate music therapy with children who have autism spectrum disorder (ASD), in New Zealand Contexts. *The Arts in Psychotherapy, 50*, 119–125. https://doi.org/10.1016/j.aip.2016.07.002

Rickson, D. J., & McFerran, K. S. (2014). *Creating music cultures in the schools: A perspective from community music therapy*. Barcelona.

Rickson, D. J., Molyneux, C., Ridley, H., Castelino, A., & Upjohn-Beatson, E. (2015a). *Music therapy for children who have autism spectrum disorder ASD: Exploring the potential for research in New Zealand using a mixed methods design*. Victoria University of Wellington.

Rickson, D. J., Molyneux, C., Ridley, H., Castelino, A., & Upjohn Beatson, E. B. (2015b). Music therapy with people who have autism spectrum disorder—Current practice in New Zealand. *New Zealand Journal of Music Therapy, 13*, 8–32. https://www-proquest-com.helicon.vuw.ac.nz/docview/1897698669?accountid=14782

Robertson, C. E., & Baron-Cohen, S. (2017). Sensory perception in autism. *Nature Reviews Neuroscience, 18*(11), 671–684. https://doi.org/10.1038/nrn.2017.112

Rojas-Bermúdez, J., & Moyano, G. (2020). Puppets as psychotherapeutic instrument: Intermediary and intra-intermediary object in psychodrama. *Journal of Applied Arts & Health, 11*(1), 135–141. https://doi.org/10.1386/jaah_00025_7

Rolvsjord, R. (2010). *Resource-oriented music therapy in mental health care*. Barcelona.

Ronconi, L., Molteni, M., & Casartelli, L. (2016). Building blocks of others' understanding: A perspective shift in investigating social-communicative deficit in autism. *Frontiers in Human Neuroscience, 10*, 144–144. https://doi.org/10.3389/fnhum.2016.00144

Rosanbalm, K. D., & Murray, D. W. (2018). *Promoting self-regulation in the first five years: A practice brief* (OPRE Brief #2017–79). https://fpg.unc.edu/publications/promoting-self-regulation-first-five-years-practice-brief

Salomon-Gimmon, M., & Elefant, C. (2019). Development of vocal communication in children with autism spectrum disorder during improvisational music therapy. *Nordic Journal of Music Therapy, 28*(3), 174–192. https://doi.org/10.1080/08098131.2018.1529698

Savarese, E. T., & Savarese, R. J. (2010). "The superior half of speaking": An introduction. *Disability Studies Quarterly, 30*(1), Online. http://dx.doi.org/10.18061/dsq.v30i1

Sayre, D. N. (2020). What does it really mean to talk about "performative" activism? *All the World's a Stage*. https://www.danasayre.com/what-does-it-really-mean-to-talk-about-performative-activism/

Schumacher, K., & Calvet, C. (2007). The "AQR-instrument" (Assessment of the Quality of Relationship)—An observation instrument to assess the quality of relationship. In T. Wosch & T. Wigram (Eds.), *Microanalysis in music therapy* (pp. 79–91). Jessica Kingsley.

Schwartzberg, E. T., & Silverman, M. J. (2013). Effects of music-based social stories on comprehension and generalization of social skills in children with autism spectrum disorders: A randomized effectiveness study. *The Arts in Psychotherapy, 40*(3), 331–337. https://doi.org/10.1016/j.aip.2013.06.001

Seligman, M. E. P. (2011). *Flourish: A visionary new understanding of happiness and well-being*. Free Press.

Sharda, M., Midha, R., Malik, S., Mukerji, S., & Singh, N. C. (2015). Fronto-temporal connectivity is preserved during sung but not spoken word listening, across the autism spectrum. *Autism Research, 8*(2), 174–186. https://doi.org/10.1002/aur.1437

Sharda, M., Tuerk, C., Chowdhury, R., Jamey, K., Foster, N., Custo-Blanch, M., Tan, M., Nadig, A., & Hyde, K. (2018). Music improves social communication and auditory-motor connectivity in children with autism. *Translational Psychiatry, 8*(1), 213–231. https://doi.org/10.1038/s41398-018-0287-3

Simpson, K., & Keen, D. (2011). Music interventions for children with autism: Narrative review of the literature. *Journal of Autism and Developmental Disorders, 41*, 1507–1514. https://doi.org/10.1007/s10803-010-1172-y

Simpson, K., Keen, D., & Lamb, J. (2013). The use of music to engage children with autism in a receptive labelling task. *Research in Autism Spectrum Disorders, 7*(12), 1489–1496. https://doi.org/10.1016/j.rasd.2013.08.013

Small, C. (1998). *Musicking: The meanings of performing and listening*. University Press of New England.

Snyder, S. L., & Mitchell, D. T. (2006). *Cultural locations of disability*. University of Chicago Press. https://doi.org/10.7208/9780226767307

Solesbury, W. (2002). The ascendancy of evidence. *Planning Theory & Practice, 3*(1), 90–96. https://doi.org/10.1080/14649350220117834

South, M., & Rodgers, J. (2017). Sensory, emotional and cognitive contributions to anxiety in autism spectrum disorders. *Frontiers in Human Neuroscience, 11*, 20. https://doi.org/10.3389/fnhum.2017.00020

Stake, R. E. (2006). *Multiple case study analysis*. The Guilford Press.

Stanutz, S., Wapnick, J., & Burack, J. A. (2014). Pitch discrimination and melodic memory in children with autism spectrum disorders. *Autism: The International Journal of Research and Practice, 18*(2), 137–147. https://doi.org/10.1177/1362361312462905

Statistics New Zealand. (2018). *2018 census*. https://www.stats.govt.nz/2018-census

Stavropoulos, K. K., & Carver, L. J. (2018). Oscillatory rhythm of reward: Anticipation and processing of rewards in children with and without autism. *Molecular Autism, 9*(4), 1–15. https://doi.org/10.1186/s13229-018-0189-5

Stern, D. N. (1977). *The first relationship: Infant and mother*. Billing & Sons Ltd.

Stern, D. N. (1985). *The interpersonal world of the infant*. Basic Books Inc.

Stern, D. N. (2010). *Forms of vitality*. Oxford University Press.

Stige, B., & Aaro, L. E. (2012). *Invitation to community music therapy*. Routledge.

Su Maw, S., & Haga, C. (2018). Effectiveness of cognitive, developmental, and behavioural interventions for autism spectrum disorder in preschool-aged children: A systematic review and meta-analysis. *Heliyon, 4*(9), e00763. https://doi.org/10.1016/j.heliyon.2018.e00763

Swain, J., & French, S. (2000). Towards an affirmation model of disability. *Disability & Society, 15*(4), 569–582. https://doi.org/10.1080/09687590050058189

Thaut, M., Hoemberg, V., & Abiru, M. (2014). *Handbook of neurologic music therapy* (1st ed.). Oxford University Press.

Thompson, G. A. (2012). Family-centered music therapy in the home environment: Promoting interpersonal engagement between children with autism spectrum disorder and their parents. *Music Therapy Perspectives, 30*(2), 109–116. http://ezproxy.massey.ac.nz/login?url=http://search.ebscohost.com/login.aspx?direct=true&db=ccm&AN=2012088717&site=eds-live&scope=site

Thompson, G. A. (2017a). Families with preschool aged children with autism spectrum disorder. In S. L. Jacobsen & G. Thompson (Eds.), *Music therapy with families: Therapeutic approaches and theoretical perspectives* (pp. 92–115). Jessica Kingsley.

Thompson, G. (2017b). Long-term perspectives of family quality of life following music therapy with young children on the autism spectrum: A phenomenological study. *Journal of Music Therapy, 54*(4), 432–459. https://doi.org/10.1093/jmt/thx013

Thompson, G. A. (2018). Dramatic role play within improvisational music therapy: Joey's story. In A. Oldfield & M. Carr (Eds.), *Collaborations within and between dramatherapy and music therapy* (pp. 31–51). Jessica Kingsley.

Thompson, G. A. (2020). A grounded theory of music therapists' approach to goal processes within their clinical practice. *The Arts in Psychotherapy, 70*, 101680. https://doi.org/10.1016/j.aip.2020.101680

Thompson, G. A., & Elefant, C. (2019). "But I want to talk to you!" Perspectives on music therapy practice with highly verbal children on the autism spectrum. *Nordic Journal of Music Therapy, 28*(4), 347–359. https://doi.org/10.1080/08098131.2019.1605616

Thompson, G. A., & McFerran, K. S. (2015a). Music therapy with young people who have profound intellectual and developmental disability: Four case studies exploring communication and engagement within musical interactions. *Journal of Intellectual & Developmental Disability, 40*(1), 1–11. https://doi.org/10.3109/13668250.2014.965668

Thompson, G. A., & McFerran, K. S. (2015b). "We've got a special connection": Qualitative analysis of descriptions of change in the parent–child relationship by mothers of young children with autism spectrum disorder. *Nordic Journal of Music Therapy, 24*(1), 3–26. https://doi.org/10.1080/08098131.2013.858762

Thompson, G. A., McFerran, K. S., & Gold, C. (2013). Family-centred music therapy to promote social engagement in young children with severe autism spectrum disorder: A randomized controlled study. *Child: Care, Health And Development, 40*(6), 840–852. https://doi.org/10.1111/cch.12121

Thompson, G., Raine, M., Hayward, S., & Kilpatrick, H. (2020). Gathering community perspectives to inform the design of autism-friendly music-making workshops for wellbeing. *International Journal of Wellbeing, 10*(5), 117–143. https://doi.org/10.5502/ijw.v10i5.1497

Timans, R., Wouters, P., & Heilbron, J. (2019). Mixed methods research: What it is and what it could be. *Theory and Society, 48*(2), 193–216. https://doi.org/10.1007/s11186-019-09345-5

Tomchek, S. D., & Dunn, W. (2007). Sensory processing in children with and without autism: A comparative study using the short sensory profile. *The American Journal of Occupational Therapy, 61*(2), 190–200. https://doi.org/10.5014/ajot.61.2.190

Trevarthen, C. (2002). Origins of musical identity. In R. A. R. MacDonald, D. J. Hargreaves, & D. Miell (Eds.), *Musical identities*. Oxford University Press.

Trevarthen, C., & Aitken, K. J. (2001). Infant intersubjectivity: Research, theory, and clinical applications. *Journal of Child Psychology and Psychiatry, 42*(1), 3–48. https://doi.org/10.1111/1469-7610.00701

Trevarthen, C., & Delafield-Butt, J. T. (2013). Autism as a developmental disorder in intentional movement and affective engagement. *Frontiers and Integrative Neuroscience, 7*, 1–16. https://doi.org/10.3389/fnint.2013.00049

Trevarthen, C., & Malloch, S. (2017). The musical self. In R. A. R. MacDonald, D. J. Hargreaves, & D. Miell (Eds.), *Handbook of musical identities* (1st ed.). Oxford University Press.

Trevarthen, C., & Malloch, S. N. (2000). The dance of wellbeing: Defining the musical therapeutic effect. *Nordic Journal of Music Therapy, 9*(2), 3–17.

Trowsdale, J., & Hayhow, R. (2013). Can mimetics, a theatre-based practice, open possibilities for young people with learning disabilities? A capability approach. *British Journal of Special Education, 40*(2), 72–79. https://doi.org/10.1111/1467-8578.12019

Tse, C. Y. A., Pang, C. L., & Lee, P. H. (2018). Choosing an appropriate physical exercise to reduce stereotypic behavior in children with autism spectrum disorders: A non-randomized crossover study. *Journal of Autism and Developmental Disorders, 48*(5), 1666–1672. https://doi.org/10.1007/s10803-017-3419-3

UN Committee on the Rights of the Child (CRC). (2009). *General comment No. 12: The right of the child to be heard*. https://www.refworld.org/docid/4ae562c52.html

Unkrich, L. (2017). *Coco.* Walt Disney Pictures.

Vaiouli, P., & Andreou, G. (2018). Communication and language development of young children with autism: A review of research in music. *Communication Disorders Quarterly, 39*(2), 323–329. https://doi.org/10.1177/1525740117705117

van Ijzendoorn, M. H., Rutgers, A. H., Bakermans-Kranenburg, M. J., Swinkels, S. H. N., van Daalen, E., Dietz, C., Naber, F. B. A., Buitelaar, J. K., & van Engeland, H. (2007, March–April). Parental sensitivity and attachment in children with autism spectrum disorder: Comparison with children with mental retardation, with language delays, and with typical development. *Child Development, 78*(2), 597–608.

van Manen, M. (1990). *Researching lived experience*. New York State University.

Walshaw, M. (2010, July 3–7). *The researcher's self in research: Confronting issues about knowing and understanding others.* Annual Meeting of the Mathematics Education Research Group of Australasia, Freemantle, WA.

Walworth, D. D. (2007, Spr). The use of music therapy within the SCERTS model for children with autism spectrum disorder. *Journal of Music Therapy, 44*(1), 2–22.

Wan, C. Y., Bazen, L., Baars, R., Libenson, A., Zipse, L., Zuk, J., Norton, A., & Schlaug, G. (2011). Auditory-motor mapping training as an intervention to facilitate speech output in non-verbal children with autism: A proof of concept study. *PLoS ONE, 6*(9), e25505. https://doi.org/10.1371/journal.pone.0025505

Warren, P., & Rickson, D. (2016). What factors shape a music therapist? An investigation of music therapists' professional identity over time in New Zealand. *The New Zealand Journal of Music Therapy, 14*, 55–81.

Warwick, A. (2019). Prelude: The unanswered question. In H. Dunn, E. Coombes, E. Maclean, H. Mottram, & J. Nugent (Eds.), *Music therapy and autism across the lifespan: A spectrum of approaches* (pp. 15–34). Jessica Kingsley.

Whipple, J. (2018). Music therapy research: Effective interventions for young children with autism spectrum disorder. In P. Kern & M. Humpal (Eds.), *Early childhood music therapy and autism spectrum disorder: Supporting children and their families* (2nd ed., pp. 49–69). Jessical Kingsley.

Wigram, T. (1992). Differential diagnosis of autism and other types of disability. *Australian Journal of Music Therapy, 3*, 16–26.

Wigram, T. (1993). Music therapy research to meet the demands of health and educational services. In M. Heal & T. Wigram (Eds.), *Music therapy in health and education*. Jessica Kingsley.

Wigram, T. (2002). Indications in music therapy. Evidence from assessment that can identify the expectations of music therapy as a treatment for autistic spectrum disorder (ASD): Meeting the challenge of evidence based practice. *British Journal of Music Therapy, 16*(1), 11–28.

Wigram, T., & Elefant, C. (2009). Therapeutic dialogues in music: Nurturing musicality of communication in children with autistic spectrum disorder and Rett syndrome. In S. Malloch & C. Trevarthen (Eds.), *Communicative musicality: Exploring the basis of human companionship* (pp. 423–445). Oxford University Press.

Wigram, T., & Gold, C. (2006). Music therapy in the assessment and treatment of autistic spectrum disorder: Clinical application and research evidence. *Child: Care, Health And Development, 32*(5), 535–542.

Wigram, T., Pederson, I. N., & Bond, O. L. (2002). *A comprehensive guide to music therapy*. Jessica Kingsley.

Williams, D. (2002). Foreword. In D. S. Berger (Ed.), *Music therapy, sensory integration and the autistic child* (pp. 11–12). Jessica Kingsley.

Williams, J. (1993). Jurassic park theme. In *Jurassic Park*. MCA Records.

Williams, L., Rycroft-Malone, J., & Burton, C. R. (2017). Bringing critical realism to nursing practice: Roy Bhaskar's contribution. *Nursing Philosophy, 18*(2), e12130-n/a. https://doi.org/10.1111/nup.12130

Willis, D. G., Sullivan-Bolyai, S., Knafl, K., & Cohen, M. Z. (2016). Distinguishing features and similarities between descriptive phenomenological and qualitative description research. *Western Journal of Nursing Research, 38*(9), 1185–1204. https://doi.org/10.1177/0193945916645499

Wimpory, D., & Gwilym, E. (2019). Musical interaction therapy (MIT) for children with autistic spectrum conditions (ASCs): Underlying rationale, clinical practice and research evidence. In H. Dunn, E. Coombes, E. Maclean, H. Mottram, & J. Nugent (Eds.), *Music therapy and autism across the lifespan: A spectrum of approaches* (pp. 97–136). Jessica Kingsley.

Winkler, R., & Hathcock, J. (1963). Welcome to my world. In *Jim Reeves, A touch of velvet*.

Winnicott, D. W. (1971). *Playing and reality*. Tavistock.

Winnicott, D. W. (2008). *Playing and reality*. Routledge.

World Health Organisation. (2019). *Autism spectrum disorders*. World Health Organisation. Retrieved August 20, 2020 from https://www.who.int/newsroom/fact-sheets/detail/autism-spectrum-disorders

World Health Organisation, & World Bank. (2011). *World report on disability*. https://www.who.int/publications/i/item/9789241564182

Yinger, O. S., & Gooding, L. (2014, July). Music therapy and music medicine for children and adolescents. *Child and Adolescent Psychiatric Clinics of North America, 23*(3), 535–553. https://doi.org/10.1016/j.chc.2013.03.003

Zwaigenbaum, L., Bauman, M. L., Choueiri, R., Kasari, C., Carter, A., Granpeesheh, D., Mailloux, Z., Smith Roley, S., Wagner, S., Fein, D., Pierce, K., Buie, T., Davis, P. A., Newschaffer, C., Robins, D., Wetherby, A., Stone, W. L., Yirmiya, N., Estes, A., ... Natowicz, M. R. (2015, October 1). Early intervention for children with autism spectrum disorder under 3 years of age: Recommendations for practice and research. *Pediatrics, 136*(Supplement 1), S60–S81. https://doi.org/10.1542/peds.2014-3667E

Index

D. Rickson, *Music Therapy with Autistic Children in Aotearoa, New Zealand*, https://doi.org/10.1007/978-3-031-05233-0